UNDERSTANDING Health

A DETERMINANTS APPROACH

Edited by

HELEN KELEHER

and **BERNI MURPHY**

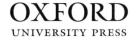

OXFORD
UNIVERSITY PRESS

OXFORD

UNIVERSITY PRESS

253 Normanby Road, South Melbourne, Victoria 3205, Australia

Oxford University Press is a department of the University of Oxford.
It furthers the University's objective of excellence in research, scholarship,
and education by publishing worldwide in

Oxford New York

Auckland Cape Town Dar es Salaam Hong Kong Karachi
Kuala Lumpur Madrid Melbourne Mexico City Nairobi
New Delhi Shanghai Taipei Toronto

With offices in

Argentina Austria Brazil Chile Czech Republic France Greece
Guatemala Hungary Italy Japan Poland Portugal Singapore
South Korea Switzerland Thailand Turkey Ukraine Vietnam

OXFORD is a trade mark of Oxford University Press
in the UK and in certain other countries

National Library of Australia
Cataloguing-in-Publication data:

Understanding Health: a determinants approach.

Bibliography.
Includes index.
ISBN 9 78019551 6616
ISBN 0 19 551661 3.

1. Public Health—Australia—Textbooks.
2. Health promotion—Australia—Textbooks.
I. Keleher, Helen, 1950–. II. Murphy, Berni.
613.0994

Typeset by OUPANZS
Printed by Bookpac Production Services, Singapore

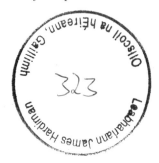

CONTENTS

LIST OF FIGURES

LIST OF TABLES

CONTRIBUTORS

Michael Ackland MB, BS, MPH, FAFPHM. Manager, Health Surveillance and Evaluation Section, Rural and Regional Health and Aged Care Services, Department of Human Services (DHS), Victoria. Mike has a lead role in the oversight of a number of key health surveillance initiatives within the DHS, including the Victorian Population Health Survey, the Victorian Ambulatory Care Sensitive Conditions study and the Victorian Burden of Disease study. He has particular expertise in the application of epidemiology to government policy and strategic planning.

Kylie Ball BA (Psych), PhD. National Health and Medical Research Council (NHMRC) Postdoctoral Research Fellow, Deakin University, Melbourne. Kylie is an investigator with the Australian Longitudinal Study on Women's Health. Her research focuses on the social and behavioural epidemiology of physical activity and diet, and the prevention of obesity.

James Balmford Grad Dip (App. Psych). Research Officer, VicHealth Centre for Tobacco Control at the Cancer Council Victoria. James's work has involved the development and evaluation of computer-based tailoring programs to facilitate tobacco cessation and prevention. He has also contributed substantially to a major literature review on community attitudes towards and exposure to environmental tobacco smoke in Australia. He is currently undertaking PhD study on refining stage models of the smoking cessation process, and prospectively examining predictors of change.

Ron Borland BSc (Hons), MSc, PhD. Co-Director of the VicHealth Centre for Tobacco Control at the Cancer Council Victoria. Ron has an international reputation for his research on environmental and regulatory determinants of behaviour change and on smoking cessation. He has published more than a hundred papers in peer-reviewed journals. He sits on the Research and Evaluation Committee of the National Tobacco Campaign. His current research interests are in the emerging field of population health, in particular on regulatory models to reduce harm from tobacco use and on strategies for maximising smoking cessation.

Cate Burns BSc, DipDiet, PhD. Lecturer, Deakin University, Melbourne. Cate teaches public health nutrition at graduate and postgraduate level. She has several research interests: food insecurity, local food access, nutrition programs for vulnerable groups, and exploring the interface between food insecurity and obesity. She is currently involved in projects working with local government to improve community food access and reduce food insecurity among the homeless. Cate is also working with migrant populations to improve food access with an emphasis on maintenance of traditional eating habits.

David Cameron-Smith BSc (Hons), PhD. Senior Lecturer in Human Nutrition, Deakin University, Melbourne. David is a leading researcher in the impact of diet and exercise on genes. He undertakes genetic research aimed at investigating how diet and exercise regulate genes controlling metabolism in skeletal muscle. Further work will aim to establish the role of genes in the regulation of skeletal muscle growth and repair.

John Catford MA, MSc, DM, FRCP, FAFPHM, FIPAA. Dean, Faculty of Health and Behavioural Sciences, Deakin University, Melbourne. John is Editor in Chief of *Health Promotion International*, published by Oxford University Press. For two decades he has been at the forefront of developments in health promotion internationally, and was co-author and editor of the Ottawa Charter for Health Promotion. Past positions have included Executive Director of Public Health and Chief Health Officer for the Victorian Government, Chief Executive of the Health Promotion Authority for Wales, Professor of Health Promotion and Founding Director of the Heartbeat Wales program at the University of Wales, United Kingdom.

Paul Dietze BSc (Hons), PhD. Senior Research Fellow & VicHealth Public Health Research Fellow, Deakin University, Melbourne and Turning Point Alcohol and Drug Centre, Fitzroy. Paul has researched the epidemiology of alcohol and other drug use and related harms for more than seven years and currently manages the epidemiology unit at Turning Point Alcohol and Drug Centre in Melbourne. He has been a key contributor to projects designed to monitor the extent of alcohol use and harm in the Australian community and currently convenes the Injecting Drug Harm Reduction Network in Melbourne and advises key government agencies including the National Expert Advisory Committee on Illicit Drugs.

Jan Garrard BSc (Hons), PhD. Senior Lecturer, Deakin University, Melbourne. Jan's career in public health research and evaluation spans several decades. She has conducted a number of evaluation studies of health promotion programs, and teaches research and evaluation methods at undergraduate and graduate levels. Jan is a keen participant in current debates about evidence-based health care, the nature of evidence, and an appropriate evidence base for public health.

Lesley Hardcastle BA, DipEd, MEdSt. Development Manager, Disabilities Studies Unit, Deakin University, Melbourne. Lesley has particular interests in examining the impact of stereotyping on equal rights for all citizens and in changing community attitudes towards people who are socially excluded. She is currently focusing her doctoral study on the employability of ex-offenders and identifying the factors that might encourage ex-offenders to re-engage with the community.

Sarah Hopkins BA (Hons), MA (Lib). Collection Services Librarian, Bayside Library Service, Melbourne. From 1997 to 2002, Sarah was the Faculty Liaison Librarian for the Faculty of Health and Behavioural Sciences at Deakin University, where she helped undergraduate students improve their searching skills, particularly in the area of online information.

Clare Hume BAppSci (Hons). VicHealth PhD scholarship student, Deakin University, Melbourne. Clare's PhD scholarship research focuses on the physical, social, and policy environments as moderators of children's physical activity. Her interests are primarily in the physical activity behaviours of primary school children, and her background includes longitudinal research in physical activity.

Damien Jolley BSc (Hons), DipEd, MSc, MSc (Epidemiology). Associate Professor in Biostatistics and Epidemiology, and Associate Dean (Teaching and Learning) in the Faculty of Health and Behavioural Sciences, Deakin University, Melbourne. Damien has worked in public health since 1980, in Australia, Papua New Guinea, and Great Britain. He is author or co-author of more than eighty refereed journal articles in the fields of epidemiology, biostatistics, and public health.

Helen Keleher RN, BA, MA, PhD, FRCNA. Associate Professor in Public Health, Deakin University, Melbourne. Helen is a public health social scientist, with research interests in primary health care, health equity, women's health, and social approaches to health promotion. She coordinates the Master of Public Health and postgraduate program in health promotion at Deakin University. She is active in advocacy for public health, particularly through the Public Health Association of Australia, of which she is immediate past Vice President (Policy). Helen is also National Convenor of the Australian Women's Health Network.

Mary Mahoney BEd, MSc (Ecology & Society), Med. Senior Lecturer, Deakin University, Melbourne. Mary coordinates the Family and Society major in the Deakin Health Sciences degree. She previously worked at Bath Spa University College, England, as Course Director of Human Ecology. Mary's research interests are focused on the intersection between policy and the health and wellbeing of people. Her most recent work has been on the application of health impact assessment (HIA) to policy development and on aspects of rural health. In 1999, Mary was awarded the Vice Chancellor's Outstanding Achievement Award for Outstanding Teaching at Deakin University.

Bernie Marshall BSc (Hons), DipEd, MPH. Senior Lecturer, Deakin University, Melbourne. Bernie has taught health promotion at undergraduate and postgraduate levels to a broad range of students and organisations since joining Deakin University in 1992. His particular areas of research and consultancy interest are in health promotion workforce development and school health. Bernie was a member of the team that developed MindMatters and is President of the Australian Health Promoting Schools Association.

Berni Murphy BEd, MPH (Health Promotion), PhD Candidate. Lecturer, Deakin University, Melbourne. Berni coordinates and lectures in the undergraduate foundation unit Understanding Health for students undertaking courses within the Faculty of Health and Behavioural Sciences at Deakin University. She has particular expertise in health education strategies and health communication. Berni has broad experience in developing and delivering innovative health promotion seminars, and has conducted health promotion research in Australia and internationally, particularly around the determinants of health. She is currently investigating the impact on health of transitioning into university settings for international students.

Rosemary Nicholson, B.Sc (Hons), MPH. Lecturer, Environmental Health, University of Western Sydney, Sydney. Rosemary holds a B.Sc (Hons) in environmental health from the United Kingdom and has recently completed a Masters in Public Health exploring capacity building for environmental health action in Australia. Rosemary's current research interests centre around community-based environmental health action.

Andrew Noblet BEd, GradDipMgt, PhD. Lecturer, Deakin University, Melbourne. Andrew's research and consultancy interests are in the areas of occupational stress and workplace health promotion. The results of his work have been presented in several peer-reviewed journals and international conference proceedings.

Maria Pallotta-Chiarolli BA, DipEd, GradDip A, MA (Women's Studies), PhD. Senior Lecturer, Deakin University, Melbourne. Maria is a senior lecturer in social diversity in health and education. She researches and writes about issues of ethnicity, gender, sexuality, and HIV/AIDS and sexually transmitted infections in education and health, particularly in relation to adolescent health. She is author or co-author of numerous publications about young people and sexuality.

Judith Raftery BA (Hons), DipT, PhD. Visiting Senior Lecturer, Department of Public Health, University of Adelaide, Adelaide. Judith is an historian with a particular interest in the history of public health and public health policy in the nineteenth and twentieth centuries. Since 1989, she has been using historical analysis as a way of teaching many aspects of public health to undergraduate and graduate students.

Daniel Reidpath PhD. Senior Lecturer, Deakin University, Melbourne. Daniel is a senior lecturer in social epidemiology. As a recent recipient of a five-year Senior Research Fellowship from the Victorian Health Promotion Foundation, he intends to study social context and health, exploring the linkages between sociocultural factors and health outcome.

Damien Ridge BMedSci (Hons), PhD. Senior Qualitative Research Fellow, Oxford University, Oxford. Damien is an expert in qualitative approaches to research, and is particularly interested in investigating the social determinants of mental health. He is currently studying the ways in which people managed to overcome depression in the United Kingdom, for the DIPEX project. Damien has recently headed an investigation into the broad issues and needs of young people in Vietnam for the United Nations.

Jo Salmon BA, BBSc (Hons), PhD. VicHealth Public Health Research Fellow, Deakin University, Melbourne. Jo's research focuses on physical activity and sedentary behaviour (e.g. television viewing, electronic games, computer use) among adults, children, and families. Her research includes physical activity assessment; psychological, social, and environmental determinants; and strategies for promoting physical activity.

Kaye Smith BA, MA (Disability Studies), PhD. Lecturer, Deakin University, Melbourne. Kaye teaches in several disability-related units including a unit that examines disability from a social perspective. Her research interests are in the areas of employment and diversity.

Christine Spratt BEd, MEd (Distance Education), PhD. Senior Lecturer, Higher Education Development Unit, Monash University, Melbourne. Christine coordinates academic staff development initiatives related to online learning. She has taught at universities in Australia, most recently at Deakin, and at Nanyang Polytechnic in Singapore. Christine has particular expertise in teaching and learning, online and distance education, and project management in settings of change in higher education; as well as in the design and development of flexible online learning environments and contemporary issues in change and change management in education, and teaching and learning with technology.

Peter Stephenson PhD. Senior Lecturer, University of Western Sydney, Sydney. Peter is an experienced environmental health practitioner, teacher, and researcher. His professional interests are in environmental health education and workforce development in Australia and overseas. For the past five years, Peter has managed national education and workforce capacity building programs for Indigenous Australian environmental health practitioners.

Jan Stewart TPTC., BEd, BA (Hons), PhD. Lecturer, School of Psychology, Deakin University, Warrnambool. Jan has been teaching psychology at Deakin University for fifteen years, during which time she has taught various units relating to health psychology. Her interests focus on health, and physical and mental wellbeing, particularly in promoting ideas of 'wellness' and positive thinking about people's lives.

Boyd Swinburn MB ChB, MD, FRACP. Professor of Public Health Nutrition, Deakin University, Melbourne. Boyd has trained as an endocrinologist and undertaken metabolic research at the National Institute of Health in Phoenix, Arizona. He has continued his research in nutrition and obesity, but is now more focused on the public health and preventive aspects. From 1992 to 2000, Boyd was the Medical Director of the National Heart Foundation of New Zealand.

Mardie Townsend BSocSci, PhD. Senior Lecturer, Deakin University, Melbourne. Mardie is currently undertaking research into the human health benefits of interaction with nature, including the effects of access to nature for the health and wellbeing of high-rise housing residents, and the use of nature-based therapies to overcome health-related behavioural problems such as substance abuse.

Cathy Vaughan BPhysio, MPH. Youth Health Advisor, Centre for International Health, Burnet Institute, Melbourne. Cathy has work experience in several countries including Pakistan, where she worked as a physiotherapist in 1996 and 1997 and Tuvalu, where she has worked with the National AIDS Committee since 1999. Cathy has particular interest in the structural determinants of health in low-income countries, particularly as they affect young people.

ACKNOWLEDGMENTS

The editors wish to acknowledge the contribution of the team at Oxford University Press, in particular Debra James, Heather Fawcett, Nina Crisp, and Anne Mulvaney, who have been most supportive and encouraging throughout the challenging process of conceptualising and creating this textbook. Thanks also go to Siobhan Bowler, our in-house editor, and Nerida Joss, our research assistant, who played critical roles in making sure we moved steadily through the various stages of developing the text to the final production of the manuscript. We appreciate that Dionne Holland and Johanna Mithen made their research assistance time available at short notice. Finally, we would like to thank our inspiring colleagues in the School of Health Sciences at Deakin University who have offered support on the journey through many social connectedness seminars (sometimes called morning tea), and who have demonstrated a commitment to this book and the key messages it seeks to share with health and other professionals.

ABBREVIATIONS

ABS	Australian Bureau of Statistics
ACIR	Australian Childhood Immunisation Register
ACSCs	Ambulatory Care Sensitive Conditions
AFRO	Africa (WHO region)
AIDS	acquired immuno-deficiency syndrome
AIHW	Australian Institute of Health and Welfare
AHPSA	Australian Health Promoting Schools Association
AMRO	Americas (WHO region)
AusDiab study	Australian Diabetes, Obesity and Lifestyle study
BBV	blood-borne virus
BCC	behaviour change communication
BEACH	Bettering the Evaluation and Care of Health
BMI	body mass index
BoD	burden of disease
CAUL	Council of Australian University Librarians
CVD	cardiovascular diseases
DALY	Disability Adjusted Life Year
DHAC	Department of Health and Aged Care
DHS	Department of Human Services
DNA	deoxyribonucleic acid
EURO	Europe (WHO region)
GATTS	General Agreements on Tariffs and Trade in Services
GBD	Global Burden of Disease
GID	Gender Identity Disorder
GNP	gross national product
HDL	high-density lipoprotein
HCV	hepatitis C
Hib	haemophilus influenzae type b
HIC	Health Insurance Commission
HIV	human immuno-deficiency virus
HPSs	health promoting schools
IDU	injecting drug use
IEC	Information Education Communication
ILO	International Labour Office
IPCC	Intergovernmental Panel on Climate Change
KAB	knowledge, attitude, behaviour change

LDL	low-density lipoprotein
LEB	life expectancy at birth
LGA	local government area
METs	metabolic equivalents
mRNA	messenger ribonucleic acid
NDSHS	National Drug Strategy Household Survey
NEHS	National Environmental Health Strategy
NGO	nongovernment organisation
NHMRC	National Health and Medical Research Council
NPHP	National Public Health Partnership
NTC	National Tobacco Campaign
NWFP	North-West Frontier Province
OAS	operator-assisted services
PBS	Pharmaceutical Benefits Scheme
PHAA	Public Health Association of Australia
PHC	primary health care
RCT	randomised controlled trial
RNA	ribonucleic acid
SES	socioeconomic status
SNAP	smoking, nutrition, alcohol, and physical activity
STI	sexually transmitted infection
UN	United Nations
UNDP	United Nations Development Program
USDHHS	US Department of Health and Human Services
WHO	World Health Organization
WTO	World Trade Organization
YLD	years of healthy life lost due to disability
YLL	years of life lost

DETERMINANTS OF HEALTH

PART 1

UNDERSTANDING HEALTH: AN INTRODUCTION

Helen Keleher and Berni Murphy

Authors in this volume set out to make research about the determinants of health accessible to undergraduate students, in a foundation textbook for students from a wide range of disciplines including **public health**, **health promotion**, nursing, medicine, behavioural and health sciences, and exercise science. The primary intention of this book is to introduce the determinants of health as a basis for understanding health and health problems. A secondary intention is that readers will use their knowledge and skills about the determinants of health in the design of effective interventions in health promotion and public health.

'Determinants of health' is a broad term for a quite complex body of evidence that comes from many disciplines. As a result, literature on the determinants of health is usually written for experienced users of research; however, this book is particularly designed for readers new to the field and especially for students in the health and behavioural sciences. Health is a popular area of study that can be addressed through various health or disease topics, or through particular approaches such as public health or the sociology of health.

Our approach in *Understanding Health* is based on the position that health practitioners from any discipline require the development of knowledge and understanding not just about health but also its underlying determinants. We believe it is essential for people working in health or related fields to have acquired the ability to draw out the interrelatedness of the determinants and their complex interplays with health and illness, as the basis of effective, equitable, appropriate, and sustainable interventions.

THE CONCEPT OF HEALTH

Health, wellness, and illness are extremely difficult concepts to define. In keeping with Koos (1954), who stated that 'health is an imponderable', we choose not to offer a definition of health, but prefer to identify a number of different approaches to understanding health:

- The medical approach—health and illness are individualised incorporating notions about the absence of disease.
- The sociological approach—health and illness have social, political, economic, and structural dimensions.
- The 1980s World Health Organization (WHO) approach—health as an ideal.
- The 1990s WHO/health promotion approach—health is related to resources and capacities.
- The socioecological approach—health is about multifaceted relationships of determinants of health with attention paid to health equity.
- Popular, cultural, or lay approaches—health is relative to situations and related to personal expectations.

While each of these models has its own validity, no single one is universally valid, or able to comprehensively define health in a way that would hold good for all people, in all communities, in all places. So rather than have this book provide neat and tidy definitions, its intent is to help you develop *understandings* about health and its determinants from a wide range of perspectives.

Understanding Health is built upon broad notions of health that recognise the range of social, economic, and environmental factors that contribute to health and that understand health in terms of people's capacity to have access to the resources they need to be healthy, and to adapt, respond to, or control the challenges and changes in the environments that surround them. This approach to health enables us to shift our focus from making the state of health itself our object of interest or measurement, to making the determinants our object of analysis and the basis of our interventions and responses.

Defining determinants

Research findings about the determinants of health have emerged since the 1990s with such strength that neither policy makers nor health systems planners can ignore this important body of evidence and the ways in which it provides depth of understanding to statistical evidence about morbidity, mortality, and the burden of disease. A determinant of health is defined by Daniel Reidpath in chapter 2, as 'a factor or characteristic that brings about a change in health, either for the better or for the worse'. Groupings of determinants of health are introduced in this book, specifically the social-ecological, environmental, cultural, and biological–genetic determinants, but these groups of determinants are highly interrelated. That interrelatedness is concerned with questions such as 'how social forces act on individuals to affect their biological processes and change disease risk' (Marmot 2001, p. 349); or how behaviour affects both social processes and disease risk; and how social and structural conditions enhance or diminish opportunities for populations to be healthy. A concern with the determinants of health focuses attention on, and helps us to gain understanding about, both individual and population health issues.

Individual and population health

Approaches to the study of determinants of health and illness come from many disciplines. A determinants approach draws on the evidence, regardless of disciplines, to understand the ways in which health is created or in which disease and ill health might arise, as well as issues about individual health and how that differs from understanding the health of populations. Individuals have their own perspectives on how to attain health and a personal understanding of their own health status; diagnosis and treatment are directed at individual health problems. **Population health**, on the other hand, is concerned with improving the health of whole populations or specific populations, particularly to reduce inequities, through policies, programs, research and interventions designed to protect and enhance health. So population health can be focused on specific populations, such as young mothers or older men, or on everyone in general, such as through road safety campaigns. The determinants of health inform our understandings of individuals and populations, with much more of an emphasis on population health than on individual health or illness issues.

Upstream, midstream, and downstream factors

We can gain a great deal of understanding about how to respond to the determinants of health by identifying 'levels' that relate to where interventions might be targeted. These levels are useful, for example, in policy development, the design of research, and for health promotion activities. Turrell et al. (1999) identify three broad levels of factors affecting health—upstream, midstream, and downstream:

- **Downstream** factors are those at micro level including treatment systems, disease management, and investment in clinical research.
- **Midstream** factors are those at the intermediate level including lifestyle, behavioural, and individual prevention programs.
- **Upstream** factors are at the macro level including government policies, global trade agreements, and investment in population health research.

Determinants of health approaches at different levels serve to deepen our understanding of not just the problems but the interventions needed to address them. Most importantly, by distinguishing these different levels, we are encouraged to direct a component of our actions upstream to ensure that we have health equity.

INEQUALITY, INEQUITY, AND HEALTH EQUITY

Equity and inequity are concepts with social and political dimensions, while health equity locates equity in a health context. **Health equity** is about enabling people to have equitable access to services on the basis of need; it also is about the resources, capacities, and power they need to act upon the circumstances of their lives that determine their health. A study of health equity is necessarily also about inequity, which arises from the way people experience those factors that determine health. We distinguish between the terms 'inequality' and 'inequity' because there are essential differences between them. Health inequality is about measurable variations in health status. Health inequity 'refers to those inequalities in health that are deemed to be unfair or stemming from some form of injustice' (Kawachi et al. 2002, pp. 1–2). Attention is drawn in this book to those whose health is the most vulnerable to conditions that adversely affect them, while drawing out those conditions that are necessary for good health. Equity and justice are shown to be central to the determinants approach of understanding health and to the models and frameworks used for interventions to respond to illness and disease conditions.

Our overall message is that health professionals need not just to understand the determinants of health and illness, but how, in particular, the vulnerable and most disadvantaged people of any society are affected by exposure to adverse determinants. Understandings about the determinants of health are increasingly prominent in opening up the evidence base for new, critical approaches to strategic planning in health promotion and public health. Instead of taking a purely theoretical stance as to why health can be compromised by adverse conditions, or a conservative approach that only looks at the treatment of health and illness, this book discusses the integration of determinants approaches into health promotion and public health. In order to tackle inequities, health professionals need to take an active role in shaping actions to mitigate the adverse effects of the determinants of health. This means that all health professionals should have the capacity to integrate actions *for* health into their practice. It means that all health professionals should understand health equity and develop core competencies of how to enable, advocate, and mediate to ensure that their clients are receiving not just the best health care but are also being given the best health choices. These are issues of justice, equity, and empowerment.

This book is not intended to provide a comprehensive introduction to the design of interventions to address the determinants of health and illness. The intention of the book is to introduce evidence about the determinants of health as a basis for effective intervention planning and design and to suggest ways in which analysis of issues using a determinants approach reveals insights into health and social issues that inform intervention design. A number of health promotion interventions are explored to illustrate how health promotion can be informed by a determinants approach. Readers of this text may well feel encouraged to consider the implications for policy and practice that arise when analysis of health problems is based on the determinants and their interrelationships. The book does contain sufficient information about public and population health to enable students to grasp the core elements of those systems.

We have not included a specific chapter on the health of Indigenous Australians. Rather, a number of authors have incorporated discussion of Indigenous health within the content of their chapters, recognising that Australia's Indigenous people have long drawn attention to the interplay between social, environmental, and biological determinants of health; and through their experience we are more acutely aware of the need to address the determinants of health through a combination of upstream, midstream, and downstream approaches.

OUTLINE OF THIS TEXTBOOK

Understanding Health has twenty-eight chapters presented in three parts: Part I—Determinants of Health; Part II—Health Promotion Action: Responding to the Determinants; and Part III—Determinants Approaches to Public Health Issues.

Part I aims to develop the foundations of health in terms of the various groupings of the determinants of health, and to draw out the relationships between the determinants of health and inequities. Special focus is placed on the social, environmental, and biological determinants of health as well as an overview of health behaviours and biomedical **risk factors** and population health. Chapter 2 concentrates on the social determinants of health and provides more expansive definitional material about what determines health. Chapter 3 explores the environmental determinants of health. It introduces the idea of environmental justice, and examines some of the challenges for managing environmental determinants of health. There is some urgency in the need for effective management of human–environment relationships. Chapter 4 explores the biological determinants and their relationships to disease outcomes with an emphasis on the emerging evidence about genetics and health. Chapters 5 and 6 draw out the interrelatedness of the determinants: chapter 5 through case studies from Asia and the Pacific; and chapter 6 by explaining Australia's systems for measuring population health, which includes a discussion of biomedical risk factors. Chapter 7 is a critique of population health as it is currently conceived in Australia with questions raised about selective and comprehensive approaches to population health. The concepts central to the book—determinants, upstream/midstream/downstream factors, health equity, and inequity are explained. Using mental health as a case study, this chapter brings together a key message of the book—that we need integrated, multilevel, multifaceted approaches to improving the health of populations.

Part II has two objectives: one is about taking an historical perspective in order to understand some of the momentum for public health and health promotion as systems have responded to health problems; the other is to explore health promotion interventions to illustrate the breadth of approaches created in response to health problems. The historical backdrop is provided in chapters 8 and 9; these two chapters also challenge normative approaches to public health history. Rather than venerating particular individuals who have played a part in public health developments, the authors emphasise the long history of community-driven responses to health problems that recognised the social and environmental contexts of health and illness. Chapters 10, 11, and 12 set out the elements of contemporary health promotion interventions. Chapter 10 begins with an account of the development of health promotion responsiveness from the Ottawa Charter for Health Promotion to the present. Chapter 11 introduces the notion of the fourth dimension in health promotion as one that incorporates new directions for policy and practice, presenting a model for understanding the range of intervention approaches. Using a case study approach, chapter 12 demonstrates how two major health promotion initiatives used determinants of health to guide the design of interventions. Chapter 13 takes a critical approach to health education and communication—the most common forms of health promotion—to demonstrate the need for health education strategies that are responsive and maximise opportunities for effectiveness. Chapter 14 encourages a critical approach to health information available online, outlining criteria to assess the quality of online information. This is pertinent and timely, as our access to, and dependence on, online health information grows.

Part III, comprising fourteen chapters, introduces challenging, familiar, and not so familiar public health issues through a determinants-of-health 'lens'. Topics covered are: alcohol; illicit drugs; physical activity; social exclusion; food insecurity; evidence and public health; ecology and place; mind–body health connections; disability; youth health; mental health of same-sex attracted men; workplace health, and ageing. While not every public health topic can be covered in a book of this size, there is sufficient breadth and detail in these chapters to allow the reader to translate a determinants approach to other public health issues, many of which will be just as important as those we have selected here.

KEY FEATURES OF THIS TEXTBOOK

- **Key concepts** are provided at the beginning of each chapter.
- **Case studies** are used throughout the book. They illustrate the analysis of health issues using a determinants approach, drawing out the vulnerability of particular people to the influence of global and local conditions. The topics covered in the case studies highlight the need for more concentrated efforts to address the inequities originating in unfair distribution of life opportunities, of access to education, or employment, or other resources.
- **Discussion topics** are provided for each chapter. These may be useful for revision and review of learning, or for the development of tutorial programs in conjunction with chapter readings from the textbook.
- **Chapter summaries** are presented at the end of each chapter.
- **Useful web sites** are provided at the end of chapters where considered appropriate.

SOCIAL DETERMINANTS OF HEALTH

2

Daniel D. Reidpath

Key concepts

- Determinants of health
- Proximal determinants of health
- Distal determinants of health
- Disability Adjusted Life Years (DALYs)
- Ecological fallacy
- Absolute and relative poverty
- Social capital

If everyone's health were exactly the same (even if it were exactly the same very poor health), this chapter would not be written. It is the variation in health that is so important. It is the fact that some people have poorer health than others do and, more importantly, that certain groups of people have poorer health than others that generates interest in the area. The characteristics that define those groups that are more likely to become sick or to die, the determinants of their health, are the focus of this and the next two chapters. The case study described in box 2.1 provides an illustration of the factors that will be highlighted in the chapter.

This case study is adapted from one used by the well-known public health activist, David Werner (1997). Before reading on, write down what it was that killed Ama, noting as many things as you can think of, and then put the list to one side. Anything you wrote down that was not a specific diagnosis of a disease is probably what is referred to in public health as a determinant of Ama's health. A **determinant of health** is a factor or characteristic that brings about a change in health, either for the better or for the worse. Determinants of health may include things as diverse as exercise, arsenic in the water supply, and sun exposure (too much may lead to skin cancer and too little may lead to vitamin D deficiency). In

Box 2.1   Case study

Ama, a small, three-year-old child, was playing with her siblings outside her home in a small, semi-urban, slum area. While chasing her older brothers she trod on a nail. Her mother washed the wound and bandaged it. The wound remained red and 'angry'. Over a week the wound did not heal, the area remained red and 'angry', with flaring up the leg. Ama began to complain that she had pain in her groin, she became weak and febrile. Ama was taken to hospital when her mother could not control her fever and she died within a few days of admission.

this chapter you will be introduced to the idea of determinants of health, examining in most detail the *social* determinants of health. In later chapters you will consider other determinants of health including environmental, biological, and genetic determinants.

Determinants of health are often divided into distal and proximal determinants. A **proximal** determinant of health is one that is proximate or near to the change in health status. By 'near' one can mean near in either time or distance, but generally it refers to any determinant of health that is readily and directly associated with the change in health status. Proximal determinants are also referred to as **downstream** factors. In contrast, a **distal** determinant of health is one that is distant either in time or place from the change in health status. The association between the change in health status and the determinant may be indirect or hard to see because of other intervening events and locations. Distal determinants of health are also referred to as **upstream** factors.

In practice, the interest in determinants of health relates almost exclusively to attempts to identify causes of health status change that are amenable to intervention. Age, for example, is a well-known determinant of health but there has been little success in halting the ageing process, so as an identified biological determinant of health, ageing is of limited value. Factors such as the level of physical activity, social isolation, and poor nutrition that may also be associated with age, and are also known to be determinants of health, are more amenable to intervention and therefore receive considerably more scientific interest.

The list of possible determinants of Ama's death (see table 2.1), although incomplete, shows the complexity of the issues involved. The last determinant listed is 'antibiotics' and it is listed as both a biological and a proximal determinant. The sociostructural factors that lead to the lack of antibiotic availability, however, are also determinants of health and are distal. 'Poor wound management' is a biological and proximal determinant, but the education that affects the parents' skills and knowledge about wound management are more socially and distally determined. How one chooses to think about the determinants of a health outcome will affect the types of interventions that one considers.

Table 2.1 The (possible) determinants of Ama's death

Septicæmia (diagnosis)

The nail (environmental—proximal)

The environment—no playground and nails on the ground (environmental, social—proximal and distal)

Lack of footwear (social—proximal)

Poverty (social—distal)

Poor housing (social—distal)

Poor wound management (biological—proximal)

Poor knowledge about wound management (social—distal)

Ama's gender, possibly affecting treatment seeking (social—distal)

Lack of education of parents (social—distal)

Poor health care facilities (social, environmental—proximal and distal)

Lack of antibiotics (biological—proximal)

The principal difficulty in writing about or understanding the social determinants of health is that while each factor may individually have an effect on health, there is a complex interaction between them. That is, social determinants do not occur in isolation. Commonly identified social determinants of health include aspects of social life such as gender, ethnicity, and wealth, and level of education (which often fall under the umbrella term of socioeconomic position). Figure 2.1 shows graphically the intersection between these determinants of

Figure 2.1 The entanglement of the social determinants of health

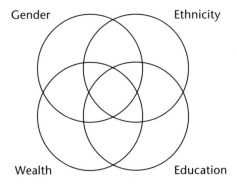

health. Inescapably, every person is either male or female (for the most part, although this is now subject to some debate), has an educational background, has a certain level of wealth, and comes from an ethnic background. Every individual is affected by all of these factors.

The following sections will introduce a few of the main social determinants of health, namely socioeconomic position, wealth inequality, ethnicity, and gender. While some of these factors are described in isolation, it should be remembered that ascribing health outcomes solely to one factor or another provides an incomplete picture.

(SOCIO)ECONOMIC POSITION

Socioeconomics describe those factors that affect a person's ability to act as a free agent, and to engage with and influence the society around them. Socioeconomics include income, wealth, level of education, and social influence. In this section the main focus is on the relationship between health and money (i.e. wealth, income, and poverty). Many of the statements that will be made about these relationships translate directly back into more general findings about the relationships between health and socioeconomic position.

Income, wealth, poverty, and health are strongly related—people who are poor tend to have worse health outcomes than people who are rich. Similarly, countries that are poor tend to have sicker populations than countries that are rich. This is probably the single most studied, and single most recurrently observed social determinant of health.

Figure 2.2 shows the distribution of health by the wealth of the fourteen World Health Organization (WHO) subregions. The subregions cover Africa (AFRO), the Americas (AMRO), Europe (EURO), the Eastern Mediterranean (EMRO), South-East Asia (SEARO), and the Western Pacific (WPRO). In the graph, *health* is quantified by a measure known as the **Disability Adjusted Life Year (DALY)** and *wealth* is quantified by the gross national product (GNP) of a country.

A per capita DALY of 0.5 (e.g. AFROD) means that on average, for every single person in the region, about half a healthy year (i.e. 'disability adjusted' life year) has been lost. A GNP of about US$2500 means that for every person living in the region, the countries produce on average US$2500 per person. Looking at any one subregion can be pretty meaningless, but the pattern is clear. As population wealth (GNP) increases, so the health status of the population (DALYs) rapidly improves. One of the Western Pacific subregions (WPROA), which includes Australia, New Zealand, and Japan, has the best health outcomes and the second-highest per capita GNP (around US$24,000). It is about six times healthier than the very poorest subregion, Africa's AFROE. What is remarkable about the graph is that, at least initially, very small increases in per capita GNP are associated with very large improvements in health until per capita GNP reaches about US$7500, when health improvements appear to

Figure 2.2   The distribution of health and the per capita gross national product for the fourteen World Health Organization subregions

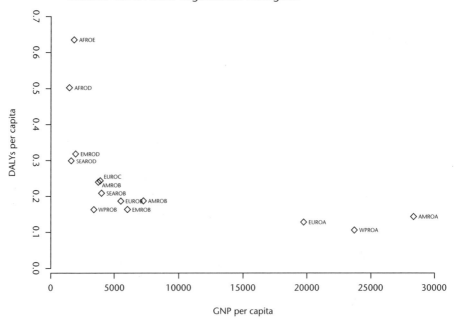

plateau sharply. This point will be returned to later in a discussion about the effects of relative and absolute poverty on health.

Another good example of the relationship between population wealth and population health can be found in work conducted by the Australian Institute of Health and Welfare (AIHW 2000, 2002b). In *Australia's Health 2000* the AIHW examines the relationship between small area data related to socioeconomic disadvantage and the DALY population health measure within those areas. The measure of socioeconomic disadvantage was derived by the Australian Bureau of Statistics (ABS) and summarises social and economic characteristics of different areas. AIHW divided small geographic areas into five groups (quintiles) of equal population size. The first quintile comprised the fifth of the population from the areas with the least socioeconomic disadvantage; the second quintile contained the fifth of the population living in the next least disadvantaged areas, and so on, down to the last quintile that comprised the fifth of the population from the areas with the greatest socioeconomic disadvantage. What is apparent in the data is a clear association between health and socioeconomic disadvantage—areas that are more socioeconomically disadvantaged have poorer health than areas that are less socioeconomically disadvantaged.

Moving from social determinants of population health to social determinants of individual health, recall the case of Ama, the small girl who died from septi-caemia. There is little in the description to say how wealthy her parents actually were. They could be very wealthy, but choose to live in a slum. However, given

Box 2.2   Ecological fallacy

Does knowing that poor suburbs have worse health outcomes than wealthy suburbs tell you anything directly about the relationship between individual wealth and individual health? Most people would think that it does. If poor suburbs have worse health outcomes than rich ones, then, they would reason, it is the poor people who have the poor health. This, actually, is not necessarily so, and the presumption that it is so, is known as an **ecological fallacy**. It could be that it is the rich people living in the poor suburbs who have the worst health outcomes. Similarly, the poor people in the rich suburbs could have the best health, but overall, the wealthier suburbs are healthier than the poorer ones.

The ecological fallacy occurs when one infers that a relationship that holds at a population level between two ecological factors such as DALYs per capita and gross national product (GNP) per capita is also true for two individual factors, such as personal health and personal wealth. The ecological fallacy is a common problem for people interested in social determinants of health, and needs to be considered when reading or listening to reports about determinants of health.

that she was living in a semi-urban slum, it seems plausible that her parents were poor. Is this an explanation for the health outcome; that is, was poverty a determinant of Ama's health? A few possibilities come to mind. Poverty limits the ability of parents to provide a safe living environment for their children—one without nails. It limits their ability to afford footwear for their children. It limits their ability to afford appropriate health care including curative care in the form of antibiotics. Poverty may well also have limited the educational opportunities of the parents, affecting their knowledge of how to deal appropriately with a deep puncture wound. Poverty is also deeply stigmatised and may affect the way others, for example health professionals, relate to Ama and her parents.

The notion that poverty 'caused' Ama's death, however, is contentious. Showing a direct and systematic relationship between poverty and any particular health outcome is almost impossible because of the distal relationship. At one level, few health researchers would actually dispute a relationship between poverty and health. The real debate, however, is around whether the observation about the existence of the relationship is even interesting. Kenneth Rothman, writing in *The Lancet*, queried whether poverty was really a matter of concern for health researchers (Rothman et al. 1998). If a determinant of health is not amenable to an intervention—and governments have often shown themselves to be remarkably resistant to addressing poverty—then it may be largely irrelevant whether it is actually a determinant of health or not. Many health authorities prefer to focus on the identification of determinants of health that are 'politically neutral' and therefore more readily amenable to intervention. Rothman was, however, wrong—poverty should be a matter of concern for health researchers—and the difficulties associated with developing suitable interventions should not be taken as evidence that poverty is not a determinant of health, or that it is not an *important* determinant of health. Developing politically palatable interventions based on addressing the determinant is, nonetheless, an unresolved challenge for many of those interested in public health.

INCOME INEQUALITY

Since the mid 1990s, another area that has captured the imagination of researchers in the area of the social determinants of health is whether it is absolute or relative wealth that is a determinant of health.

Look again at figure 2.2. There is enormous variation in the health outcomes of populations with average per capita GNP of US$2500 and those with an average per capita GNP around US$7500. There is a sharp, almost linear improvement in health with a relatively small improvement in wealth. There is almost no variation, however, between the health outcomes of populations with an average per capita GNP around US$7500 and those with an average per capita GNP of US$25,000. This suggests that absolute poverty is what is really important. Once populations lift their average GNP per capita above the US$8000 mark, there is little health to be gained by any additional wealth. This is the succinct argument for absolute wealth as the important determinant of health.

There is a problem with the absolute poverty argument, however. The USA is one of the richest countries on earth. Through welfare and charity even the poor receive money greater than that enjoyed by many in developing countries. Yet the health outcomes of the economically poorest in the USA rival, and in some cases surpass, some of the worst health outcomes in the developing world.

Box 2.3   Absolute and relative poverty

Absolute poverty: In some countries, such as the USA, government agencies have adopted the idea of a 'poverty line'. If one earns below this line then one is, in absolute terms, considered poor. Australia does not have an official poverty line, but one may, nonetheless, have a sense that if the annual household income of a family of two adults and two children is below $15,000 then they are, in absolute terms, poor.

Relative poverty: This idea is quite different. A person worth $1 million is, in absolute terms, wealthy. However, if that person lived in a society in which everyone else was worth $2 million, then our hapless millionaire would, in comparison to others, be poor. Relative poverty is about how the wealth is distributed between the members of a society, and not about the absolute amounts held by each person.

This suggests that absolute wealth may not be the only issue. It appears that being relatively poor is also bad for one's health.

Although the finding is not universal, research conducted in the USA, the United Kingdom, and Australia (among other places) has shown that, in general, health outcomes are worse for people living in areas of high wealth or income inequality than in areas of low wealth or income inequality. In other words, health outcomes are better when there are no vast differences between the rich and the poor. Bruce Kennedy and his colleagues in the USA, for example, found that states with very high levels of income inequality, such as Louisiana and Mississippi, also have high mortality rates (Kennedy et al. 1996). In contrast, those states with the lowest levels of income inequality, such as Utah and New Hampshire, have much lower mortality rates.

The explanations for this finding have resulted in a quite heated debate between the proponents of two possible interpretations. There is a 'psychosocial' interpretation associated with researchers including Richard Wilkinson (1996) and Michael Marmot (1999) and a 'neomaterialist' interpretation associated with researchers including John Lynch and George Kaplan (Lynch, Davey Smith, Kaplan, and House 2000). The **psychosocial** interpretation posits that unequal societies are unfair societies, and people express their perception of the unfairness

Box 2.4   The psychosocial versus the neomaterialist

John Lynch provides a metaphor to explain the difference between the **psychosocial** and **neomaterialist** positions. Imagine two passengers flying about twenty hours from Australia to the United Kingdom. One passenger is travelling economy class, the other is travelling first class. At the end of their journeys, if they were asked to rate their health, the first-class passenger would, on average, rate her health higher. She received better food, sat in a wider and more comfortable seat, and slept in a fully reclining chair. The economy-class passenger sat in a cramped seat with poor legroom, ate bad food, and slept little. Under a psychosocial interpretation, the differences in the health outcomes can be explained in terms of the negative emotions brought about by the economy-class passenger's perception of the unfairness of the inequality in treatment and service. Under a neomaterial interpretation, passengers travelling economy class report worse health because their material conditions (cramped seats, bad food, and no sleep) are worse. The psychosocial treatment could include the abolition of first class, because this would remove the perception of relative disadvantage by people in economy class. The neomaterial position would be to improve the conditions of those in economy class.

Source: Lynch et al. 2000, pp. 1200–4

of the wealth inequality as psychosocial stress. Although some amounts of stress appear to be positive for health, prolonged exposure to stressful environments (such as an unfair society) is causally related to higher mortality and morbidity. In contrast the **neomaterialist** explanation argues that people living in more unequal societies have poorer health outcomes because unequal societies invest less in social infrastructure such as housing, transport, and health services. The health outcomes are therefore a result of a combination of lack of resources to buy health and the lack of resources to provide health.

SOCIAL COHESION

For the proponents of a psychosocial model, the social determinant at the heart of the observed health disparities in unequal societies is one of social cohesion. Unequal and unfair societies are societies in which respect, trust, and 'social capital' are absent, and in these circumstances there is little sense of social belonging. If one lives in such a society, it is easy to imagine (though this doesn't mean it is true) that life would be more of a struggle and health would suffer.

Box 2.5   Social capital

Social capital is a term that became of intense interest to many health researchers looking at social determinants of health in the late 1990s. There is no single definition of social capital, but its use generally encompasses terms like 'trust' and 'reciprocity'. The political scientist Robert Putnam described it in terms of the features of social organisations, such as trust, that improved the efficiency of the society. In studying social capital there have been debates about whether it is an attribute of individuals (i.e. person *a* owns more social capital than person *b*; just as *a* can own more money than *b*) or whether it is somehow an attribute of places or groups.

The evidence in support of this view is found in studies showing strong associations between wealth inequality and trust, trust and reciprocity, wealth inequality and reciprocity, and all of these and health. For example, Ichiro Kawachi and colleagues found a strong association between the percentage of people in each state in the USA who answered 'yes' to the assertion that 'most people would try to take advantage of you if they got the chance' and the state level mortality rates (Kawachi et al. 1997). States with low levels of trust, that is states in which a higher percentage of people believed that others would try to take advantage of them, were the same states with the highest mortality rates. This kind of ecological association between trust ('social capital') and mortality rates is used as evidence for social cohesion as a determinant of health.

Between 1901 and 1991 there was a steady rise in **life expectancy** for people living in England and Wales of around two years every decade. During the decades in which World War I and II occurred, however, the rise in life expectancy rose to between six and seven years. Thus, in decades of major conflict, the health of the population improved. This observation is remarkable and counterintuitive. It is counterintuitive because social cohesion and major conflict appear to be, on initial consideration, antithetical and most people would probably expect life expectancy to decline during times of war. Wilkinson (1996) suggests a number of factors that may have contributed to improvements in life expectancy including a greater sense of intra-societal cohesion and camaraderie; in effect, a society pulling together in the face of shared adversity. For the neomaterialists, the explanations lie in the improvements in living conditions associated with labour reform and the rationing of food, clothing, and fuel, which ensured that everyone received at least something.

The reality is probably 'both'—a combination of the psychosocial and neo-materialist positions. The sharing of social resources and a sense of trust and belonging are unlikely to be unrelated. If people do not trust each other to share, why would anyone want to pool resources? It was recently shown that, in the USA, those states with the highest proportion of African Americans in the population were also those states with the highest mortality rates among the white population. This was true even after one took account of the level of poverty in the states (because those states that have the highest proportion of African Americans in the population—the southern states—also tend to be the poorest states). Why do white mortality rates go up as the proportion of African Americans in the population increases? A ready, and facile, explanation would be that somehow African Americans are killing whites. This is too glib and a more plausible explanation is that the deeply ingrained racism of the USA has effectively created a divided society in a perpetual state of internal conflict. In order for the white population to avoid sharing resources with the African American population (and vice versa), they have to withdraw investment from social infrastructure. The disinvestment affects both populations. The lack of trust driven by racism affects the social infrastructure, which in turn affects health. Both psychosocial and neomaterial explanations for the poor health outcomes are available. This example of ethnicity, social cohesion, and health provides a foretaste of the next section, in which we look specifically at ethnicity as a social determinant of health.

ETHNICITY

Before discussing ethnicity, *race* as a determinant of health needs to be considered. In the sociological literature, 'race' is generally regarded as an entirely artificial construct used by one group to claim dominance and superiority over another. In the health literature it has also been used as a term to specify biological distinctions between groups of people. The evidence for the effects of race on health is limited. For example, in malarious areas of Africa the sickle cell trait occurs. The sickle cell trait is a genetic variation in hæmoglobin that provides some protection for its carriers against infection by the malaria parasite. More often, however, observed disparities in the health outcomes of different 'races' says less about biological distinctions between groups of people than it does about the manner in which societies are structured.

In the USA, for example, African Americans have much poorer health outcomes than white Americans. This is true even after one has taken account of socioeconomic disadvantage. These observations are not credibly explained in terms of biological distinctions and are much more likely to be artifacts of social structure. For this reason, 'ethnicity' is generally a better umbrella term than race. Having said that, even the term ethnicity has been criticised because of the manner in which health researchers utilise the categories of black, white, Indigenous, Chinese, Hispanic, and so on, as if these terms actually describe culturally (and sometimes genetically) homogenous groups. 'Indian', for example, is supposed to be a useful label of ethnic group membership, but it is a word that can be applied to a billion people who are culturally very diverse.

Notwithstanding the difficulties associated with the use of 'ethnicity', and the care that needs to be taken in the study of the association between health and ethnicity, there is ample data to suggest that ethnicity does have an effect on health outcome. In *Australia's Health 2000* (AIHW 2000), for example, the health of Australia's Indigenous population is shown to be much worse than that of the non-Indigenous population. From 1995 to 1997, more than half of the deaths of Indigenous males occurred in people younger than fifty. If one examines the whole of the Australian population, however, more than 70 per cent of male deaths occur in people older than 65.

Indigenous Australians have higher rates of death than non-Indigenous Australians from cardiovascular disease, cancers, respiratory disorders, injury and poisoning, digestive disorders, mental disorders, genito-urinary disorders, and infectious and parasitic diseases. Even if one were to attempt to argue that this reflected some biological predisposition to poorer health, the argument is just not sustainable across all the causes of death. A more likely explanation for the poor health outcomes of Indigenous Australians probably relates to broad issues of poverty, and political and socioeconomic marginalisation. Indeed, Indigenous minorities, from Japan and Guatemala through to Canada and the USA, have poorer health outcomes than the dominant majority of the population. In all these countries, the Indigenous groups are the subjects of political and socioeconomic marginalisation.

The discriminatory response to ethnic minorities can be extreme, and there is data to suggest that in the USA people receive different treatment in health care facilities according to their ethnicity (e.g. Funk et al. 2002). Given an African American and a white American attending a hospital following a heart attack, the white American is more likely to receive better treatment than the African American.

For the reasons outlined in the earlier discussion on the entanglement of the social determinants of health, deciding which health outcomes are attributable to ethnicity as opposed to those attributable to other social factors such as employment, education, and wealth, is complex. Membership of minority ethnic groups is often associated with lower income, higher rates of unemployment, lower rates of high school completion or university education, and concentration in particular job sectors. All these can be social determinants of health.

> ## Box 2.6   The healthy migrant effect
>
> Interestingly, one area in which membership of an ethnic minority appears to be related to better health outcomes is among voluntary migrants to Australia. Generally, migrants who did not enter Australia under a refugee or humanitarian program have better health outcomes than people born in Australia. This appears to be an artifact of the selection process for migration. When people are accepted for migration to Australia, they have passed a series of health checks that ensure they are fit, healthy, and unlikely to be an undue burden on the Australian health care system. Thus, they have better health outcomes because they were healthier to begin with.

GENDER

As with the race/ethnicity distinction, a distinction needs to be made between gender and sex. 'Sex' refers to the biological distinction attributable to possession of the XX or XY chromosomes. 'Gender' is defined by the Australian researcher, Pascale Allotey, in the following way: Gender captures socially and culturally constructed aspects of being 'male' or 'female' that reflect relations between individuals at a personal level and the values and norms that permeate the broader social structures (Allotey and Ravindran 2003). Debates about the sex/gender distinction obscure the significant interaction, however, between biology, society, and the environment, to affect health outcomes. The position Allotey takes is that biology provides diverse potentials, and that cultures and societies limit, select, and channel these potentials into what is constructed as appropriate or acceptable.

Gender can affect health at multiple levels. Where one can write of the poor having worse health outcomes than the rich, there is less point in identifying one gender as having worse health outcomes than the other. However, it is worth noting ways in which gender can affect health outcomes and how gender can pattern health outcomes. Examples of this include the following:

- The ratio of male births to female births is around 509 males to every 491 females. In some societies, such as in parts of India and China, in which the girl child is seen as costly and burdensome, this ratio can be heavily skewed by infanticide and sex-determined terminations of pregnancy. Under these circumstances the ratio can be in excess of 600 males born for every 400 females.

- Because of the difference in the value of a girl child over a boy child, in some cultures the girl child is less likely to be taken to a health care facility when she is sick than a boy child, and more likely to receive a home remedy. This may, for example, have been one of the reasons for delaying seeking treatment for Ama.
- In the marketing of alcohol and tobacco—two known factors associated with poor health outcomes—advertising companies take advantage of gender to target and place their products, portraying them as desirable or advantageous for one sex or the other.
- The types and causes of violence that are experienced by men and women are patterned by gender. Men who are physically assaulted will generally have been attacked by a stranger, who is almost always male. Women who are physically assaulted will generally be attacked by someone known to them.
- In broad terms, men are more likely to engage in high-risk behaviours and are therefore overrepresented in the statistics on car crashes, alcohol-related injuries and deaths, and drug-related morbidity.
- The act of seeking treatment for health problems is strongly affected by gender. For example, women who suffer from a chronic disease are far more likely than men to approach disease-specific support groups.
- Occupations are heavily gendered. The occupational hazards to which workers are exposed are, therefore, quite different.
- 'Women are sicker, men die quicker.' Chronic diseases are a common concern for older women. While women are living relatively longer than men, they have higher rates of cancers, degenerative heart disease, osteoporosis, and other chronic conditions. Combined with the poor economic status of the elderly, this creates multiple jeopardies for health.

Gender as a social determinant of health is also entangled with other social determinants such as income inequality between males and females, and their often disparate roles within the household and broader society.

CONCLUSION

Before finishing this chapter, pause for a moment and think about why one might be interested in looking at social determinants of health instead of, say, biological determinants of health. In choosing to consider the distal rather than the proximal determinants of health, one is invited to look beyond the individual and think about how we structure our societies and whether that is good for our health. In always focusing on the proximal determinants of health, there is a danger in accepting that those distal social structures that affect health are somehow inevitable and immutable (i.e. fixed and unchanging). Should we, for instance, accept Ama's death as inevitable? Should we focus on the biological, and seek to improve the quality of medical care available to her? Alternatively, should we look beyond Ama (tragic as her death may be) and ask whether there are ways of changing the nature of society so that where one fits within the social structures does not create inequities in the distribution of health?

SUMMARY

- This chapter has introduced the ideas of determinants of health and focused on some social determinants of health. These included socio-economic position, income inequality, race and ethnicity, and gender. These by no means cover the field of social determinants.
- Social determinants of health are health determinants attributable to the structure and functioning of society. This means that transportation can be a social determinant of health, because it is a social structure that affects physical activity, which in turn appears to affect nutritional intake and cardiovascular health.
- Workplace relations are a social determinant of health because they affect aspects of health associated with occupational health and safety and job stress.
- Social norms around sexual behaviour are social determinants of health because they can affect people's approaches to risky sexual behaviour, and can result in stigma and discrimination, and social marginalisation.
- When thinking about what a social determinant of health is, there is an implicit opportunity to think very broadly about issues surrounding health and the factors that affect health.

DISCUSSION TOPICS

1 How might education be thought of as a social determinant of health? How is it related to other determinants of health?
2 Discuss how structure and functions of the social determinants of health affect the health of Australia's Indigenous people.

ENVIRONMENTAL DETERMINANTS OF HEALTH

Rosemary Nicholson and Peter Stephenson

Key concepts

- Environmental health
- Ecologically sustainable development
- Equity and environmental health justice
- Physical settings
- Life support systems

The essential links between human health and wellbeing and the environment in which we live have long been recognised. For centuries, these links have been central to the Indigenous cultures of the world (Smith and Desai 2002), yet over the past 150 years developing and industrialised nations have lost sight of this connection. In our relentless quest for economic wealth we have increasingly abused our own life support systems. We have overfarmed, overfished, and generally depleted our natural resources. We have treated the ecosystem as a bottomless pit into which we have relentlessly dumped increasing quantities of industrial and human wastes. As a result we are now witnessing the environmental and health effects of this global destruction of our life support systems (Kickbusch 1989a).

In this chapter we aim to provide an overview of the extent and nature of these impacts and of the current relationship between the state of the environment and human health. We begin by looking at some of the traditional and emergent or 'modern' environmental threats facing the world's populations. Sociopolitical considerations and issues of equity are brought to bear on these concerns. We then explore some of the environmental determinants of health typically associated with urban environments, rural and remote environments, the workplace and the home, drawing on both Australian and international examples. The chapter concludes with a discussion of five key environmental determinants of health: air, water, biodiversity, land, and food.

BACKGROUND

The World Health Organization (WHO) currently estimates that some 25 per cent of the disease burden worldwide is environmentally induced (WHO 1997b), although recent work of researchers at Cornell University suggests the true figure to be 40 per cent—and rising (Pimental et al. 1998). Whether or not the WHO estimate is conservative, there is no disputing that figures of this magnitude confirm the close association between the state of the environment and the level of risk to human health. While administratively governments continue to treat health and the environment as separate entities, the links between the state of the physical environment and human health are irrefutable (Soskolne and Bertollini 1998).

Hancock and Perkins' (1985) 'mandala' of health (figure 3.1) serves as a graphic illustration of the inextricable linkages between human health, the social and cultural environments, and the broader ecosystem. The mandala depicts human health in its broadest possible context. This bio-psycho-social-environmental model places the individual at the centre of concern. Four critical factors influence the health of the individual and their family (or social unit). These are human biology, personal behaviour, the psychosocial environment, and the immediate physical environment. Our work environment, built environment, lifestyle, and health

Figure 3.1 Mandala of health: a model of the human ecosystem

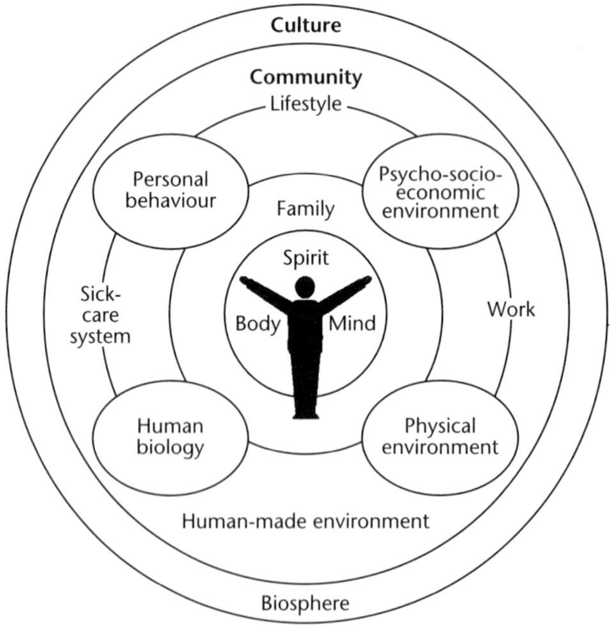

Source: Hancock and Perkins 1985

care system together comprise the human-made environment that influences our health. These are, in turn, shaped by our cultural values, attitudes, beliefs, and the condition of the global ecosystem, or biosphere, of which we all form a part.

Notwithstanding the accepted linkages, the outcomes sought by the environmental and health sectors can be in conflict with one another. An example can be found in the tension between the need for food supplies and concerns relating to the dangers of persistent organic pesticides (POPs) both to human health and to the ecosystem (WHO 1993a). Similarly the logging of remnant forests provides much needed employment while at the same time contributing to global **environmental health** issues through serious disruption of local ecosystems. Conversely the two sectors may work towards the same outcome but for different purposes. Examples of such congruence include the management of solid and liquid wastes or concerns for the environmental and human health impacts of a society highly dependent on the use of private motor vehicles.

Australia's National Environmental Health Strategy (NEHS) seeks *inter alia* to bridge the gulf between environmental management and public health. Quoting from Bidmeade and Reynolds (1997), the NEHS notes that: 'The interdependence of public health and environmental protection should be strongly emphasised in governmental practice and decision making, and a dichotomy between the two should not be allowed to exist' (enHealth Council 1999, p. 36).

Chapter 7 of the NEHS identifies the environmental health challenges presented by a range of issues at the human–environment interface, describes current activities aimed at addressing these issues, and identifies associated current and future environmental health needs. These issues can all be linked with human health and therefore 'dominate the core business of environmental health management'. They include water and air quality, food safety, contaminated land, waste management, vector-borne diseases, and the built environment.

Sustainable development is emerging as the accepted basis for integrating environment and health issues (Brown et al. 2001). In Australia, this is often known as **ecologically sustainable development**, or ESD. Nationally, and in most Australian states, ESD is expressed as five principles guiding humans in relation to their environment:

- equity between generations (give our grandchildren the freedom to make their own choice)
- equity within generations (maintain this generation's freedom to choose)
- the precautionary principle (ensure no risk of serious harm)
- protect environmental integrity (protect biodiversity and intact ecosystems)
- monitor progress (towards a sustainable human–environment relationship).

GLOBAL ENVIRONMENTAL CHALLENGES

Many of today's greatest environmental health challenges relate to the human health impacts of the global 'ecosphere' (Kickbusch 1989; Brown, Ritchie, and

Rotem 1992; WHO 1992, 1997b; Pimental et al. 1998; Soskolne and Bertollini 1998; McMichael 2001a; World Information Transfer 2002). We are now grappling with the complexities of living in an era of unprecedented population density, cultural diversity, food and resource consumption, and global connectivity. As the NEHS suggests: 'Changes to local and global environments are interactive and have a significant ability to impact on human health. Environmental health programs need to take into account that global environmental protection requires local action and that local actions impact globally' (enHealth Council 1999, p. 9).

This accords with the view taken by MacArthur and Bonnefoy (1998), who emphasise the need for global ecologically sustainable solutions to local environmental health issues. Local activities that impact both on human health and on global ecological **sustainability** include those associated with motor transport, industry, and the storage and packaging of food. Motor vehicles contribute to local air pollution, local health problems and also to global warming. Industry may give rise to local pollution, consumes energy, and produces waste. Food packaging is resource-intensive and increases solid waste, and refrigeration impacts on energy use. Ironically the health industry itself contributes significantly to issues of envi-

Table 3.1 Local effects of loss of global sustainability

GLOBAL CHANGE	AUSTRALIAN LOCAL EFFECTS
Air	
Ozone depletion	Melanomas (world's highest level), Tasmania
Global warming	Floods, droughts, changed pollination patterns
Water	
Irrigation	Salting, acidification of soils
Forest clearances	Increased erosion, drop in rainfall
Land	
Productive land	Reduced by 10 per cent every year, 60 per cent degraded
Life	
Biodiversity	More mammals extinct than any other continent
People	
Population	Waste production per head second in Organization for Economic Cooperation and Development
Energy	
Energy Use	Greenhouse gases increasing by 16 per cent (8 per cent allowed by 2008 in the Kyoto Agreement)

Source: Brown 1999

ronmental degradation (which then, in turn, impact adversely on human health) through its heavy consumption of energy and natural resources and (arguably unsustainable) waste management practices (Guest et al. 1999). Other examples from the Australian perspective are reproduced in table 3.1.

In short, current environmental health trends are driven by an array of interconnected causes associated with rapid industrial expansion and an increasingly global economy (Stephens 2000; Stewart 2002). These causes include cultural values, increasing urbanisation, technical, scientific and economic development, and genetic engineering (WHO 1997b). Poorly understood interactions between global ecological risks and the health impacts of social, cultural, and economic activities have resulted in environmental health issues that no longer lend themselves to simple cause-effect interventions. The human health effects are typically cumulative, long-term, and complex (Kickbusch 1989).

'Traditional' versus 'modern' environmental health threats

Historically, environmental threats to human health have tended to result from issues of *under*development (poor housing, inadequate water quality, and the absence of sanitation) and have been primarily contained within the local environment. These 'traditional' threats, while now largely under control in the more affluent areas within developed nations, are still very much in evidence in the poorer countries of the world and among socially disadvantaged and disenfranchised population subgroups of developed nations. 'Modern' threats, on the other hand, arise as a result of overconsumption and pollution associated with unsustainable *over*development (WHO 1997b). While Third World nations continue with their struggle to combat the escalation of traditional environmental health threats, the primary environmental health concerns of industrialised nations are now the *modern* and more *global* hazards. These are brought about by a continued focus on economic development with scant attention to the consequences to the global ecosystem.

EQUITY AND ENVIRONMENTAL HEALTH JUSTICE

Different communities vary in their susceptibility to environmental threats and in their response to such threats. The term **environmental health justice** describes the right of all people to a safe, healthy, productive, and sustainable environment. This principle is of particular concern to, for example, Indigenous Australians, whose life expectancy continues to be of the order of sixteen to eighteen years less than the population average (Guest et al. 1999). Indeed nearly every quality of life indicator for Indigenous Australians remains significantly lower than those of most, if not all, non-Indigenous citizens. An array of environmental determinants sit alongside a host of other social, political, and historical influences in accounting for this unacceptable health status of Australia's first nation peoples.

The relationship between relative wealth and exposure to environmental health risk, both in Australia and worldwide, is well documented (WHO 1991; Hancock 1994; Baum 2002). In the words of Labonte, 'there is something toxic about the steepness of the slope of hierarchic inequalities' (1997, p. 19). There is also a well-established positive correlation between environmental quality and the literacy levels, income distribution, civil liberties, and political rights of citizens. In short, environmental problems 'bear down disproportionately on the poor' (Agyeman and Evans 2002). The WHO report, *Health and Environment in Sustainable Development, Five Years after the Earth Summit*, acknowledges that: 'Impoverished populations ... are at greatest risk from degraded environmental conditions. The cumulative effects of inadequate and hazardous shelter, overcrowding, lack of water supply and sanitation, unsafe food, air and water pollution and high accident rates impact heavily on the health of these vulnerable groups' (WHO 1997b, p. 198).

Hancock condemns this situation, both for its social injustice and for its impact on ecological sustainability, pointing out that:

> It is no coincidence that the poor live downwind, downstream and downhill (unless the hillsides are dangerous, in which case they live uphill!). Nor is it a coincidence that it is the citizens of the poorest countries, and the poorest residents of any country, who live on the most environmentally unsustainable and marginalised land, and who out of poverty, are often forced to use their land and resources in environmentally unsustainable ways.
>
> Hancock 1994, p. 38

While air and water pollution remain priority environmental health issues worldwide, the global environmental health concerns of industrialised nations are neither shared by the majority of citizens of underdeveloped countries, nor by the socioeconomically underprivileged sectors of their own populations (Hancock 1994; Labonte 1997). The priority concerns of these communities are necessarily more immediate and more local even though the causes of their drought or flood conditions, shortages of basic needs, and high risk of infectious and parasitic disease may, at least in part, be global (WHO 1993b, 1997b). The populations of developing countries undergoing rapid industrialisation are at risk from the combined threats of both traditional and modern environmental health hazards (WHO 1993c, 1997b). Furthermore, 'modern' issues such as ozone depletion and climate change respect neither national nor regional boundaries and therefore threaten the population health of both developed and developing countries.

Ozone depletion and increased exposure to ultraviolet radiation

The release of human-made halocarbons such as chlorofluorocarbons (CFCs) into the atmosphere has resulted over the past thirty or more years in significant stratospheric ozone depletion and the much-publicised hole in the ozone layer over the Antarctic. As a result the quantity of ultraviolet-B (UV-B) radiation entering the atmosphere has risen by up to 10 per cent in some parts of the world (McMichael and Kovats 2000). UV-B is a known cause of skin cancer and cataracts and may also adversely affect the human immune system (Guest et al. 1999). UV-B may also have other, more indirect, effects through its adverse impacts on aquatic and terrestrial biota (WHO 1997b). Most at risk are the Caucasian populations of mid- to high-latitude countries and in particular children and outdoor workers.

Global warming and changing weather patterns

Increasingly we are witnessing the worldwide environment and health impacts of human-induced climate change in the form of drought, flooding, severe storms, and extremes of temperature. These conditions are brought about by the release and atmospheric accumulation of greenhouse gases such as carbon dioxide, methane, chlorofluorocarbons, and ozone (Ewan et al. 1990; Martens and McMichael 2002; Smith and Desai 2002). The direct health effects of changing weather patterns are most pronounced in the very young, the very old and the chronically sick, all of whom are placed at additional risk from cardiovascular and respiratory conditions exacerbated by heat stress. Climate change and global warming are directly associated with the spread of insect pests and infectious disease vectors and with reduced food production (UN 2002).

Many of the warmest years on record occurred in the 1980s and 1990s. The Intergovernmental Panel on Climate Change (IPCC) has predicted that this will continue and that average surface temperatures are likely to increase by between 1.4°C and 5.8°C between 1990 and 2100 (IPCC 2001). The IPCC has reported that we will also experience changes in rainfall patterns, sea level rises, and changes in the frequency and intensity of some extreme climatic events. The IPCC has documented glacier retreat, sea-ice diminution, earlier bird nesting, earlier flowering, and altered timing of insect migration as evidence of effects. The small Pacific island states (including Kiribati, Fiji, and the Cook Islands) will experience impaired agriculture and freshwater sources along with population displacement within fifty years as sea levels rise.

Any steps to reduce global warming, for example, through green alternative fuel sources, reduction in consumption of fossil fuels, and reductions in pollution from car emissions, are likely to have positive health effects. Environmental protection programs are addressing a wide range of environmental issues including reductions in pollution levels, energy use and efficiencies, water use and efficiencies, waste minimisation, watershed conservation, and sustainable agriculture. However, low-income countries are more likely to feel the negative effects of global warming, as they do not have the economic power to force stronger countries to change those environmental policies that contribute to the problem.

PHYSICAL SETTINGS

Global causes of local environmental health issues and local impacts on the global environment call for the implementation of public protection and health promotion strategies that recognise the human health impact of physical **settings**. To quote MacArthur (1999, p. 9): 'Although many of the new threats are global the problem, and the response, will often be regional or local, even individual'. The Ottawa Charter for Health Promotion (WHO 1986b) makes specific reference to the human health impacts of the settings of our everyday lives—the places where we 'live, work, play and love'. (See chapter 10 for further discussion of the Ottawa Charter.)

WHO draws a clear distinction between the broader *contextual* settings of cities, suburbs, villages, and islands and the *elemental* settings of which they are comprised. Elemental settings include schools, homes, workplaces, hospitals, marketplaces, and similar local environments which, by virtue of their regular use, impact significantly on the health of local communities. Contextual settings play a major role in determining a community's level of access to services, and educational and employment opportunities.

Urban environments

McMichael (1993, p. 260) describes the cities of the world—the seats of wealth and power—as 'the star performers in human culture' while at the same time noting the appalling health status and social deprivation of the rapidly growing numbers of urban poor.

The evolution of the city can be traced back to settlements of farming communities eventually able to generate sufficient food to support the subsequent growth of urban populations. But despite their prominent positions as seats of government and centres of religion, learning, art, and scientific discovery, our cities have come to epitomise socioeconomic, environmental, and health iniquity. There are sixteen cities worldwide with a population in excess of ten million (UNDP 2000), and an estimated sixty cities with a population in excess of five million. At the upper end of the scale is Tokyo (population twenty-nine million) and Mexico City (population twenty-five million). The extent of urban development in the poorer countries of the world is such that by 2025 the combined urban population of developing countries could be as much as four times that of the developed world (McMichael 1993).

Hardoy et al. (2001) note that the quality of urban areas, with their complex mix of natural elements and built environments, are greatly influenced by their individual geographical settings; the scale and nature of human activities and structures within them; the wastes, emissions, and environmental impacts that these generate; and the competence and accountability of the institutions elected, appointed, or delegated to manage them. Today's urban health issues are at the same time diverse, complex, essentially interconnected, and socially based.

In a recent United Nations Development Program (UNDP) study, 135 city mayors were each asked to rate the problems of their particular city. Baum (2002) summarises their top responses as:

- overcrowding
- transport, mobility, and pollution
- increased levels of air, water, and land pollution
- large populations of 'underclasses', without full citizen rights and living in hazardous areas in squatter settlements and shantytowns
- inadequate sanitation, sewerage, and solid waste disposal
- lack of clean water
- increasing socioeconomic iniquity
- social isolation and decline of social capital
- increasing crime and violence
- unemployment, especially of young people
- inadequate social services.

Environmental problems such as those contained in this list become particularly serious in the face of rapid expansion in urban population and production with little or no consideration for the environmental or human health implications; or for the political and institutional framework that is needed to ensure that such environmental problems are addressed (Hardoy et al. 2001).

Rural and remote environments

The major environmental risks to the health of rural communities include indoor air pollution from burning of solid fuel for heating or cooking (a common cause of childhood pneumonia in Third World countries), poor sanitation, pesticide toxicity from agricultural and horticultural activities, water scarcity, and vector-borne diseases such as malaria (Lvovsky et al. 2000). For example, many of the 800,000 dams estimated to have been constructed worldwide, while of undoubted benefit to human health, have also brought about negative environmental health impacts. Dams increase local access to water for drinking and irrigation and are integral to the generation of hydroelectric power. But their construction also frequently involves widespread social displacement, interferes with migrating fish species, causes siltation and salination, and facilitates the spread of disease vectors and human parasites (WHO 1993b; Brewster 1999). The incidence of malaria in children living in close proximity even to small dams in Ethiopia has been found to be as much as seven times that of those in more distant villages (Brewster 1999).

Rural and remote communities in Australia have, over recent years, suffered the financial and consequent health effects of agricultural decline and depopulation exacerbated by an extended period of drought. Areas once able to boast relative affluence are now instead experiencing high rates of unemployment and financial hardship, contributing to high levels of stress and a dramatic increase in the incidence of suicide (Baum 2002).

In the case of Indigenous populations in rural and remote Australia, researchers have, over many decades now, repeatedly highlighted the importance of managing the physical environment for the protection of health and wellbeing (see Gracey 1987; Hearn et al. 1993). Despite this, a great number of environmental determinants of health in Indigenous communities remain poorly addressed and the health impact of poor environmental conditions on Australia's Indigenous populations is significant (Stephenson 2001). The findings of the 1995 *Western Australian Aboriginal Environmental Health Survey* illustrate this point clearly. The survey report provided empirical data on the status of environmental health conditions in 155 rural and remote Western Australia Aboriginal communities. In summary:

- Ongoing design and maintenance problems prohibit the effective functioning of water supply and sanitation systems in just over one third of Western Australia communities.
- Seventy per cent of the total survey sample had significant or serious, and sometimes multiple, problems with various aspects of their housing.
- Rubbish was not collected at all in over one third of communities and, in others, the methods of disposal were often inadequate.
- Pests were problematic in 44 per cent of communities and the hygiene and maintenance of communal toilets unacceptable in 25 per cent of cases.
- On-site environmental health workers could not be identified in 72 per cent of communities surveyed and external environmental health worker support services were unavailable to 52 per cent of communities. (Western Australia Health Department 1995).

The *Atlas of Health-Related Infrastructure in Discrete Indigenous Communities* (Bailie et al. 2002) is the latest publication to illustrate the urgent need for improvements to environmental health-related infrastructure in Indigenous communities nationwide. This data, combined with that of the 1995 Western Australian survey, clearly identifies the building of healthy Aboriginal and Torres Strait Islander communities as one of the most important environmental health challenges facing Australia today.

Work environments

Worldwide, the International Labour Office (ILO) estimates that workplaces claim on average 500 lives each day. The number of nonfatal accidents is calculated to be around 1000 times this figure (Kleish in Pantry 1995). Coupled with the increasing impacts of workplace stress (Skiold 2000), these statistics serve to highlight the magnitude of the risk to health posed by the work environment. Most at risk of serious or fatal injury are those who work in agriculture, forestry, mining, or construction (Takala 1995; WHO 1997b).

The precise nature of physical, biological, or chemical hazards, and the associated threats to human health, varies enormously from one industry to another. And it is not only employees who are at risk. During the 1970s a chemical explosion at a factory in Bhopal, India killed or injured thousands of outsiders. Similarly, in the 1980s, the Chernobyl disaster impacted far beyond the confines of the nuclear reactor. The full extent of the health impacts of accidents of this scale can probably never be known.

In countries such as Australia, employers are bound by occupational health and safety legislation to ensure the physical integrity of, for example, buildings, mines, and construction sites. Machines must be adequately guarded; potentially dangerous noise levels attenuated; hazardous biological, chemical, and radioactive substances safely handled, transported, and contained; tripping and slipping hazards ameliorated; and excessive heat, dust, odours, and fumes removed through effective ventilation and filtration. Thereafter additional safeguards include the implementation of safe working procedures together with the use of personal protective equipment.

Outdoor workers are more likely to be exposed to UV-B radiation and extremes of temperature, while the comfort of indoor work environments varies enormously from noisy and hot (or cold) factories to plush offices. The sedentary nature of office work, and the increasingly high demands on office workers are known contributory factors to stress-related depression, cancers, and cardiovascular disease. Long hours spent in front of the computer screen contribute to worker fatigue, itself a determinant of safety.

Home environments

A healthy physical home environment is dependent on sound housing design and construction, regular maintenance, an adequate supply of clean water, good sanitation, heating or cooling, sufficient ventilation, refrigerated food storage, and suitable arrangements for the storage and removal of refuse. As WHO states:

> Housing is of central importance to quality of life. Ideally it minimises disease and injury, and contributes much to physical, mental and social wellbeing. Over and above its basic purpose to provide shelter against the elements and a focus for family life, the home environment should afford protection against the hazards to health arising from the physical and social environment.
>
> WHO 1997b, p. 113

The proximity of housing to industry, main roads or other sources of traffic noise or pollution (e.g. railway lines or aircraft flight paths) also impacts on the health of inhabitants. Defective housing design and maintenance invites infestations of rodent and insect vectors, which, in turn, increase the opportunity for the transmission of infection. Cold and damp conditions exacerbate chronic respiratory disease, particularly in the very young, the very old, or those previously disposed to such conditions. At the other end of the temperature scale, heat stress represents another potentially serious health threat. Guest et al. (1999) note in particular the correlation between substandard housing conditions and some more widespread psychosocial disorders including violence, crime, delinquency, vandalism, drug and alcohol abuse, and breakdown of the family unit.

Mostly throughout Australia and the rest of the developed world, the high standard of living means that the relationship between health, housing, and community infrastructure is less obvious. However, for many Aboriginal and Torres Strait Islander communities in Australia higher rates of infections, injuries, and general health problems are directly attributable to poor living conditions and a lack of basic amenity (New South Wales Health 2003). In response to repeated studies identifying the inadequacies of Indigenous housing and infrastructure, current Indigenous housing policies, programs and priorities are geared towards improving 'health infrastructure'.

DEGRADED LIFE SUPPORT SYSTEMS

Despite international conventions highlighting the urgency for action, environmental degradation continues unabated across the globe—the global temperature is still rising, the ozone hole is widening, irrigation and the resultant shortages of water, soil salinity and contamination, and the depletion of forests are all increasing. Food production per head is falling, species are disappearing, human population numbers continue to rise (although the rate of population increase is slowing), and fossil fuel use is increasing (although the proportion of renewable energy use is rising) (Brown et al. 2002).

The WHO *World Health Report 2002: Reducing Risks, Promoting Healthy Life* details a range of priority risk factors that have an influence on health or wellbeing. The top ten leading risks include important factors that relate to the physical environment such as unsafe water, sanitation and hygiene, air quality, transport, and climate change. In the remainder of this chapter we will concentrate on air, water, land, and food, as key environmental determinants of health.

Air pollution

Air pollution from industrial and domestic sources, motor transport emissions, and the large-scale burning of bushland for agricultural clearing have all contributed to a decline in air quality within and across air sheds. As a truly transboundary environmental issue, city and rural dwellers in developing countries are now exposed to atmospheric pollution on the scale of the infamous London 'pea souper' of the early 1950s while photochemical smogs pervade car-congested cities worldwide (McMichael 1993).

Specific threats to human health are caused by a combination of gaseous material and respirable particles. Atmospheric pollution is a known cause of a range of respiratory diseases including asthma, bronchitis, and lung cancer and has also been linked to cardiovascular disease (Guest et al. 1999). Some of the key influences of atmospheric pollution include:

- *Small respirable particles* (less than 2.5 microns): are likely to penetrate deep into the respiratory system. Particles of this size are typically found in the exhaust fumes from motor vehicles, particularly those fuelled by diesel, and are often chemically active.
- *Sulphur dioxide:* mostly comes from sulphur-containing coal burnt in industry and power stations. It contributes to the severity of photochemical smog and causes acid precipitation, in turn associated with damage to vegetation and fish stocks.
- *Ozone:* the major constituent of the photochemical smogs evident in major cities during the summer months. Peak levels generally occur in summer due to the effects of sunlight and increased temperatures. Ozone is a respiratory irritant that can reduce lung function, and cause coughing, shortness of breath, and chest pain (Guest et al. 1999).

Water pollution

The three main categories of water pollution are liquid organic wastes (such as domestic human effluent), liquid inorganic wastes (i.e. agricultural run-off and industrial effluent), and waterborne or water-based pathogens (i.e. introduced and naturally occurring diseases, viruses, and worms in waterways) (Hardoy et al.

Table 3.2 Examples of drinking water contaminants and impacts on health

CONTAMINANT	SOURCE	HEALTH IMPACT
Pathogens	Animal waste from surrounding catchment Cross-contamination of untreated sewage	Diarrhoeal disease Intestinal worms
Persistent Organic Pollutants (POPs)	Bio-accumulated in aquatic (and other) food chains	Cancer Nervous system disorder
Lead	Mobilised through acidification of water	Cumulative nerve poisoning (young children particularly vulnerable)
Arsenic	Industrial effluent Naturally occurring constituent of soil	Cancer Peripheral neuropathy Vascular disease
Nitrites	Fertilisers Industrial waste	Impede oxygen carrying capacity of blood (identified risks to bottle-fed infants in underdeveloped countries)

2001). Accordingly, the high cost of providing clean and safe drinking water has become a major issue worldwide as urban populations increase in size. The problem of degraded water supplies, as exemplified by the *Cryptosporidium* and *Giardia* scare in Sydney in late 1998, is by no means unique to the Third World.

Although arguably not altogether clear-cut, WHO (1997b) notes the existence of a distinct North:South dichotomy whereby industrialised nations are more concerned with managing the risk of biological and chemical pollution while the populations of developing countries, with their more agriculturally related economies, are more at risk from waterborne bacteria, parasites, and vectors of microbial disease. Worldwide and on an annual basis, we are witnessing one billion deaths from malaria, the majority from the Amazon region, Africa, south Asia and South-East Asia, 200 million schistosomiasis infections, notably in sub-Saharan Africa, and tens of thousands of cases of dengue fever. Poor water quality and inadequate supplies of water for drinking and sanitation in densely populated areas in underdeveloped and developing countries are also closely linked with outbreaks of cholera and endemic diarrhoeal disease—still the world's number one killer. Examples of contaminants of drinking water supplies and their human health impact are provided in table 3.2.

Land contamination and degradation

Urban and suburban development on contaminated land can pose serious, and frequently long-term and chronic, health risks to children in particular (WHO 1992, 1997b; UNEP, UNICEF, and WHO 2002).

Soil may be contaminated by an array of chemicals and pathogens. Soil contaminants can potentially impact on human health either through direct contact or indirectly through the consumption of food or water. Contaminants fixed or loosely bound in soils can also be distributed by wind as in the case of remnant asbestos or tailings from lead mines. Wind erosion can also disperse toxic chemicals or heavy metals related to industrial or agricultural activity, at the same time stripping nutrients from the soil (Pimental et al. 1998). Alternatively, soil particles themselves can act as irritants or allergens. Dust particles and microbes from cleared land can be blown into the air causing ocular and respiratory irritation and aggravating allergies and asthma in susceptible individuals. Examples of contaminants of land and their human health impacts are provided in table 3.3.

Contaminated food

Physical, chemical, and biological contaminants, as well as some natural constituents, can render food hazardous to human health. In 1990, WHO recorded 240 million reported incidents of food-borne disease worldwide. The main sources of food-borne infection are animals bred and slaughtered for human consumption. Food can also be contaminated by the environment or even by other foods, although

Table 3.3 Examples of land contaminants and impacts on health

CONTAMINANT	SOURCE	HEALTH IMPACT
Arsenic	Mining procedures Pesticides Industry emissions	Liver and kidney damage Dermatitis Paralysis of muscles Cancer
Asbestos	Mining and processing Brake linings Roofing material Fire retardant in buildings	Cancer Chronic respiratory disease Chromosomal damage in miners
Lead	Industry emissions Paint Leaded fuel Water pipes	Poisoning Death Neurological impacts Behavioural disorders
Mercury	Industrial waste	Neurological damage Poisoning Kidney damage
Polychlorinated biphenyls (PCBs)	Electricity transformers Fire retarding products	Cancer causing Nerve skin and liver damage Reproductive and immune system disorders

often the source of infection is the food handler. The risk of contamination can be reduced considerably through careful control of the environments in which, and procedures whereby, food crops are cultivated, animals reared and slaughtered, and food processed and handled prior to human (and animal) consumption.

Under favourable (usually warm and moist) conditions high protein foods in particular will support the growth of toxic bacteria such as *Salmonella spp* and moulds such as *Aspergillus flavus* (a common contaminant of nuts and cereals). Food-borne parasitic infections from protozoa, tapeworms, and roundworms such as *Trichinella spiralis* are endemic to many tropical locations. Toxic chemicals from agricultural fertilisers, pesticides and herbicides, food containers, or land contaminated by industry, can all potentially find their way into food. Many bio-accumulate, becoming more concentrated, and hence more toxic, as they pass up the food chain. The use of chemical food additives to improve the colour, texture, and taste, and maintain quality of food represents an additional human health burden, while the precise nature and extent of human health effects of food irradiation and genetically modified food ingredients are yet to be determined (Miller Jones 1998).

SUMMARY

- Human health depends now as much as ever on the sustainability of the environmental system in which we live. The health of the environment is under ever-increasing risk and the long-term picture for rising environmental sources of ill health is bleak. And yet morbidity and mortality levels in industrialised nations are in decline with twenty years being added to Western life expectancies in the past fifty years (AIHW 1998).
- The optimistic view is that if 'health' programs and services could do it for the social determinants of health, then their 'environmental' equivalents can do it for environmental determinants.
- The key message of this chapter is that the challenge for managing environmental determinants of health is an urgent one and lies in the effective management of the human/environment relationship. In a previous publication we suggested that this can only be achieved through:
  - preserving the physical condition for life: *environmental security for human biology*
  - protecting communities from local and global environmental risks to health: environmental security for human population
  - managing place-based economics, social, and environmental risk: physical security for workplaces and human settlements
  - re-establishing human/environment sustainability: long-term security for global self-supporting systems. (Brown et al. 2001).
- The goal of environmental health policy and action in this era of globalisation is to reduce both social risks to environmental sustainability and environmental risks to social sustainability (Brown et al. 2002).
- In order to address environmental determinants for health in a sustainable way, national and international policies must be implemented at all scales from the local to the global. Environmental health practice is a key area for identifying and managing environmental threats to human health well into the future.

DISCUSSION TOPICS

1 Develop case studies to explain how the 'goal of environmental health policy and action in this era of globalisation is to reduce both the social risks to environmental sustainability and environmental risks to social sustainability'.

2 Find out about an international policy/protocol implemented to address a global environmental concern such as greenhouse gas emissions, land clearing, or commercial fishing in international waters.

3 In what ways might such an international policy or protocol be expected to positively impact on health?
4 What are the likely implications, both locally and in the global community of a country such as Australia, for failing to comply with this policy/protocol?

USEFUL WEB SITES

enHealth Council: www.enhealth.nphp.gov.au
Indigenous Communities Environmental Health: http://iceh.uws.edu.au
International Council for Environmental Initiatives (ICLEI): www.iclei.org
International Institute for Sustainable Development: http://iisd1.iisd.ca
International Healthy Cities Foundation: www.oneworld.org/cities
United Nations Environment Program (UNEP): www.unep.ch

4 BIOLOGICAL DETERMINANTS OF HEALTH

Boyd Swinburn and David Cameron-Smith

Key concepts

- Biological determinants of health and disease
- Models of disease causality
- The role of genes
- Race and ethnicity as determinants of health and disease
- Morbidity and mortality in relation to age
- Gender differences in health and disease
- Understanding biological markers of risk

The biological determinants of health and disease refer to a wide range of hetero-geneous, intra-individual factors that drive, mediate, or moderate the pathways towards health or disease. At a fundamental level, genes provide much of the underlying biological variations between individuals and interact with most of the other individual, social, and environmental factors that influence health and disease. Phenotypic features such as stature, fatness, and skin colour are often markers of the interactions between genes, behaviours, and environments. Two major biological determinants are age and gender. Age, in particular, has such huge effects on causes of morbidity and mortality that most disease-related data are shown as age-specific or age-adjusted rates to account for this confounding influence.

The genetic and physiological systems within the body are dynamic, complex, and highly interconnected, with whole systems balancing and competing against each other. Indeed, it is not dissimilar to the complexity and dynamism of the social and environmental systems external to the individual. The tools we have at our disposal to measure the factors involved in health and disease and their relationships, although rapidly improving, are nonetheless crude. When we measure a factor (such as high blood pressure) that predicts a disease outcome (e.g. stroke), we tend to consider the high blood pressure to be a 'determinant' or independent cause of the disease, whereas it would be more properly described as a 'mediator'. This is because there are multiple underlying distal factors (such as a high salt intake, physical inactivity, central adiposity, genetic factors) that are the 'determinants' of high blood pressure itself. Initial models of health and disease causality tended to be linear (e.g. high salt intake → high blood pressure → stroke) but they then become more and more complex as other determinants of salt intake, blood pressure, and stroke are added to the model. The entire causality diagram ends up as a mass of boxes and arrows depicting many interconnected determinants and is often referred to as the '**web of causation**' (Krieger 1994). Therefore, it is more appropriate to consider the 'determinants' as measurable **nodes** (the connecting point where several lines come together) within a 'web of causation' rather than as independent causes of health and disease.

This chapter will explore some biological determinants and their relationships to disease outcomes (which are more easily measured than health outcomes) using a number of examples to illustrate those relationships. Cardiovascular diseases will be used to illustrate some of the issues involved in determining causality because these diseases are very common and their biological, social, and environmental determinants have been intensively studied.

GENES

The major international effort to sequence the human genome ended in 2001 when a consortium of publicly funded institutions and a private company jointly announced that the entire human genome had been sequenced. This announcement, made by the then President of the USA, Bill Clinton, was heralded as the greatest discovery in medical science—one that would revolutionise the quest to conquer complex diseases. Few doubt that major discoveries will come and that the human genome holds the key to many diseases. However, the identification of small differences in deoxyribonucleic acid (DNA) between a healthy and a diseased individual is equivalent to searching for a needle in many haystacks. For example, thousands of scientists are searching for the gene that causes cancer. One might ask, 'Why is this so difficult and why hasn't it been done?' The answer is that the link between genes and disease is complicated by the nature of the disease itself, the genetic variations from one individual to another, the technology that scientists have at their disposal, and scientists' limited understanding of the biochemical pathways involved in the development of complex diseases.

The human genome

The human genome is a remarkably complex sequence of nearly five billion DNA bases, located on twenty-two pairs of autosomal chromosomes and two sex chromosomes (XX for females and XY for males). Within each chromosome, the vast majority of the DNA provides scaffolding and structure, while less than

5 per cent makes up genes. Genes are the small segments of DNA that code for proteins. It is estimated that the human genome has 30,000 active genes.

Genes lie dormant within the enormous strands of DNA until a signalling molecule activates the DNA to unlock the message coded within. Ingeniously, each gene has sequences that bind to proteins that transfer messages from the outside world. Generally, signals such as hormones trigger gene activation by recruiting signalling proteins that pass into the nucleus of the cell, bind to the DNA and activate the complex cellular machinery to make many copies of the genes (figure 4.1). These copies are made in the form of **messenger ribonucleic acid** (mRNA). Each mRNA is an accurate replica of one of the DNA templates. The mRNA moves out of the nucleus and is used as the code for the synthesis of new proteins. For this, the RNA bases are read in groups of three that correspond to one of the twenty amino acids. These amino acids are joined sequentially to make a new protein.

The synthesis of mRNA occurs simultaneously for many genes. Scientists are only just beginning to grapple with the impact that different physiological stimuli have on the activation of genes and protein synthesis. What should be appreciated is that this process is remarkable in that each gene is 'read', mRNA produced, and new protein synthesised minute by minute, with many adjustments being made to precisely regulate the function of every cell in the human body. Genes respond rapidly to changing physiological conditions. For example, when a person exercises, activated muscle must be equipped with thousands of metabolic **enzymes** (i.e. the proteins produced by a cell and that act as catalysts in specific cellular reactions) and contractile proteins (i.e. the proteins in muscle

Figure 4.1　From genes to proteins: the process of decoding genetic information in DNA to be used in the synthesis of proteins

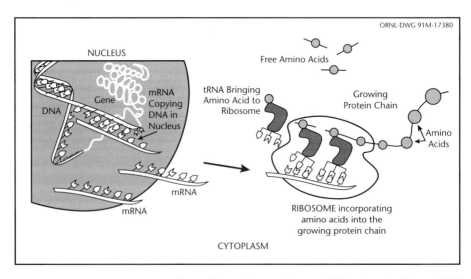

Source: Human Genome Program US Department of Energy 1992

(actin and myosin) that slide past each other to cause contraction) to efficiently perform the required task. To do this, following a bout of exercise, many thousands of genes are activated and the coded proteins are synthesised. These are needed to repair damaged muscle and to ensure that the muscle is ready for the next bout of exercise. With time, muscle cells build up proteins required for metabolism and contraction, enabling the muscle to become more efficient and better equipped to perform the exercise.

The genes of humans are about 98 per cent identical to the gene sequences of apes, and only slightly less similar to those of rats and mice (about 95 per cent identical). Given the minor differences, it is surprising that humans have so many unique physical and metabolic characteristics. Between individuals, there are many small and subtle differences in sequences of genes that determine each individual's unique characteristics. Differences in genes that are common within the population (i.e. occurring in >1 per cent of people) are called **polymorphisms**. Most genes in the human genome are polymorphic, with differences as small as one or two **DNA bases**. In the vast majority of cases, these polymorphisms are 'silent', having no obvious effect on human physiology or health. However, occasionally, very small differences affect physiological pathways to significantly change disease risk or responses to changing physiological conditions (i.e. exercise, a high fat meal or fasting).

One example of a polymorphism that has a positive effect on human physiology is the polymorphism in the angiotensin converting enzyme (ACE) gene. ACE is important in the regulation of blood pressure and the control of blood flow. A common polymorphism found in the population is either the presence or absence of a 287 base-pair section of the ACE gene. It was first observed that many mountaineers and elite soldiers had this polymorphic insertion in the ACE gene, suggesting that the extra section of the ACE gene increases the capacity for physical performance (Jones et al. 2002). In a follow-up study, British Army soldiers were analysed before and after basic training (Montgomery et al. 1998). The recruits with the insert ACE gene polymorphism had eleven-fold greater gains in the ability to perform repetitive arm curl exercises with a 15 kg barbell compared with those who had the deleted ACE polymorphism (Montgomery et al. 1998). It is not yet clear what the extra section of the ACE gene does; however, this example demonstrates that subtle changes in one gene can influence physical performance.

The vast majority of human disease states may be associated with the inheritance of many polymorphisms. Geneticists begin the hunt to find which polymorphisms contribute most to the development of a complex disease, such as hypertension, obesity, and type 2 diabetes, by firstly establishing that the disease has a genetic component. The contribution of genes is established by assessing the heritability of the disease. Large-scale epidemiological studies track the inheritance of the disease through families (family studies); or in individuals who share many common genes and have been raised and are living in the same environment (twin studies); or in individuals who share many common genes but who have been raised in different environments (adoption studies). Such studies establish the relative contribution of genes versus the 'environment' in the development of disease states. Having established that genes are important, regions of the DNA are scanned for polymorphisms that are linked to the disease state.

Less common than polymorphisms are mutations. A **mutation** is a change in the sequence of a gene that results in the protein produced being severely altered or nonfunctional. In many cases, mutations occur over large sections of a chromosome and affect the synthesis of many different proteins. Mutations giving rise to the classic inherited diseases (e.g. cystic fibrosis, muscular dystrophy) are inherited from one or both parents. Some mutations, such as those that cause some forms of cancer, arise spontaneously when errors occur in the replication of chromosomes as cells divide and replicate during growth.

Gene–environment interaction patterns

There are a variety of models for understanding the relationships between genetic make-up and environmental factors (Kendler and Eaves 1986). Note that these models usually describe everything external to the genes (including behaviours of the individual) as 'environment', whereas the true environment is external to the individual.

The *additive model* is the simplest, and is based on the assumption that for two individuals at different genetic risks for a disease (such as stomach cancer), the risks for both increase proportionally as they go from a protective to a high-risk environment (e.g. a low to high intake of smoked and pickled foods). The *multiplicative model* is based on a differential response between individuals such that a diet of smoked and pickled foods greatly increases the risk of stomach cancer in the genetically predisposed person but barely alters the risk in the genetically resistant person. This can be seen as genetic control of sensitivity to the environment or environmental control of gene expression. The multiplicative model is probably the more common model in human gene–environment interactions. A third model is based on the assumption that the genes influence the *exposure* to a high-risk environment (a genetic preference for the taste of pickled and smoked foods), rather than influencing the relationship between the foods and the development of the cancer.

An example of single gene disease—sickle cell anaemia

Simple models are usually a good starting point for understanding human health and disease; however, in reality they are often too simplistic to account for the observed differences in disease rates between individuals and between populations. One disease where a clear two-way relationship between genes and environments has been identified is sickle cell **anaemia**. In this condition, a single genetic abnormality results in an amino acid substitution on the β-globin subunit of haemoglobin. A person who is **homozygous** (i.e. both genes are the abnormal sickle variant) for the sickle cell gene has a significant, chronic anaemia (low haemoglobin levels) because the abnormal haemoglobin causes the red blood cells to deform into a sickle shape and prematurely break up. A person who is **heterozygous** (one normal gene, one sickle gene) is asymptomatic and has no anaemia. Interestingly, the heterozygous state confers a degree of resistance to infection with malaria, which is a distinct advantage in high malaria areas. The prevalence of the sickle cell trait in African Americans is about 8 to 10 per cent, whereas in the West African countries of Nigeria and Ghana, where malaria is endemic, the prevalence is about 25 to 30 per cent. The malarial environment therefore promotes an increased frequency of the genetic abnormality, even though the homozygous sickle cell state clearly confers a selective disadvantage.

Examples of multi-gene diseases

Most of the disease burden in high-income countries such as Australia, and increasingly in low-income countries, is attributable to chronic, noncommunicable diseases such as cardiovascular diseases (CVD), diabetes, some cancers, arthritis, and mental illness. Many of these diseases have significant genetic contributions, but it is the combination of dozens, if not hundreds, of key genes that determine the genetic contribution. However, the gene–environment pattern is often a multiplicative one, where the high-risk environment brings out genetic susceptibilities. This is illustrated in the gene–environment interactions that occur in weight gain and obesity.

Figure 4.2   Two population distribution curves for body size (body mass index)

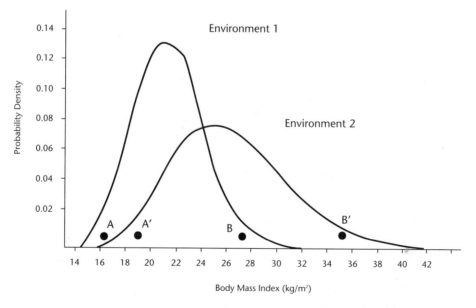

Adapted from Rose 1992

A population living under conditions of food scarcity and with minimal technology available for work, transport, and entertainment would have a relatively lean population distribution curve (see Environment 1 in figure 4.2) (Rose 1992). The variation in body size is a mixture of genetic, behavioural, and environmental factors, but it is fairly narrow. By contrast, the distribution curve for a population living in a modern, 'obesogenic' environment (see Environment 2 in figure 4.2) is much wider, flatter, and skewed to the right. The genetically lean people in each environment (hypothetically shown as A and A') show small differences in body size compared to those genetically predisposed to obesity (hypothetically shown as B and B'). The obesogenic environment therefore allows the 'obesity' genes to be expressed. In general, one can say that environmental differences predominantly determine the differences in obesity **prevalence** between populations and that, within a population living in the same environment, genetic differences predominantly determine differences in body size between individuals (i.e. the *presence* of obesity).

Race and ethnicity

Differences in disease rates between populations may be attributed to racial or ethnic differences. Race implies a set of biological characteristics, whereas ethnicity also includes other dimensions such as cultural, social, and economic factors, and is now widely accepted as the more appropriate descriptor. One area where ethnicity has had a prominent place in a list of disease determinants is type 2 diabetes. This is typically an adult-onset, obesity-related disease that is characterised metabolically by liver and muscle resistance to the action of insulin. Some populations have extremely high rates of diabetes, with the most studied ones being the Pima Indians in Arizona and the Micronesian population of Nauru. In both of these populations, over half of the middle-aged adults have type 2 diabetes (Knowler et al. 1978; Coyne 2000). Further evidence for a genetic influence on diabetes comes from studies that show that populations with a higher Native American genetic admixture have higher rates of diabetes (Gardner et al. 1984).

While the genetic predisposition to diabetes cannot be ignored, social and economic influences may also be powerful in these populations. The Pima have suffered from the marginalisation, deprivation, and poverty common to almost all Native American populations. The association between low socioeconomic status and obesity is strong in high-income countries, especially for women. This may in part be explained by reduced access to the healthier but more expensive foods (such as fruit and vegetables and lean meat), reduced opportunities for recreational physical activity, and a low priority placed on health promoting behaviours. Chronic stress may also result in the overproduction of the hormone cortisol that can contribute to the development of central adiposity (Bjorntorp and Rosmond 2000). By contrast, Nauru, a small isolated island in the mid-Pacific, experienced a period of extreme wealth from mining its phosphate resources in the centre of the island and this promoted obesity through a marked reduction in physical activity and increase in energy intake. Clearly, these populations do have a large proportion of people with a genetic predisposition to diabetes; however, the social and economic circumstances that have allowed the expression of these genetic factors are also extraordinary.

AGE

Age is probably the most potent determinant of specific risk factors, morbidities and mortality. Table 4.1 shows the steep increase in **death rates** in older people in Australia—over three-quarters of deaths occur after the age of 65 (AIHW 2002b). This is the characteristic pattern of a high life expectancy population. Currently in low-income countries (and previously in all populations), a different pattern is seen with much higher infant mortality, higher childhood and maternal mortality, and fewer people dying in older age. The types of diseases that give this high mortality pattern are mainly infectious (and obstetric) in nature. Infectious diseases are particularly dangerous in those with underdeveloped immune systems (the very young), malnutrition (often children), and other compromising diseases. By contrast, the list of killers in table 4.1 shows that the

Table 4.1 Leading causes of death by age and percent of total deaths in Australia

AGE (YEARS)	PERCENT OF TOTAL DEATHS (MALE, FEMALE)	LEADING CAUSES OF DEATH	PERCENT OF DEATHS IN AGE GROUP (MALES, FEMALES)
<1	1.1, 0.9	Perinatal conditions	49, 50
		Congenital anomalies	25, 25
1–14	0.6, 0.4	Injury and poisoning	51, 36
		Cancer	14, 17
15–24	1.8, 0.7	Injury and poisoning	73, 61
		Cancer	7, 12
25–44	6.5, 3.3	Injury and poisoning	52, 32
		Cancer	12, 33
45–64	16.7, 10.9	Cancer	41, 55
		Cardiovascular diseases	29, 18
65–84	54.3, 45.2	Cardiovascular diseases	38, 41
		Cancer	35, 30
85+	19.0, 38.5	Cardiovascular diseases	48, 56
		Cancer	18, 11

Adapted from AIHW 2002b

Figure 4.3   The age-specific prevalence of obesity (defined as having a body mass index >30kg/m²)

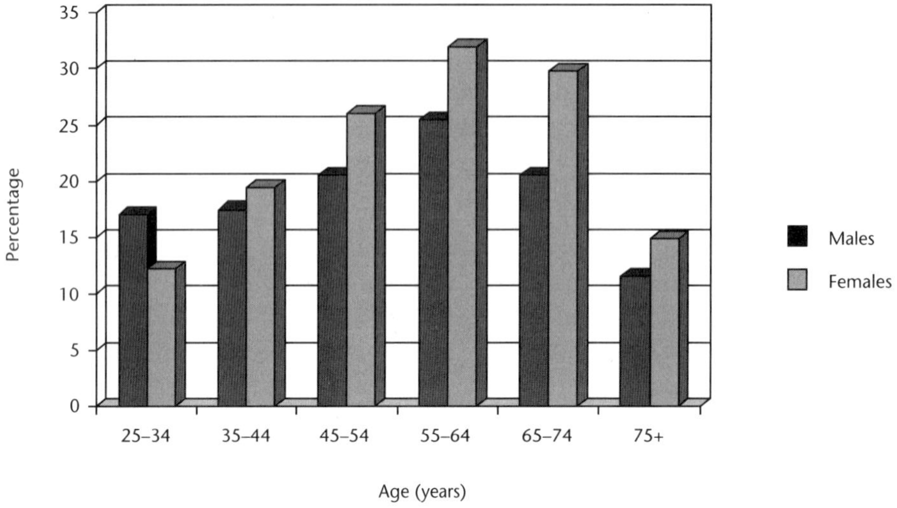

Source: Adapted from Dunstan et al. 2000

dominant causes of death are cardiovascular diseases and cancers (approximately two-thirds of total deaths) and that these are typically diseases of older people.

Cross-sectional relationships between age and various diseases and their risk factors also show marked age effects. For example, the relationship between obesity prevalence and age shows a relatively linear increase up to about age 60 and then a decrease (figure 4.3) (Dunstan et al. 2000). There are several factors that explain this apparent decline in obesity in old age. First, individuals may lose weight as a result of concurrent diseases such as cancer, age-related loss of appetite, poor dentition, therapeutic weight loss for diseases like diabetes, poorer access to foods and so on. Second, the apparent decline partly reflects a 'healthy survivor' phenomenon, whereby people with obesity die prematurely and so the older population as a whole is thinner. Third, the apparent decline may represent time trends in the obesity epidemic in that older people have had less lifetime exposure to obesogenic environments. (Here, obesogenic means the sum of influences that the surroundings, opportunities, or conditions of life have on promoting obesity in individuals or populations.)

GENDER

Some of the broad gender differences in health and disease patterns can be seen in table 4.1, with a higher male mortality rate throughout life and longer female life expectancy (82.1 years versus 76.6 years) (AIHW 2002b).

Injuries

Initially the differences are minimal, but between 15 and 44 years, males have about twice the mortality rate of females with injuries and poisonings largely accounting for the difference. The major causes in this category are suicides (where males outnumber females by 3–4:1) and motor vehicle crashes (where males outnumber females by more than 2:1) (AIHW 2002b). While the overall prevalence of mental disorders is similar between males and females, males tend to have more problems with aggressive behaviours and substance abuse.

Osteoporosis

Apart from obvious gender-related diseases such as breast and prostate cancers, there are gender differences in other common diseases. Osteoporosis is much more common in females, especially with the loss of the protective effects of oestrogens after menopause. Males are generally protected against osteoporosis by larger body size and testosterone effects.

Cardiovascular diseases

Coronary heart disease (heart attack) is the other common disease with a large gender difference, with higher rates occurring in males (figure 4.4) (AIHW 2002b). Interestingly, there is no gender difference for the other major cardiovascular disease (i.e. stroke), which has the same underlying disease process as coronary heart disease except that it occurs in the blood vessels supplying the brain rather than the heart muscle. This disease process is called **atherosclerosis** and it is characterised by a gradual build-up of cholesterol and other material underneath the lining of the artery (figure 4.5). The first signs of atherosclerosis can often be seen in young adults at autopsy and are 'fatty streaks' of cholesterol under the lining of medium and large arteries. The cholesterol is deposited there by scavenger cells (**macrophages**) that pick up the transport particles (**lipoproteins**) that carry cholesterol and other fats through the blood. Often these particles have been damaged by oxidation and their removal is part of the body's normal clearing mechanisms. A large number of these lipoprotein particles (such as in people with high blood cholesterol levels) or a high proportion of damaged particles (as occurs with the increased oxidation induced by smoking) can swamp the body's clearance capacity. The cholesterol therefore remains under the arterial lining, setting off an inflammatory process that results in a further build-up of material (including inflammatory cells, connective tissue, and calcium deposits).

Some of the factors that promote atherosclerosis include a diet high in saturated fat (which increases the so-called 'bad' or low-density lipoprotein/**LDL cholesterol** particles), a lack of exercise (which reduces the so-called 'good' or high-density lipoprotein/**HDL cholesterol** particles), smoking, and high blood pressure (which damages arterial lining). Decades of even moderate exposure to these risk factors

Figure 4.4 Death rates from coronary heart disease (CHD) and stroke in Australia 1950–98

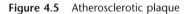

Source: AIHW 2001b

Figure 4.5 Atherosclerotic plaque

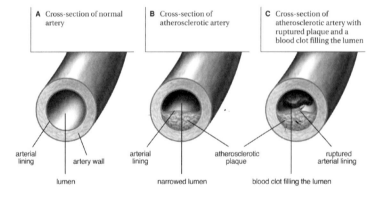

promotes atherosclerosis and the gradual accumulation of atherosclerotic plaque, setting the stage for a cardiovascular event (heart attack or stroke).

A cardiovascular event occurs when a blood clot forms over the atherosclerotic plaque (often in response to a tear in the lining of the artery) and blocks the blood supply to the heart muscle or the brain. If the lack of blood flow affects a large enough area of the heart or brain, death will result. Even a small heart attack can trigger a cardiac arrest in which the heart stops beating effectively. A high intake of saturated fat promotes not only atherosclerosis but also clot formation (thrombosis) and cardiac arrest. Given that this long and complex set of biological and behavioural pathways is affecting both the coronary arteries supplying the heart and the cerebral arteries supplying the brain, one might ask, 'Why do males under the age of 75 have three times the risk of a heart attack compared to women when their risk of stroke is similar to that of women?'

The gender differences for several key risk factors and protective factors for cardiovascular disease are shown in table 4.2. Men have a slightly higher risk profile in relation to smoking, high blood pressure, high LDL ('bad') cholesterol, diabetes, and vegetable and fruit consumption. They have a slightly better risk profile in relation to physical activity and a low-risk alcohol-drinking pattern in the 60-plus age group. Body fatness shows a mixed picture, with males having a higher prevalence of overweight and obesity (measured by a body mass index of >25 kg/m^2)) but a lower prevalence of central adiposity (measured by an abdominal girth >102cm for males and >88cm for females). A major risk factor that shows a distinct gender pattern is the level of HDL ('good') cholesterol. Females have a high prevalence of adequate HDL levels (<1.0 mmol/l), and this is a deciding factor in the gender differences in coronary heart disease.

Table 4.2 Gender differences in risk factors and protective factors for cardiovascular diseases (prevalence rates except for saturated fats)

DETERMINANTS	MALES (%)	FEMALES (%)
Risk factors		
Smoking (current smokers)	18	13
High blood pressure (>140/90)	31	27
High LDL ('bad') cholesterol (>3.5 mmol/l)	50	42
Overweight + obesity (body mass index >25 kg/m2)	67	52
High abdominal girth (m >102cm, f >88cm)	27	34
Diabetes	8	7
Saturated fat intake (% of energy)	13	13
Protective factors		
Physically active (>150 minutes/week)	56	44
Alcohol intake (low risk pattern in 60+ age group)[1]	67	62
Vegetable and fruit consumption (>five serves/day)	39	47
Adequate HDL ('good') cholesterol (>1.0 mmol/l)	81	95

1 Low-risk drinking pattern is small to moderate intake without binge drinking. The 60+ age group is used as this is where the benefits accrue.

Sources: Mathers et al. 1999; Dunstan et al. 2000; AIHW 2001, 2002b

Interestingly, the development of atherosclerosis in the coronary arteries seems to be particularly influenced by too high levels of LDL cholesterol and low levels of HDL cholesterol, whereas the same process in the cerebral arteries is particularly sensitive to high blood pressure (i.e. hypertension). This may explain why there are marked gender differences for coronary heart disease but not for stroke even though the disease process in the arteries appears similar. A similar dissociation between these two diseases is seen in the Japanese, who have very low rates of coronary heart disease but high rates of stroke. Their risk profiles show low LDL cholesterol levels (probably due to a diet that is high in fish and vegetables and low in meat and dairy fat) but high rates of hypertension (probably due to a high salt intake). The low blood levels of LDL cholesterol mean that the atherosclerotic process is slow to develop even in the presence of high rates of smoking and hypertension.

[handwritten margin note: Cholesterol determining Heart Disease.]

UNDERSTANDING BIOLOGICAL MARKERS OF RISK

Association or causation?

As mentioned at the start of this chapter, biological risk factors are best thought of as measurable nodes or junction points within a web of causality. How do we know if their relationships to health and disease outcomes are real or spurious? There are several criteria, first articulated by Bradford Hill (1965), that help to establish causality between a measured risk factor and a health outcome:

- consistency of findings (similar relationships found in different populations and using different study designs)
- strong relationship (high relative risks or odds ratios and strong correlations showing exposure to the risk factor is associated with high rates of the disease)
- temporal sequence (exposure to risk factor is prior to disease occurrence)
- dose response (a greater intensity or duration of exposure is associated with a greater risk of disease)
- specificity (confounding factors have been eliminated as explanations for the relationship)
- biological plausibility (explanatory mechanisms are known and credible)
- experimental evidence (changing the exposure experimentally changes the outcomes).

It has been demonstrated, for example, that there is a statistical relationship between baldness and heart disease in men. Obviously, the absence of hair does not cause heart disease, but both are probably related to one or more unmeasured third factors that could be, for example, hormonal or genetic. However, it may be that there is no apparent third factor, such as in the statistical association between a diagonal earlobe crease and higher rates of heart disease. By contrast, an elevated LDL cholesterol level fulfils all of the above criteria for causality and is widely accepted as being a causal factor in atherosclerosis.

More recently discovered risk factors for heart disease, such as a high blood homocysteine level, are the focus of intense research. The fitting together of the pieces of the homocysteine story to fulfil the above criteria is an interesting story in scientific detective work (Bolander-Gouaille 2000). In the early 1960s, extremely high levels of homocysteine were found in the blood and urine of some mentally retarded children and the cause was identified as a genetic defect in the enzyme cystathionine-β-synthase, the enzyme that breaks down homocysteine into cystathionine (figure 4.6). More than half of these children had experienced a heart attack or stroke and a quarter died before the age of 30. This led to the hypothesis that a moderately elevated homocysteine level in the general population could moderately increase the risk of cardiovascular diseases. More than sixty studies have tested this hypothesis and have shown a 5 to 70 per cent increase in the risk of coronary heart disease and a 10 to 116 per cent increase in the risk of stroke in subjects with high homocysteine levels (variation in estimates is related to differences in study design) (Ford et al. 2002). This evidence establishes homocysteine as a 'predictor' of cardiovascular disease events, but does not establish whether it is involved in the causal pathway. These epidemiological studies

Figure 4.6 Homocysteine metabolism

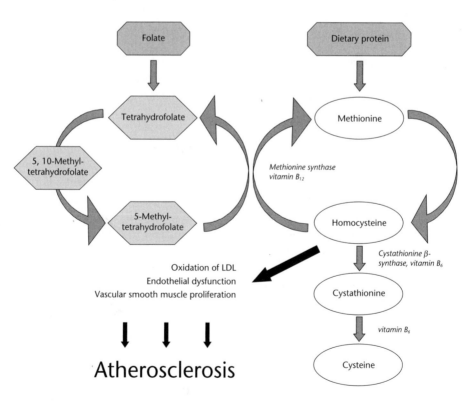

Adapted from O'Grady et al. 2002

confirm the consistency and strength of the relationship, the appropriate temporal association, and the dose response nature of the relationship. Statistical analyses have confirmed the specificity as far as possible by adjusting for potential confounding factors.

Mapping the pathways related to homocysteine has provided the important criterion of biological plausibility. Homocysteine is a sulphur-containing amino acid derived by demethylation from the essential amino acid methionine (figure 4.6). It can be remethylated to methionine by an enzyme (methionine synthase) that needs vitamin B12 as a **co-factor** (i.e. a nonprotein substance that must be combined with the protein portion of an enzyme before the enzyme can act). The **methyl donor** in this reaction is a folate-based compound, 5-methyl-tetrahydro-folate. Alternatively, it can be metabolised to cystathionine and then cysteine by enzymes that are dependent on vitamin B6 as a co-factor. Therefore, insufficient intakes of folate and vitamins B6 and B12 will potentially lead to moderate elevations in blood homocysteine levels. Clinical trials have shown that increased intakes of these vitamins (especially folate) can indeed reduce homocysteine levels in people with moderately elevated levels. Many studies have also identified the potential mechanisms by which homocysteine promotes atherosclerosis and thrombosis. These include oxidative damage to the endothelial cells that line the arteries, promoting oxidation of LDL-cholesterol particles and promoting the proliferation of smooth muscle cells (Bolander-Gouaille 2000). Therefore the only causation criterion that remains unfulfilled is the existence of experimental evidence, that is, whether reducing homocysteine levels (such as with folate supplementation) will reduce the rates of heart attacks and strokes. Large and expensive randomised clinical trials are currently under way to determine this.

Independence or dependence?

Often the scientific question being asked about the relationships between risk factors and diseases is whether or not they are 'independent'. For example, before an endocrinologist decides whether to pursue hormonal links between baldness and heart disease, he or she would want to be sure that the relationship is not simply due to the fact that older men tend to bald and are at higher risk of heart disease or, in other words, that the relationship is dependent on age. Age is therefore added into the statistical analysis (or adjusted for) so that the relationship is shown to be independent of age. The multiple links between measurable risk factors sometimes makes it difficult to know whether or not to adjust for age or other factors. For many years, obesity was not considered to be an important risk factor for heart disease because it had only a weak statistical relationship after adjustment for the classical risk factors. However, because obesity causes high blood pressure, diabetes, high LDL cholesterol and low HDL cholesterol (i.e. these classical risk factors mediate the relationship between obesity and heart disease), statistically adjusting for these factors takes away most of the relationship. Statistical adjustment for confounding factors can therefore produce inappropriate results in some instances.

Relative or absolute risk?

A moderately elevated blood pressure increases the risk of a cardiovascular event (mainly heart attack or stroke) by two to three times (i.e. the relative risk is between two and three). A 30-year-old woman with no risk factors has a tiny chance of a cardiovascular event over the next five years (say, 0.5 per cent) because of her age and gender. If she has high blood pressure, her risk will be doubled to 1 per cent (still very small). However, a 60-year-old man with diabetes might have a 15 per cent chance of a cardiovascular event. Having high blood pressure will double that risk to 30 per cent, which is a substantial increase in 'absolute risk' and would warrant much more aggressive treatment than that recommended for the 30-year-old woman with the same raised blood pressure. She would have the same relative increase in risk (two-fold), but this would be from a very low absolute risk level. This type of quantitative information is available in the form of risk tables that take into account age, gender, diabetes, smoking, blood pressure, and cholesterol levels. These tables greatly assist clinical decision making about how aggressively a particular risk factor should be treated.

Physiology or pathology?

The distinction between normal physiological processes and abnormal pathological processes is often blurred, especially in the area of risk factors for chronic disease. A pathologist can look at a cervical smear test and categorise almost all cells into two populations—normal cells or cancer cells. A few cells may be in genuine transition from normal to cancer cells (a distinction that diagnostic techniques are not able to make); however, generally, the distinction between normal and abnormal is clear in pathological processes like cancer. On the other hand, if a risk factor for a disease (e.g. homocysteine levels, blood pressure, body mass index, or cholesterol levels) shows a single distribution pattern without a clear distinction between high and low, then it is likely that it reflects normal physiological processes rather than pathological ones. People at the upper end of a normal distribution are at a high risk of diseases but distinguishing clearly between them and 'normal' risk is impossible—for example, is a blood pressure reading of 122/82 any different to a reading of 118/78 if 120/80 is arbitrarily defined as the upper limit of normal? The need to classify these continuous risk factors into dichotomous values of 'normal' or 'abnormal' is often driven by the clinical need to decide 'yes' or 'no' to treatment (Rose 1992).

Type 2 diabetes shows a clear transition from physiological response to pathological process (Lillioja et al. 1988). Figure 4.7 is a composite of population distribution of blood glucose levels showing two clear populations—nondiabetic and diabetic. The straight lines are the relationship between insulin and glucose levels that reflect the underlying processes in the progression from normal to diabetes. The normal state at the left of the diagram shows low glucose and insulin levels. With increasing age, weight gain, and physical inactivity, the body becomes increasingly resistant to the effects of insulin and thus glucose levels rise somewhat. This stimulates an increase in insulin secretion to compensate for the resistance to insulin action in skeletal muscle and liver and to keep glucose levels in check. At the peak of the glucose–insulin relationship, this physiological adaptation has reached its maximum capacity. The next series of events are clearly pathological as the β-cells in the pancreas increasingly fail to secrete the large amounts of insulin needed to overcome the resistance. Consequently, glucose level rises substantially, and this in turn is toxic to the β-cells. Thus, a vicious cycle is established that results in clinical diabetes. It is this vicious cycle that creates the two clear populations of nondiabetic and diabetic. For other risk factors, such as high blood pressure and cholesterol levels, the two populations of diseased and nondiseased are only apparent after the person has an event such as a stroke or heart attack.

Figure 4.7 Frequency distribution curves for Pima Indian women showing two distinct distributions of nondiabetic and diabetic

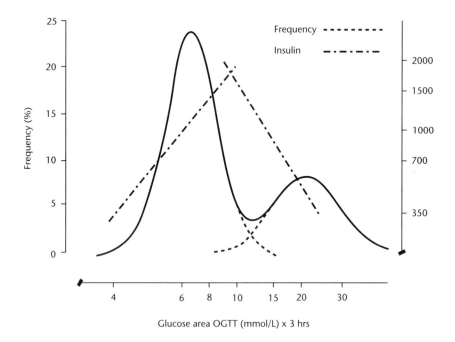

Glucose area OGTT (mmol/L) x 3 hrs

Source: Lillioja et al. 1988

SUMMARY

- The biological determinants of health and disease are various and highly interconnected with each other and with an individual's behaviours and environments.
- Making the aetiological linkages between various measurable factors and health and disease outcomes is not straightforward as the story is constantly changing. That's what makes it so fascinating.
- The role of known biological determinants of health and disease is under constant reanalysis and reinterpretation as increasingly sophisticated analytical techniques enable scientists to delve with greater precision into the mechanisms of disease development and progression. This research continues to focus on the major biological determinants that are discussed in this chapter. These include the role played by: genes, particularly gene–environment interactions; age; and gender.
- Future scientific research will enable a greater understanding of the role of biological markers in disease risk, with the aim of establishing: association or causation; independence or dependence; relative or absolute risk; and physiology or pathology.

DISCUSSION TOPICS

1 In reporting the increased risk of a disease (say, breast cancer) in relation to an exposure (say, number of pregnancies or smoking), should you quote absolute risk or relative risk or both? What is the effect of quoting one or the other, or both?

2 What are the causation factors you need to consider in understanding the high prevalence of diabetes in the populations of Nauru, Native Americans in Arizona, and Indigenous Australians? What social and economic factors might contribute to the high diabetes rates? What information do you need to determine how much of the high prevalence rates are due to socioeconomic factors and how much due to genetic or metabolic factors?

3 Imagine you have been asked to advise the government about how to address this high prevalence of diabetes. How might your advice about strategies be affected by your understanding of its causation?

DETERMINANTS OF HEALTH: CASE STUDIES FROM ASIA AND THE PACIFIC

Cathy Vaughan

> ## *Key concepts*
>
> - Globalisation
> - Determinants of disability
> - Determinants of HIV/AIDS
> - Structural determinants of health and illness

The interconnectedness of our world is increasingly apparent—be it through the global media, advertising, the Internet, or the international threat of terrorism, the barriers of time, distance, language, and **culture** are being eroded. Likewise, making distinctions between domestic and international health problems is often no longer possible or relevant. In the 'global village', the health problems of one country should be of concern to all of us.

As the preceding chapters have made clear, a range of determinants are important to consider in understanding health. These are equally important for understanding health in countries with less developed economies, as they are in industrialised countries such as Australia. The health of communities in less economically developed countries is seen, at times, solely through the lens of 'tropical' or 'exotic' diseases. However, health for most of the world's population is less determined by the biology of 'exotic' pathogens, than it is by social, cultural, environmental, political, and economic factors. When discussing health in low- and middle-income countries, it is also important to consider the wider structural determinants of health such as economic globalisation, structural adjustment programs, speculative currency markets, historical factors including colonialism, communication technologies, and the global media. All of these factors have a tremendous impact on the health of populations globally.

GLOBALISATION

The term **globalisation** is one that is highly debated, and has come to mean different things to different people. Bettcher and Lee (2002) define globalisation as a set of processes leading to the creation of the world as a single entity, relatively undivided by national borders or other types of boundaries (e.g. cultural, economic, temporal). It has been argued that the underlying 'driver' of globalisation is an economic process of trade and finance deregulation based on speculative currency markets. This process has elevated economics, based on the neoliberal free market model, to be the dominant discipline within global policy making, including international health policy. While the processes of globalisation are not new, the speed of change and reach of global capitalism is a recent development. For the first time, the entire world is now either capitalist or dependent on capitalist economies with few agrarian societies remaining.

The impact of globalisation on the determinants of health is enormous. Some authors argue that globalisation has had a predominantly positive influence on the health of populations (Feachem 2001), while many have highlighted the increasing exclusion and inequity within and between nations (Navarro 1998; Baum 2001; Frenk and Gomez-Dantes 2002; Kawachi and Kennedy 2002) and the concentration of wealth and power within a small group of (almost entirely) men who are not held to account for the impact of their actions (Kickbusch and Buse 2001).

In this chapter we will explore in depth two quite different case studies to illustrate the broad range of health determinants and their impact on individuals and communities in low-income countries.

DETERMINANTS OF DISABILITY: A CASE STUDY FROM PAKISTAN

The main causes of poor health, chronic diseases, and long-term impairments in both high- and low-income nations throughout the world are poverty and inequity, inadequate sanitation, poor nutrition, substandard housing, environmental pollution, lack of access to health services including immunisation programs, industrial and road traffic accidents, violence, and war. In Australia, people with disabilities face problems of discrimination and access to facilities, basic health care, education, and employment options. For people with disabilities living in low-income countries, the challenges can be even greater.

The North-West Frontier Province (NWFP) of Pakistan is a spectacular part of South Asia. The frontier contains wild landscapes ranging from the rugged peaks of the Hindu Kush in the north to the harsh deserts of the south. Peshawar, the capital city of the province, is a bustling hive of activity straight out of an ancient Silk Road tale. Its colourful bazaars are filled with tall, turbaned tribesmen, and the magical old city fills visitors with a sense of its rich and proud history. However, life in Pakistan can be very hard. Life expectancy at birth for

Pakistanis is relatively low (60 years, compared with 79 years for Australians), and Pakistan's infant mortality rate is the highest in South Asia. More than one-third of children under five years of age are underweight. Thirty-one per cent of the population live on less than US$1 per day. The adult literacy rate for men is 58 per cent, and for women only 28 per cent (UNDP 2002).

In NWFP, the statistics tell the story of an even tougher existence. In addition to the serious poverty experienced by many Pakistanis living in the frontier, NWFP is home to another group of particularly vulnerable people. Peshawar is at the end of the Khyber Pass, and since 1977 this narrow mountainous path has provided passage to millions of Afghan refugees fleeing their war-torn country. Pakistan is host to more refugees than any other country in the world (more than two million). Most of them live in NWFP. Infrastructure and services for both Afghans and Pakistanis in the province are stretched to the limit.

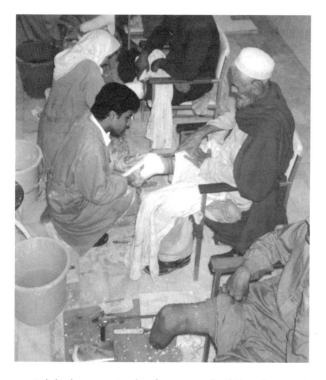

Prosthetist-orthotists at the PETCOT rehabilitation centre in Peshawar, making artificial legs for amputees

Bilal, the man in the foreground of the above photograph, is a refugee from Afghanistan who had been living in Pakistan for almost three years when this photograph was taken. Bilal and his son fled to Pakistan on foot to escape fighting near their village. His son stepped on a landmine near the city of Jalalabad. Bilal lost the lower half of his right leg in the accident. His son died. It took several days for other refugees to get Bilal to Peshawar for medical care. He was lucky to survive the journey.

Bilal's health is substantially affected by a range of determinants other than the biological factors normally the focus of health care workers. It is true that his wounds took longer to heal because of his age and the infection that developed en route to Peshawar, but other crucial determinants of Bilal's health and function include:

- *Economic vulnerability.* Bilal arrived in Pakistan without money or possessions. His wife had died many years previously, and his remaining children were still in Afghanistan. He had some relatives living in already overcrowded conditions in one of the camps near Peshawar who took him in. Bilal had been a resourceful farmer prior to the war, but now as an older man without land or his health, he found himself without employment options and dependent on aid agencies.
- *Physical barriers.* Peshawar has few paved roads, and even fewer ramps. There are no escalators or lifts. Bilal used crutches to move around—a hot and dusty job much of the year, and a physically exhausting battle through the mud when it rains.
- *Limited access to information and services.* Bilal spoke several languages, but was illiterate. Inability to access information was also a major determinant of his health. For example, it was almost three years after losing his leg before Bilal found out he would be eligible for a low-cost prosthesis.
- *Violence and war.* The war in Afghanistan has drastically affected Bilal's health in many ways. His serious injuries, his poor nutritional state at the time of the accident, his separation from family and carers, his significant psychological trauma... the list goes on. War-related injuries and trauma affect not just Bilal, but millions of people worldwide. Violence and war is one of the major contributors to ill health globally.

LANDMINES

Landmines are powerful and unforgiving devices. Unlike other weapons of war, most of which must be aimed and fired, landmines are 'victim' activated. They are specifically constructed to shatter limbs. The detonation of a buried mine rips off one or both legs of the victim and drives soil, grass, gravel, metal and the plastic fragments of the mine casing, pieces of the shoe, and shattered bone up into the muscles and lower parts of the body.

International Committee of the Red Cross 1998, p. 3.

Landmines as a determinant of community health make for a powerful case study in themselves. Most often, landmines are considered a determinant of health for an individual. This is, of course, accurate. The physical injuries (most commonly shattering of limbs, amputation, blindness, and major blood loss) and mental health consequences are severe.

However, the consequences at a family and community level also require consideration. Survivors of landmine blasts usually need repeated surgery and extensive rehabilitation.

In a country such as Pakistan, where resources are already scarce, caring for landmine victims draws resources from other essential health services, and therefore tends to worsen the health status of the population overall.

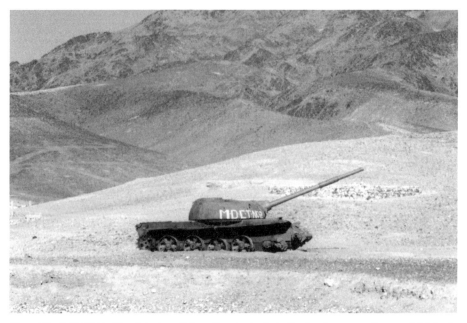

The white 'MDCT No.2' painted on this rusting tank alerts the local community near Jalalabad, Afghanistan, that Mine Detection and Clearance Team number 2 has cleared this area. Areas not yet safe are marked with stones painted red.

Landmines are also linked to waterborne diseases where access to safe drinking water is mined; malnutrition because minefields cannot be cultivated and food cannot be imported on mined roads; increase in infectious diseases because vaccination teams are unable to operate near mined areas; the spread of blood-borne disease due to the hugely increased need for blood transfusions; and family disintegration due to mine injuries to parents and breadwinners. Refugees are particularly vulnerable—displaced persons are unaware of where the mines are (either on fleeing or returning to their homeland). Landmines make post-conflict reconstruction expensive, difficult, and dangerous.

The Ottawa Treaty (formally the Convention on the Prohibition of the Use, Stockpiling, Production and Transfer of Anti-Personnel Mines and on their Destruction) was opened for signature in December 1997; the United Nations General Assembly passed a resolution encouraging all states to ratify the convention; and the International Campaign to Ban Landmines movement was awarded the 1997 Nobel Prize for Peace. However, the world's major producers—including the USA, Russia, and China—have still not signed the Ottawa Treaty.

Historically most mines have been produced in industrialised nations and exported to low-income countries thousands of miles away. Landmines are one very clear example of the international transfer of health risks associated with contemporary transnational trade (other important examples include the export and marketing of tobacco, the dumping of unsafe or ineffective pharmaceuticals, cross-border environmental destruction and pollution, and trade in contaminated foodstuffs). It should be noted that in many situations substantial trade barriers are simultaneously enforced by the World Trade Organization (WTO) limiting access to the means to protect and improve health: 'Many political borders serve as semi-permeable membranes, often quite open to diseases and yet closed to the free movement of cures' (Farmer 1996).

UNDERSTANDING THE DETERMINANTS OF HIV/AIDS

The United Nations Program on AIDS (UNAIDS) estimated that by the end of 2002, about 42 million people across the globe were living with human immuno-deficiency virus (HIV), the virus that causes acquired immune deficiency syndrome (AIDS). Since the beginning of the epidemic, over twenty-seven million people have died from AIDS with 3.1 million deaths in 2002 alone. HIV/AIDS has reached almost every nation on earth.

The phrase often heard is that 'AIDS is everyone's epidemic', but this picture of AIDS has been described as a 'necessary fiction'—necessary in order to break down widespread complacency that HIV infection could only happen to 'other people', and to raise community awareness that biologically anyone can become infected with HIV. However 'everyone' is a fiction nonetheless, as it does not describe the complex interaction of biological, social, cultural, political, and economic determinants that shape the epidemic (Parker 1996).

The number of people infected with HIV across the planet is overwhelming. Moving beyond the absolute numbers, it is important to note that the global distribution of HIV—both between and within countries—is anything but equal. AIDS is not 'everyone's epidemic'. The world over, HIV/AIDS is now primarily an epidemic of the poorest and most marginalised sectors of society. This is a cause for great alarm. Those in our communities most affected by HIV, are often those with the least resources to respond.

The syndrome of immune-related diseases we now know as AIDS was first described in 1981. Scientists identified HIV in 1983. Since that time, there have been many lessons learned—often at great human cost—about effective responses to the epidemic.

HIV is spread in three ways: through sex; through blood (including blood transfusions, needles, and syringes); and from mother to child. While all humans can become infected with HIV, there are biological factors that increase a person's vulnerability to infection. For example, if a person has another sexually transmitted infection (STI), such as gonorrhoea or chlamydia, the risk of them becoming infected with HIV during sex is considerably higher. If a person has a blood disorder that means they need frequent blood transfusions, they are also at higher risk. If a woman living with HIV has health problems during pregnancy and/or breastfeeding, there is a greater chance of the infection being passed to her baby. These biological factors are important, but it is clear that a focus on biological risk factors alone will not halt the spread of the epidemic.

The risk of HIV infection is also intimately related to behaviours. These behaviours include having sex without a condom when it is unknown whether a sexual partner is infected with HIV, and having multiple sexual partners (it is important to remember that most people—in both high- and low-income countries—do not know their own HIV status). Sharing equipment used for injecting drugs is also a high-risk behaviour. However, responses to HIV that only encourage individuals to change their behaviours have also been found to be ineffective.

For example, HIV prevention programs emphasising condom use alone are based on the premise that rational choices are made in risk assessment and decision making in sexual contexts. Is it reasonable to assume that decision making around sex is always rational? The assumption of rational choice does not adequately account for sexual double standards, gendered power relations, or indeed desire. This assumption also does not consider the fact that in many circumstances people have to weigh up many different social and situational risks when making decisions about sex. The risk of having sex without using a condom may be balanced against the risk of gender-based violence, the risk of not having enough money to feed the children, or the risk of being alone. HIV is not spread through 'exotic' cultural practices, but because of normal responses to everyday problems such as substantial economic hardship and uncertainty (Parker et al. 2000).

To achieve sustainable behavioural and other change, our responses to HIV must go beyond giving people information and telling them to change their behaviour. Programs must address the wider social, cultural, and economic environment to ensure the circumstances of people's lives allow healthy behaviours.

Young people and HIV: a case study from the Pacific

Every day, 6000 young people between the ages of 15 and 24 become infected with HIV (UNICEF et al. 2002). Young people aged between 15 and 24 account for two-thirds of new HIV infections every year. There are many reasons why young people are particularly at risk. Adolescence is frequently seen as a period of sexual experimentation, and in most societies sexual intercourse first occurs during adolescence. Youth may also be a period of experimentation with alcohol and other drugs. However, young people are vulnerable not just because they are having sex or injecting drugs. The context in which these activities occur often contributes to an increased risk of HIV infection. The central Pacific island nation of Tuvalu provides a useful case study to explore this context in more detail.

Tuvalu is one of the smallest and most isolated countries on earth. The total land area of the nine inhabited atolls that make up Tuvalu is only 26 square kilometres. The population is approximately 10,000 people. On first appearances, it would seem that unlike the rest of the world, HIV could not become a problem in Tuvalu. Funafuti, the capital, surrounds a glorious turquoise lagoon. Everywhere coconut palms sway gently in tropical breezes. Friendly villagers peacefully go about their daily work in unhurried Pacific style. Geographic isolation discourages most tourists. For the outsider, Tuvalu really does seem like a tropical paradise. Many people live a subsistence lifestyle, based on fishing and farming small plots of land. Traditional government remains important, and many other traditions—particularly singing and dance—are as important to the community today as they were generations ago. The Christian church is one of the most powerful institutions in the country. There is no commercial sex work, there is no injecting drug use. There is not even television. Surely there is no risk of HIV gaining a foothold way out here?

Yet there are people living with HIV in this tiny country, and the risk of this situation worsening is very real. To understand the reasons for this, it is important to consider a range of determinants of health, particularly as they affect young people living in this community.

- *Biological determinants*. The presence of another STI significantly increases the risk of a person becoming infected with HIV. Doctors in Tuvalu report cases of syphilis, gonorrhoea, and other STIs, particularly among young men. In neighbouring Fiji, two-thirds of reported cases of gonorrhoea occur in young people between 15 and 24 years of age (United Nations 1996).

- *Behavioural factors*. Condom use among young people in Tuvalu is not high. Although condoms are supplied free of cost, and there are plenty available on the main island, condoms can only be obtained from a limited number of sites, and these are not open after hours. Lack of privacy and confidentiality is another major deterrent. If a young person is seen going to the hospital or clinic, other people are very curious to know why. In a small community, gossip is a very real barrier to accessing condoms, information, and other sexual health services.

- *Social determinants*. A significant number of young people in Tuvalu are sexually active before marriage, despite restrictions imposed by family, culture, and the church. The common double standard of tacit approval for sexual experience in young men while expecting abstinence in young women, is also seen in Tuvalu. While premarital sexual activity is accepted as being 'men's ways', young Tuvaluan women known (or suspected) to be sexually active are subject to gossip, social ostracism, and in some instances violence. Most sexual activity occurs within an ongoing relationship, but the double standard means that relationships must be kept secret. Young women in hidden relationships may be subject to sexual coercion in unprotected environments. The lower social status of women, particularly relating to sexual decision making, also increases the risk of HIV for young women in Tuvalu (as in many other countries—globally, young women are particularly vulnerable to HIV, as shown by their increased rate of infection compared to males in the same age group).

- *Alcohol*. This is a major determinant of sexual health in Tuvalu. Excessive alcohol use is associated with increased sexual risk behaviour, with some young people reporting that they only have sex after drinking and are unable to use condoms when drunk. Young women also find that excess alcohol consumption in young men can lead to increased coercion and even physical intimidation for sex. This is in agreement with the findings of researchers from many other countries (Dowsett and Aggleton 1999).

- *Cultural taboos*. These make it very difficult to talk about sex and sexuality in Tuvalu. This is a particular challenge for public education and awareness raising programs.
- *Economic determinants*. Tuvalu has been largely a local subsistence economy based on fishing and small family *pulaka* (swamp taro) plots for centuries. Colonisation, and later the introduction of the cash economy, impacted negatively on the local food economy. The impact of these changes has rapidly increased in recent years with global capitalist forces reaching Tuvalu. As more and more people become dependent on imported goods (such as tinned and frozen foods, motorcycles, cars, and Western clothes) there is an increasing demand for cash. Land and agricultural resources are limited, so Tuvaluans compete for a place in the global market with their labour. Tuvaluans are internationally renowned as hard working and skilful seafarers. Remittances sent home from these young men working the high seas is the only source of cash income for many families, and this money makes up a significant percentage of the nation's gross domestic product (GDP).

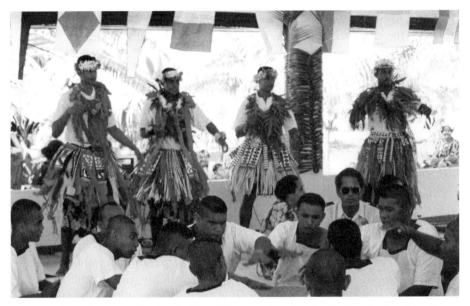

Young seafarers from the Tuvalu Maritime School performing *fatele* (dancing), celebrating their graduation. That evening these same young men could be seen celebrating in a very different way—enthusiastically dancing to Britney Spears, cans of Victoria Bitter in hand!

Tuvaluan seafarers travel to ports all over the world, and are away from their families for often a year at a time. In foreign countries, these young men may or may not have access to condoms, they may or may not speak the local language, and they are often in places where the prevalence of HIV is higher than at home. The risk of infection is high. More than two-thirds of Tuvaluans who have been infected with HIV have been seafarers. It is a tragic reality that these young men, who contribute so much to their country, are now paying with their health. Migratory labour patterns are one of the key determinants of vulnerability to HIV infection worldwide.

These are some of the main factors influencing HIV risk for young people in Tuvalu. There are many others including the introduction of video and the Internet, limited employment and educational opportunities, limited access to sexual health services, and isolation. It is a complex picture that clearly cannot be addressed by one strategy alone.

As stated in Woodward et. al (2000): 'Efforts to protect and improve health are left mostly to the health sector. Yet the major determinants of ill health, including poverty, lack of education, and environmental degradation, are beyond the direct control of health services.' The Tuvalu National AIDS Committee is a multisectoral organisation, made up of representatives from several government ministries (e.g. health, education, planning), non-government organisations (e.g. Tuvalu National Council of Women, Tuvalu Family Health Association, Tuvalu Red Cross Society), church groups, youth groups, and the Tuvalu Overseas Seamen's Union. Various individuals and organisations have taken the lead in planning and implementing different components of the national response—to address the wide-ranging determinants of health, many partners in the community outside the health sector need to understand HIV risk and find ways of integrating HIV-related activities into their work. This is true around the world, not just in the small island states of the Pacific.

STRUCTURAL DETERMINANTS OF HEALTH

These case studies have highlighted factors that can increase threats to health in two quite different situations. The determinants already outlined in this book (biological, environmental, and social) are no less important in low- and middle-income countries. In addition, there are broader structural factors to consider in understanding health in our interconnected world.

Many countries are poorer than they were thirty, twenty, or even ten years ago (UNDP 2002). Global inequities have reached obscene levels. More than one billion people exist on less than US$1 per day, with the richest 200 people in the world having combined incomes of more than the 2.3 billion people. The dominant neoliberal economic model of profit at all costs ('greed is good'), is intimately linked with this rise in global inequity. The international institutions of the current economic world order such as the WTO, the World Bank, and the International Monetary Fund (IMF), are controlled by the world's richest nations (the G8 nations[1] have almost 50 per cent of the voting power of the IMF and World Bank) and increasingly influenced by transnational corporations. Most decisions made by the WTO are reached behind closed doors, with low-income countries excluded. These institutions deeply affect the determinants of health worldwide, yet low- and middle-income countries are unable to influence the institutional decisions, which overwhelmingly reflect the interests of the rich and powerful nations.

Paul Farmer (1999) describes the social and economic inequities that determine who will be at risk of negative health consequences and who will be shielded, as 'structural violence'. In considering how best to address this structural violence that determines the health of so much of the 'global village', health professionals need to develop skills in advocacy, political analysis, economics, international relations, and law.

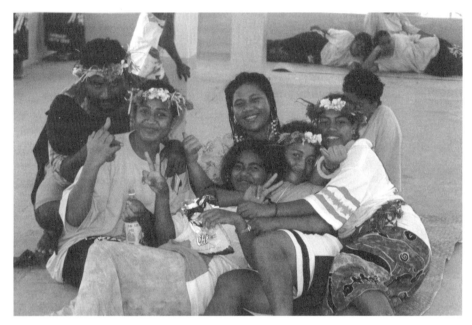

Young Tuvaluans from the Nanumea Youth Group celebrating another year of hard work. Young people—supported by international donors and agencies—have been at the forefront of the response to HIV/AIDS in the Pacific Islands.

In the context of massive structural violence and the concentration of power in the hands of a wealthy few, it would be easy to assume that communities in low-income countries are despondent and powerless. Nothing could be further from the truth. Worldwide, local communities are responding to their own health issues in innovative and effective ways. The resilience of tiny communities such as those of the Pacific island nations, in the face of such an uneven global playing field, is enormous; the optimism and quiet determination of individuals such as Bilal, inspiring. However, it is not enough for health professionals to be inspired or impressed. Health cannot be separated from broader struggles for responsibility, fairness, and **social justice** (Parker 2002). As health professionals, we are privileged members of a global elite who need to consider our role in the current world system. Understanding health in our increasingly interconnected world is to understand that we must challenge inequity to be relevant. Understanding global health today entails health professionals acknowledging their responsibility and opportunity to make the WHO policy of 'Health for All' a revitalised reality.

SUMMARY

- Poverty and inequity are prime determinants of health globally. Inequity within and between nations has increased rapidly in the last twenty years.
- Factors associated with globalisation that have an impact on health are numerous and interact in complex ways. The control of these health determinants is often beyond the realm of individual nations or states, and requires joint action by the wider international community.
- The range of health determinants considered important in health program planning in industrialised nations are also key determinants of health in low-income nations.
- Transnational trade is often associated with the international transfer of health risks.
- Globally the HIV/AIDS pandemic does not follow international political borders, but rather economic margins.
- The biological and behavioural factors that increase risk of HIV infection and many other negative health outcomes are in turn shaped by economic, political, social, cultural, and structural determinants.
- The interconnectedness of all peoples in our current 'globalised' environment means the Australian community is affected by, and should be interested in, the health of communities around the world.

DISCUSSION TOPICS

1 A review of UNDP indicators and reports provides useful insight into the health inequities existing between nations. Go to the UNDP web site (www.undp.org) and follow the links to these reports and summaries of the indicators.

2 Compare and contrast the data from different countries such as Pakistan, Tuvalu, Papua New Guinea, and others in the Pacific region, Africa, and Asia. What conclusions can you draw from studying these reports?

3 Consider the possible impact of globalisation on the following: a tiny Pacific nation such as Tuvalu; a small rural community in Australia.

4 In what ways might low literacy rates impact on the health of Pakistani people?

5 Consider a regional conflict currently being reported in the media. Use a determinants perspective to review the likely health implications for people living in close proximity to this conflict.

NOTES

1 The Group of Eight Nations (G8, originally G7) are the USA, France, Germany, the United Kingdom, Italy, Japan, Canada, and Russia. The G8 summit of government leaders is held annually and is a forum for this exclusive 'club' to set transnational trade, finance, and policy agendas.

6
MEASURING POPULATION HEALTH STATUS IN AUSTRALIA

Michael Ackland and John Catford

> ## Key concepts
>
> - Mortality and morbidity
> - Burden of disease
> - Health and disease registers
> - Indigenous health
> - Health services
> - Risk factors
> - Preventive services

Knowledge of the health of populations underpins all public health programs and services worldwide. This chapter is in two sections. The first section introduces some of the main sources of health status information and draws on them to give examples of how healthy Australians are. The second section shows how some of the information collected on people who receive health care can be helpful in understanding health problems, and gives an overview of the important health behaviours and biomedical risk factors that promote or reduce health status.[1]

There is a vast array of approaches to measuring population health including the documentation of vital statistics such as births and deaths, conducting health surveys, collecting administrative health services data, and using complex epidemiological techniques such as those used in calculating the burden of disease. Surprisingly often, these approaches generate information that is of considerable interest, but of marginal relevance and application to those responsible for designing, funding, and implementing public health programs. It is important that when we are measuring health, the information can be used in some practical way to assist in improving population health outcomes. So it is essential that we know not only how to measure health and where to find useful data, but what difference this information will make to improving health and supporting the health system.

REPORTED HEALTH

Government health departments and health authorities dedicate significant resources to measuring population health. Much effort can be saved, and most likely more practical information obtained, by asking health professionals who are working in local communities: 'What is going on in your patch?' Current best practice in public health recognises the value of local experienced experts in identifying health issues that require some form of intervention. However, in the absence of simple, reliable, and valid data or information systems it becomes impossible to adequately target interventions or to evaluate the impact of programs that may or may not be effective.

Further use of the experienced observer can be derived through special studies where experts visit communities and make observations about specific behaviours or health attributes. This can be done informally or through structured research techniques. Such observational studies can provide invaluable qualitative data about population health and behaviours (especially the 'upstream' determinants of health) that would not usually be available through more formal surveys or information systems.

One of the simplest ways to measure health is to ask people how healthy they are. Questionnaire surveys of different population groups are commonly used to collect information from respondents on their self-perceptions of health. The Australian Bureau of Statistics (ABS) conducts a variety of national surveys on a regular basis, important examples being the 1995 and 2001 National Health Surveys, and the 1997 National Survey of Mental Health and Wellbeing of Adults. The next National Health Survey is planned for 2004–05. Most states and territories also conduct periodic population health surveys.

A strength of these surveys is that they may provide an ongoing systematic approach to collecting information that allows trends in health to be mapped over time (health surveillance) and action to be taken as a result. Emerging health problems may be identified early enough for new and effective interventions to be implemented. For example, trends in poor nutrition and levels of physical inactivity that can be causes (or precursors) to preventable chronic diseases may be detected in specific communities, allowing targeted health promotion programs to be initiated. Surveys can also be important in improving our understanding of **inequalities** in health across population groups.

A common method for conducting population health surveys in many state health departments is to use computer-assisted telephone interviewing (CATI). However, significant biases can occur with this method, as it requires people to have a home with a telephone and be available and have the time to take the call. For example, people living in poverty, disabled persons, and Indigenous people, are less likely to be respondents to CATI surveys. There are further well-known

Figure 6.1   Self-assessed health status, Australia 1997

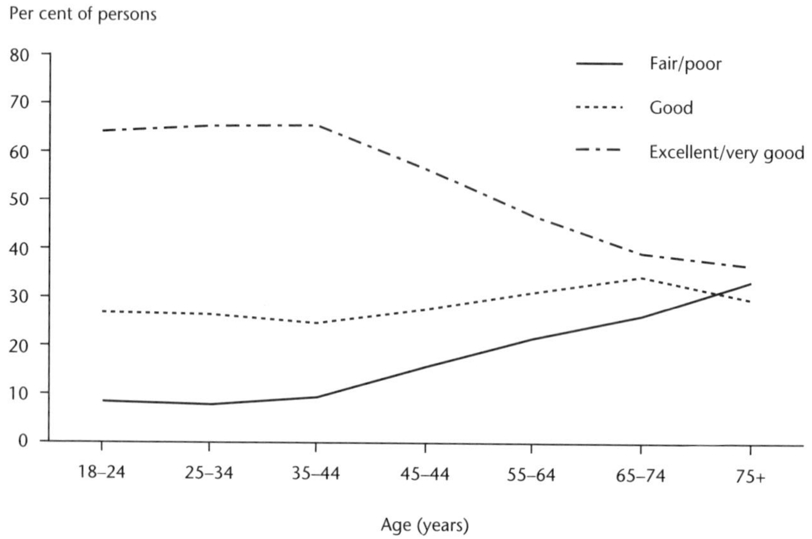

Per cent of persons

Age (years)

Source: AIHW 2002b

biases in self-assessed health, for example in females where weight is consistently underreported, and for males height is consistently overreported.

Figure 6.1 shows an analysis of self-assessed health from the 1997 National Survey of Mental Health and Wellbeing. Just over half of people aged 18 years and over reported their overall health as excellent or very good in 1997, and a further 28 per cent reported that they were in good health. Proportions were similar for both sexes. Similar findings and trends across age groups were found in the 2001 Victorian Population Health Survey conducted by the Victorian Department of Human Services (DHS 2002a).

Vital statistics: births and deaths

One of the legacies of the nineteenth-century public health movement is that by law all births and deaths must be registered with state Registrars of Births, Deaths and Marriages. These so-called *vital statistics* are collated and reported by the ABS. These statistics provide important demographic information on changes in age–sex specific population levels, and are elementary indicators of population health that are readily overlooked in developed countries such as Australia. In many parts of the world where famine, malnutrition, warfare, and poverty can be huge problems, birth rates, infant mortality, and death rates are dramatically affected. These statistics will be reflected in summary population data that are frequently depicted as *population pyramids*. In Australia, the ABS is responsible for documenting population levels (and growth projections) and collects these data through its housing and population census program.

Figure 6.2a Population pyramid, Australia 1971

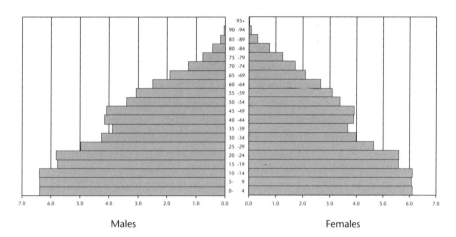

Males   Females

Source: ABS 1999

Figure 6.2b Population pyramid, Australia 2001

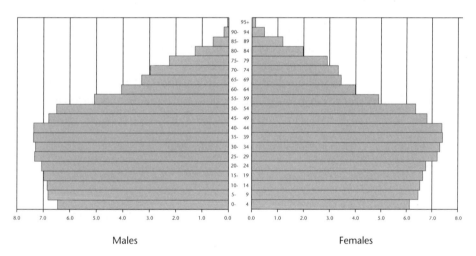

Males   Females

Source: ABS 2001

Figures 6.2a and 6.2b illustrate two population pyramids for Australia (1971 and 2001), showing two quite contrasting age–sex population profiles. These data show that over a thirty-year period there has been a significant ageing of the Australian population due to increasing life expectancy with an accompanying decline in births. These facts have a major impact on the health system, placing increased demands on services directed to the treatment of both acute and chronic diseases that are prevalent in older persons.

Live births

Australia faces a continuing decline in the annual number of live births. In 1971 276,362 births were registered, while in 2000 there were 249,636 births (ABS 2001a). Crude birth rates for 1971 (21.7 per 1000 population) and 2000 (13.0 per 1000 population) demonstrate the contrast more dramatically.

Perinatal mortality

Perinatal deaths include stillbirths and deaths of infants within the first twenty-eight days of life. The main causes of perinatal deaths are respiratory conditions, congenital malformations, chromosomal abnormalities, and disorders related to length of gestation. In countries with severe social deprivation, poverty, and malnutrition, perinatal death rates are generally very high. Perinatal deaths also tend to be higher among very young and older mothers. The perinatal death rate in Australia has declined significantly over the last decade from 11.3 deaths per 1000 births in 1990 to 8.3 deaths per 1000 births in 2000 (ABS 2001b).

Mortality

Age and sex patterns of death and causes of death provide the most fundamental indicators of population health status. In 2000, there were 128,291 deaths recorded in Australia, comprising 66,817 males and 61,474 females. Coronary heart disease and cerebrovascular disease accounted for more than 30 per cent of all deaths, while all cancers accounted for another 30 per cent.

Over the last century Australia has seen a steady decline of around 62 per cent in age-standardised death rates. It is important to note that death rates in males have been consistently higher than for females, and for eighty years there

Figure 6.3   Trends in mortality, Australia 1907–2000

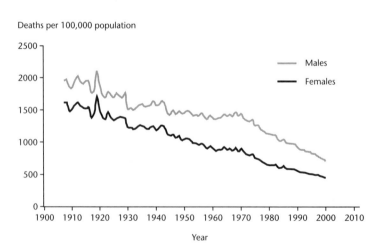

Source: AIHW 2002b

has been remarkably little overall convergence in this 'health gap', though data for the last twenty years do indicate a greater rate of decline in deaths for males than for females. It is useful to compare these data with trends in life expectancy data illustrated later in this chapter.[2]

Health and disease registers

Another indicator of a well-planned and well-resourced health system is the use of specific registers to record the details of people who have particular health problems or diseases. These registers can be used to assess the scale of the condition (prevalence), whether new cases are increasing (incidence), which groups of the population are most affected (e.g. children, low-income families, factory workers), and what the outcomes are (e.g. survival times). Epidemiological studies can also be designed using disease registers to investigate possible causes of disease (e.g. lung cancer associated with smoking or asbestos exposure).

Table 6.1 Selected congenital malformations, Australia 1981–97

ICD-9 CODE	CONGENITAL MALFORMATION	NUMBER	NEW CASES PER 10,000 BIRTHS
740.0	Anencephalus	1153	2.8
741	Spina bifida	2294	5.5
742.3	Hydrocephalus	1609	3.9
745.1	Transposition of great vessels	1474	3.6
745.4	Ventricular septal defect	6703	16.2
749	Cleft lip and/or cleft palate	6180	14.9
750.3	Tracheo-oesophageal fistula, oesophageal atresia, and stenosis	1243	3.0
751.2	Atresia and stenosis of large intestine, rectum and anus	1362	3.3
752.60, 3–5	Hypospadias	8350	20.2
753.0	Renal agenesis and dysgenesis	1473	3.6
754.30	Congenital dislocation of hip	8613	20.8
756.61	Diaphragmatic hernia	1158	2.8
758.0	Down syndrome	5123	12.4

Source: AIHW 2002b

Congenital malformations registers

Congenital malformations (physical abnormalities that are present at birth) are a significant cause of morbidity (disease, disabilities, and handicaps) and mortality in childhood. All states and territories require notification of congenital malformations and the data are compiled in a national database. These data provide the basis for monitoring and evaluation of a number of clinical and public health prevention programs. A good example is the recommendation from the National Health and Medical Research Council (NHMRC) for pregnant women to take extra folate (a water-soluble vitamin) in their diet to prevent neural tube defects (spina bifida) in their baby. Table 6.1 shows the national incidence rates for the leading congenital malformations.

Cancer registers

Australia has a comprehensive system in place for monitoring cancers through state- and territory-based cancer registers. It is a legal requirement for clinical and demographic data to be collected on all people with newly diagnosed cancers. The AIHW manages a National Cancer Statistics Clearing House and has records of all new cases of cancer from 1982 onwards. In addition, data on deaths from cancers are compiled from death certificates by Registrars of Births, Deaths and Marriages, and when combined with cancer register data allow statistics to be produced on cancer incidence, survival, and mortality.

Notifiable infectious diseases registers

All states have a Health Act of Parliament, which requires the mandatory notification of selected infectious (or communicable) diseases. In Victoria these conditions are described under the Health (Infectious Diseases) Regulations 2001, requiring medical practitioners (general practitioners or hospital doctors) to notify the Department of Human Services (DHS) of the occurrence of any new cases at the time of diagnosis (e.g. meningitis, Legionnaire's disease, food poisoning, tuberculosis, HIV/AIDS, gonorrhoea). The active surveillance of these conditions allows the earliest possible response to outbreaks of infectious diseases with the implementation of appropriate public health interventions (e.g. withdrawal of a contaminated food from supermarkets and shops).

Life expectancy

Life expectancy is one of the most useful objective measures of health status available. It presents the average number of years of life someone can expect to live from a given age when applying current death rates. In countries where good records of vital statistics (births and deaths) are maintained, life tables can be constructed providing indicators of life expectancy for the whole population by gender at any age. The quality of these data is often inadequate in developing countries, and even for the Australian Indigenous population there are remarkably poor data available on this most elementary indicator of health.

Life expectancy at birth (LEB) is a most commonly used metric for the purpose of comparing population health status across different strata of the population. Australians enjoy a steadily improving life expectancy, and while females experience a higher LEB than males, in recent years males have been 'catching up'. In 2000, LEB for Australian males was 76.6 years, and for females 82.1 years. On an international scale, the LEB for Australians is among the highest in the world with Japan (LEB males 77.5, females 84.7), Sweden (LEB males 77.3), and France (LEB females 83.1) having the highest life expectancies.

Figure 6.4 shows the most recent data reported from Victoria, and while the gender-specific trends are clear, it is also apparent that there are some other important differentials in life expectancy. Notably, the LEB for rural Victorians remains consistently about one year less than the LEB for those living in metropolitan Victoria. The data suggest that there have been some slight improvements in LEB for rural Victorians, but this is clearly a health inequality that still needs to be addressed by the public health community.

Figure 6.4   Life expectancy at birth in rural and urban Victoria, 1988–99

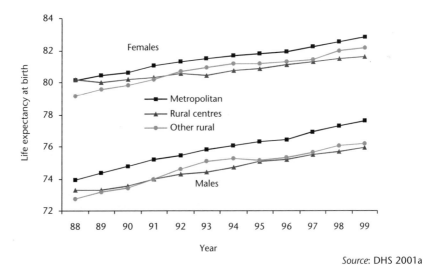

Source: DHS 2001a

Indigenous health

The health and health inequalities of Indigenous Australian people present one of the greatest challenges to the Australian public health system. It is widely known that many Indigenous people live in isolated communities and are extremely marginalised from society due to their very poor socioeconomic status. Nevertheless, we have extremely poor information about the health and determinants of health for Indigenous populations.

Many of the approaches to reporting health status information which have been illustrated in this chapter simply fail to provide the kind of information for Indigenous people that is available for non-Indigenous people. The Australian

Figure 6.5 Age-specific death rates, Australia 1997–99

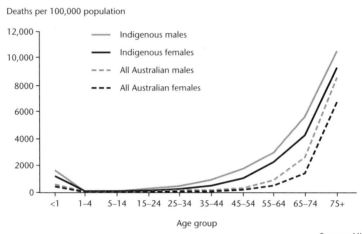

Deaths per 100,000 population

Source: AIHW 2002b

Figure 6.6 Perinatal death rates, Australia 1996–98

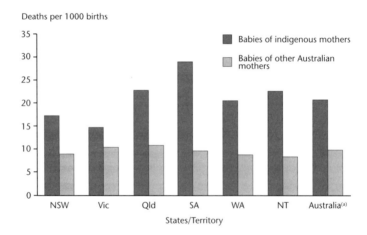

Deaths per 1000 births

Source: AIHW 2002b

health system continues to remain out of reach for vast numbers of Indigenous people and there is evidence that Indigenous people have the poorest health status in the country. Some of the most striking data available to illustrate this major health inequality are contained within recently published age-specific mortality data (figure 6.5) and perinatal deaths data (figure 6.6).

Indigenous people are more likely than other people across all age groups to be hospitalised for most diseases and conditions. This may in part reflect the inaccessibility for Indigenous people of our primary care systems, such as general practitioners and community health services, but is very likely to be an indicator of an increased susceptibility to diseases such as cardiovascular disease, kidney

Figure 6.7   Diabetes mellitus age-specific death rates, Australia 1997–99

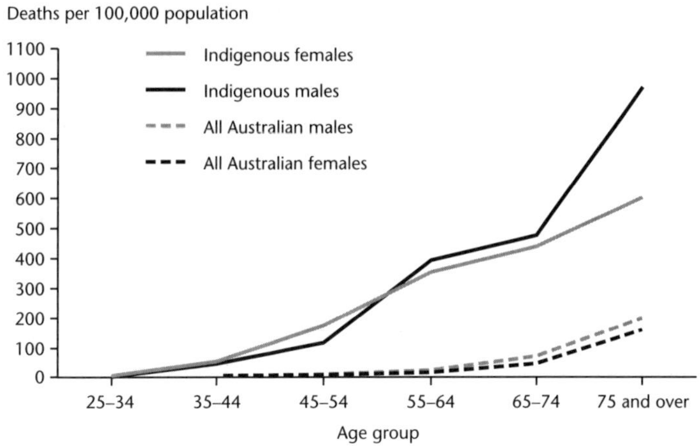

Deaths per 100,000 population

Source: AIHW 2002b

disease, respiratory diseases, and, in particular, diabetes. Indigenous people who have type 2 diabetes often develop the disease earlier than other Australians and often die at younger ages. Figure 6.7 provides an illustration of the excessive diabetes-related mortality experienced by Indigenous males and females.

The inequalities of health status experienced by Indigenous Australian people are stark, and arise from complex interrelationships of social, economic, cultural, and political determinants of health.

The burden of disease

Over the last decade, burden of disease (BoD) studies have been conducted in a number of countries in an attempt to provide new and more practical approaches to measuring health status. This work followed the initial research undertaken for the Global Burden of Disease Study published in 1996 by epidemiologists at the Harvard School of Public Health and the World Health Organization (Murray and Lopez 1996). This initial work was developed specifically to inform global health planning.

Studies recently conducted in Australia (DHS 1999; AIHW 1999b) use the Disability Adjusted Life Year (DALY) as a summary measure of health status. It is beyond the scope of this text to detail the methods used to calculate DALY estimates, however, some basic concepts are presented to the reader. More detailed information is readily accessible in the DHS 1999 and AIHW 1999b references.

The DALY is a summary measure of mortality and disability designed to link information on disease causes and occurrence to information on both short-term and long-term outcomes including impairments, functional limitations (disability), and death. It is based on the underlying concept of time lost: a combination of years of life lost (YLL) due to premature mortality in the population and years of healthy life lost due to disability (YLD). The extent of loss of healthy life due to nonfatal conditions can only be estimated with information on the incidence of the condition over a specified time interval, average duration of the condition, and some quantification of the severity of the condition. The latter attempts to account for the equivalent loss of healthy years of life through the existence of a disabling state or condition, an issue that is still controversial, especially with disability advocacy groups who perceive this approach as potentially devaluing the significance of certain disabilities. Therefore: DALY = YLL + YLD, that is, one DALY is the equivalent of one lost year of 'healthy' life, be it from early death or disability.

A major advantage of the Australian burden of disease studies is that they have, for the first time, provided an objective overview of all major disease states with a range of potential applications that include:

- comparing health status between sectors of the population and providing meaningful estimates of health inequalities
- bringing nonfatal outcomes to the attention of policy makers (especially important for mental health conditions)
- providing a tool for analysing the benefits of public health interventions
- providing one form of evidence to assist with the setting of priorities for health planning
- provoking community dialogue about locally important health issues that may often be overlooked in other forms of health status reporting.

Figure 6.8 provides a simple diagram of the national distribution of DALYs across the main disease groups for males and females in 1996. The major contribution of cardiovascular disease, cancers and mental disorders should be noted, especially in the context of Australia's National Health Priority Areas, which include, as well as these three major disease groups, diabetes, asthma, and injuries. It was estimated for 1996 that the total DALYs for males was 1,331,311 and for females 1,178,963.

Figure 6.8   Burden of disease (DALYs) by sex and main disease groups, Australia 1996

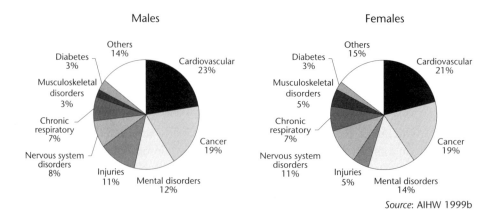

Source: AIHW 1999b

In the Australian context, noncommunicable diseases (e.g. cancers, heart disease, stroke, diabetes, asthma) account for 87 per cent of the total burden of disease, communicable diseases 5 per cent, and injuries just over 8 per cent (AIHW 1999b). This pattern is very typical of the distribution of disease burden across other developed market-economy countries. However, the contrast with global figures from WHO is striking. Worldwide noncommunicable diseases are equal to communicable diseases (each amounting to 43 per cent of the disease burden) with injuries accounting for the remaining 14 per cent. The reasons for this are clear if one considers the effects of large-scale poverty, social deprivation, and warfare on the health of huge populations within developing countries. These living conditions cause infectious diseases such as gastroenteritis and respiratory infections, which are the major killers of young children, and are prominent among Indigenous populations.

The relative lack of prominence of communicable diseases in BoD estimates within Australian populations provides no cause for complacency. These data in fact highlight the importance of existing communicable disease control measures, including immunisation (vaccination) programs, as a mainstay to public health in this and other developed countries.

Figure 6.9, also derived from the national BoD study, illustrates the relative contributions of YLL and YLD for the major disease groups across Australia. These patterns were consistent in the Victorian study, and have been important in providing

Figure 6.9 Burden of disease (YLL, YLD, and total DALYs) for major disease groups, Australia 1996

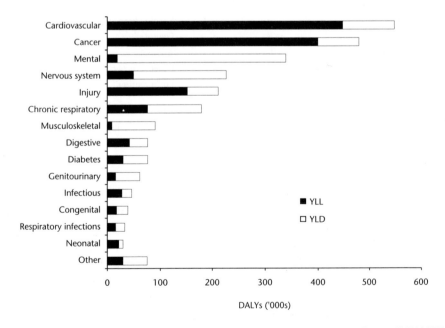

Source: AIHW 1999b

renewed political and strategic policy attention to the relative importance of conditions with a major disability component (e.g. depression and psychotic disorders). These contrast to established high-priority diseases (e.g. coronary heart disease and some cancers) that are known because of their high levels of mortality.

By examining trends from available sources of data, both the national and Victorian studies have been able to produce projections of the estimates of BoD over the twenty years from 1996 to 2016. Figure 6.10 shows the projected changing rank-order of diseases over this period for Victoria. These data have proved invaluable in convincing health planners to look into the future, so that appropriate interventions can be put in place sooner than later, providing the best chance of improving population-wide health outcomes. It should be noted that for males, diabetes, prostate cancer, and heroin dependence are prominent in their increasing importance. For females, the picture is quite different with dementia projected to become the most significant cause of disease burden, and lung cancer increasing dramatically in importance.

Figure 6.10   Ranking of DALYs 1996 and 2016

Males	1996	2016	Females	1996	2016
Ischaemic heart disease	1	1	Ischaemic heart disease	1	2
Stroke	2	10	Stroke	2	9
Lung cancer	3	4	Breast cancer	3	3
Emphysema (COPD)	4	11	Dementia	4	1
Diabetes	5	2	Depression	5	4
Bowel cancer	6	8	Osteoarthritis	6	6
Depression	7	9	Emphysema (COPD)	7	7
Prostate cancer	8	3	Diabetes	8	8
Suicide	9	13	Asthma	9	11
Road traffic accidents	10	29	Bowel cancer	10	10
Dementia	11	5	Lung cancer	11	5
Hearing loss	12	7			
Heroin dependence	16	6			

Source: DHS 1999

A final illustration of how BoD information can be used is in the context of local community health planning. It may be apparent that while the initial work of Murray and Lopez (1996) was pitched at providing a global picture of health, it would require a considerable leap in faith to apply their same model to local government area (LGA) data. Victoria has in fact led the world in constructing a comprehensive set of DALY estimates for each LGA in the state. This of course provides a very real test of the sensitivity and reliability of all aspects of the methodology, and the value of the outputs can readily be criticised as being only as good as the data used in the analyses.

Figure 6.11 provides a sample output from this work, and clearly shows some marked differentials in the burden of disease experienced across six LGAs compared with Victoria (in this case for males). This simple chart contains a huge amount of information, and together with other sources of data, has been used by the identified local governments as a rich source of evidence to stimulate a new approach to health planning at a local community level. Again, these data highlight some important differentials in health within a population and are having a direct application to setting up improvements within state and local public health systems. For local community level planning, there remains a continuing need to gather data at local community level, below that of LGAs.

Figure 6.11 DALY rates per 1000 males in selected local government areas (LGAs) 1996

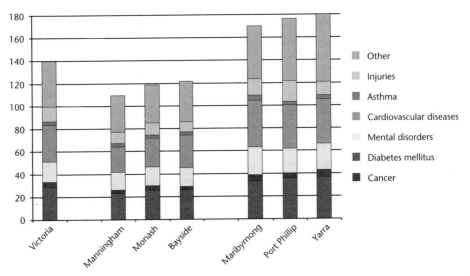

Source: DHS 1999

HEALTH SERVICES AND RISK FACTORS

The overarching aim of health services should be to improve both the quality and the quantity of life. By studying the use of treatment and preventive health services we can, in some situations, get a better understanding of the health status of the population. This section of the chapter outlines the sort of information that is available from health service contacts, and provides some examples. We then examine some of the risk factors (health behaviours and biomedical) that increase the likelihood or risk of health problems. These form part of the spectrum of health determinants that are discussed in other chapters. Some of the impacts that risk factors can have on health and disease are described, as well as patterns of occurrence in the Australian population.[3]

Treatment services

Hospitalisations

In all states and territories, health departments collect vast amounts of administrative data on all episodes of care within the hospital system. With increasing demands on hospitals to account for their expenditure through accurate data management, these data sets have increased in their quality and reliability over recent years. For each hospital admission within the public and private sector in most states, data are recorded to identify clinical diagnoses, procedures, and clinical outcomes. International coding standards are used to ensure quality and consistency in the data collected. In Australia the most current coding classification system in use is from the first edition of the International Statistical Classification of Diseases and Related Health Problems, 10th revision, Australian Modification, otherwise known as ICD-10-AM. This is based on the original ICD-10 classification system developed by WHO and a classification of procedures based on the Australian Medicare Benefits Schedule.

Injuries

Hospitalisations data are a principal source of data that allow the **epidemiology** (the study of the patterns and causes of disease in populations) of injuries to be monitored. These data, together with collections from hospital emergency departments, provide high-quality information that is the backbone of much of the research into injury prevention programs nationally. Agencies such as the AIHW National Injury Surveillance Unit and the Monash University Accident Research Centre have effectively used data from hospitals to support the introduction of legislation in Australia, which has led the world. Provisions in such legislation include the mandatory wearing of seat belts and cycle helmets, child-proof bottles and containers (to prevent poisoning), and maximum temperatures in domestic hot water systems (to prevent scalds).

Preventable admissions

Hospitalisations data have also been used to assist public health policy-making through the analysis of Ambulatory Care Sensitive Conditions (ACSCs). These are conditions where effective community-based primary care (including primary and secondary prevention programs) results in reduced rates of hospital admission—and improved outcomes. Conditions such as asthma, diabetes complications, and heart failure are classic ACSCs.

Figure 6.12 shows recent Victorian data on admission trends for asthma over a number of years (DHS 2001). It illustrates convergence in admission rates for rural and metropolitan Victoria, with a resulting overall reduction in demand for hospital beds for people with asthma over time. These data provide an important indicator of the success of initiatives directed at improving asthma management practices (e.g. adherence to asthma management plans) across the state, and especially in rural Victoria.

Figure 6.12   Asthma admission rates for rural and metropolitan regions, Victoria
1993/94–1999/2000

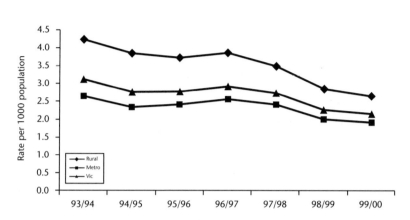

Source: DHS 2001

While these data can be very useful, there are also problems in overreliance on hospitalisations data to document health status. This is obvious if one considers that the majority of people seeking care from the health system never reach a hospital, and that indeed, a significant (but unknown) proportion of people with health problems may never see a general practitioner, or have a complete record of their health documented.

Health systems administrative data are only likely to provide a superficial or proxy view of health status. Information derived from hospitalisation trends data will generally be most useful and reliable for epidemiologists due to the ongoing stability in quality of hospital-based data capture systems. Linkage of hospitalisations data to other health data systems (e.g. mortality data and cancer register data) provides an opportunity to significantly improve the quality of accessible health information.

Primary care episodes

Surprisingly there is no systematic approach for recording details of episodes of primary care (e.g. general practitioner contacts) in Australia, equivalent to that described for hospitalisations. The Health Insurance Commission (HIC) collects information on patterns of service delivery and procedures performed through the Medicare payments system, but information on the details of diseases and patterns of morbidity presenting to general practitioners is not available.

The best available information of this kind is provided through a continuous national study of general practice activity in Australia known as BEACH (Bettering the Evaluation and Care of Health). A random sample of around 1000 general practitioners provides information on about 100,000 patient encounters every year. This study is conducted by the General Practice Statistics and Classification Unit, a collaboration between the AIHW and the University of Sydney.

Other services

Other major health services from which some information on the health of Australians can be obtained include mental health services, veteran's affairs services, alcohol and other drug treatment services, Medicare services (administered and collected by the HIC), the Pharmaceutical Benefits Scheme (PBS), and dental health services. There are also a number of important population health screening services, which are covered in the following section.

Preventive services

Cancer screening registers

There are a number of health services focused on the prevention of ill health in Australia that contribute important information about health status and health systems performance. For example, a number of cancer screening programs operate, with both cervical cancer screening and breast cancer screening (mammography) being the most established. These programs have depended on highly effective clinical data registers and computer-generated recall systems to result in improved prevention and early detection of these cancers with consequent reductions in mortality. Screening programs for other cancers are yet to be established in Australia. A screening program for bowel cancer is in the early developmental stages, but for prostate cancer, there is currently no screening test available that satisfies national screening criteria.

In Australia in 1997–98, 54.3 per cent of women aged 50 to 69 were screened for breast cancer, falling short of the national target of 70 per cent (National BreastScreen Program). For cervical screening, performance is better with 64.8 per cent of Australian women aged 20 to 69 screened in 1998–99 (National Cervical Screening Program). In 2002, a national screening target was yet to be set for cervical screening.

Australian childhood immunisation register

There is also a recently introduced system in Australia for registering the immunisation status of children. Since 1996, the HIC has operated the Australian Childhood Immunisation Register (ACIR), and with the assistance of state health departments, vaccination data are collected for Australian children under seven years of age. This has facilitated the fine-tuning of nationwide immunisation programs that remain one of the most successful public health disease prevention initiatives ever implemented.

The principal diseases that are the focus of Australia's current Standard Vaccination Schedule (2000–02) are diphtheria, tetanus, pertussis, measles, mumps, rubella, poliomyelitis, haemophilus influenzae type b, hepatitis B, pneumococcal disease, influenza, and most recently meningococcal disease. Table 6.2 is derived from the ACIR and shows the uptake of immunisation against specific diseases for 2001, by states and territories for children aged 12 to 15 months.

Table 6.2 Children aged 12 to 15 months[(a)] fully immunised against specific diseases, by states and territories, 2001

	NSW	VIC	QLD	WA	SA	TAS	ACT	NT	AUST
Number of children	20,721	15,119	11,641	6074	4375	1453	990	778	61,151
Diphtheria, tetanus, and pertussis (%)	91.0	92.2	91.8	90.1	91.5	93.1	92.9	88.9	91.5
Poliomyelitis (%)	90.9	92.3	91.8	90.0	91.5	93.2	92.8	89.6	91.4
Haemophilus influenzae type b (%)	94.3	95.3	94.4	93.6	95.0	95.6	95.4	94.0	94.6
Fully immunised (%)[(b)]	90.7	92.1	91.4	89.5	91.4	92.6	92.7	88.6	91.2

(a) Aged 12 to 15 months at 31 December 2000

(b) Fully immunised = No. children vaccinated/No. children on register x 100

Derived from Australian Childhood Immunisation Register (ACIR) data

Source: AIHW 2002b

Figure 6.13 Notifications of haemophilus influenzae type B infections, Victoria 1991–98

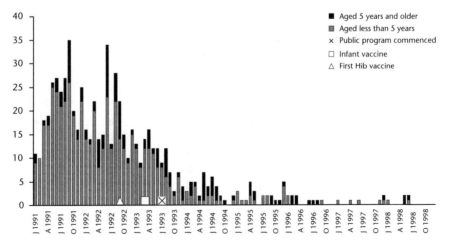

Source: DHS Victoria

Invasive haemophilus influenzae type b (Hib) provides a dramatic example of the effectiveness of immunisation. Hib is a bacterium that causes a wide range of clinical illnesses, especially in young children. Conditions such as meningitis, acute epiglottitis, and septicaemia due to Hib are associated with significant mortality, especially in children less than five years of age. The case fatality ratio for Hib in Australia is between 2.5 and 3.5 per cent; in addition, around 4 per cent of survivors of the disease will suffer profound neurological disability.

In 1993, funding arrangements were put in place for a comprehensive Hib vaccination program to be introduced Australia-wide. This single public health intervention resulted in a 94 per cent reduction 'overnight' in the number of cases of Hib in children under five years. The impact of this vaccination program is illustrated in figure 6.13, showing the most currently available data from Victoria. These data are derived from Victoria's notifiable diseases register, referred to earlier in this chapter.

The NHMRC is continually reviewing its recommendations for schedules of vaccination as new combined vaccines come onto the market, and as new threats from communicable diseases emerge.

Health behaviours

The major risk-taking and health-promoting behaviours requiring public health interventions in Australia are smoking, nutrition, alcohol consumption, and physical activity, commonly referred to as 'SNAP'. Other lifestyle behaviours such as use of illicit drugs, occupation, and sexual practices are also very important public health issues that contribute significantly to the overall burden of disease on society. Figure 6.14 shows the established relationships between various common chronic disease states and risk factors. For anyone in a clinical setting, it can

Figure 6.14   Risk factors common to major chronic diseases

	Cardio-vascular disease*	Diabetes	Cancer	Chronic-obstructive pulmonary disease
Risk factor				
Smoking	■	■	■	■
Alcohol	■		■	
Physical inactivity	■	■	■	
Nutrition	■	■	■	
Obesity	■	■	■	■
Raised blood pressure	■	■		
Dietary fat/blood lipids	■	■	■	
Blood glucose	■	■	■	

* Including heart disease, stroke, hypertension

often be difficult to establish whether a particular risk factor (such as poor diet) has caused a disease (such as bowel cancer).

At a population level, the contribution of risk and protective factors to health and disease can be calculated. If we know the proportion of people who have the risk factor in question (e.g. the percentage of smokers and ex-smokers) and the extra risk that this imposes (e.g. the relative risk of lung cancer in smokers compared with nonsmokers) it can be estimated that around 80 per cent of all lung cancer cases can be attributed to smoking. This is known as the 'attributable fraction'.

Figure 6.15 offers a further perspective and shows, at a glance, the relative importance of risk factors as they contribute to all mortality and morbidity from diseases across the population (DHS 1999). These data have been calculated using attributable fractions. In terms of total attributable burden, behaviours including smoking, low fruit and vegetable intake, physical inactivity, and alcohol consumption are the most significant.

The following sections provide some snap shots of information regarding patterns of occurrence of the SNAP risk factors in the Victorian and Australian populations. The reader is referred to the AIHW web site (www.aihw.gov.au) and its publication *Chronic Diseases and Associated Risk Factors in Australia 2001* (AIHW 2001a), for more detailed information, which is beyond the scope of this chapter. The Victorian Department of Human Services web site (www.dhs.vic.gov.au) provides more information derived from annual surveys of the Victorian population (Victorian Population Health Survey) as well as the Victorian Burden of Disease study.

Figure 6.15   Burden of disease attributed to selected risk factors, 1996

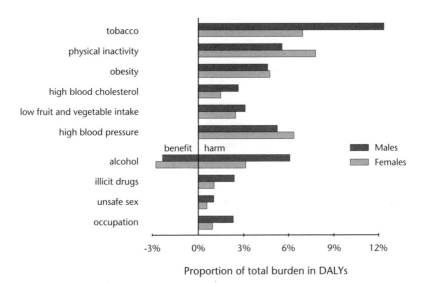

Source: DHS 1999

Tobacco smoking

The use of tobacco in the form of cigarette smoking is widespread and is the risk factor associated with the greatest BoD. Estimates from the 2001 National Drug Strategy Household Survey (AIHW 2002a) indicate that around 3.1 million Australians (19.5 per cent of people aged 14 years and over) smoke tobacco on a daily basis.

The 2001 Victorian Population Health Survey (n=7,500) measured tobacco consumption patterns among Victorians aged 18 and above and found that more than half (51.3 per cent) had smoked tobacco products at some time in their lives (DHS 2002a); 24.5 per cent of Victorian adults identified themselves as current smokers, with the highest prevalence of current smokers in the 18 to 24 year age group (males 44.2 per cent and females 27.6 per cent). Males were more likely to identify themselves as current smokers for every age group except 55 to 64 years.

Figure 6.16 shows patterns of smoking in adolescents aged 12 to 17 years since 1984, and reveals alarmingly that the highest rate of smoking is among girls aged 16 to 17 years. Of concern is the fact that the onset of smoking-related lung cancer occurs many years after initial exposure to tobacco. The Victorian Burden of Disease Study (DHS 1999) projects a relative increase in the morbidity and mortality from lung cancer in females over the next twenty years.

Figure 6.16   Proportion of adolescents (aged 12 to 17) who are smokers, 1984–96

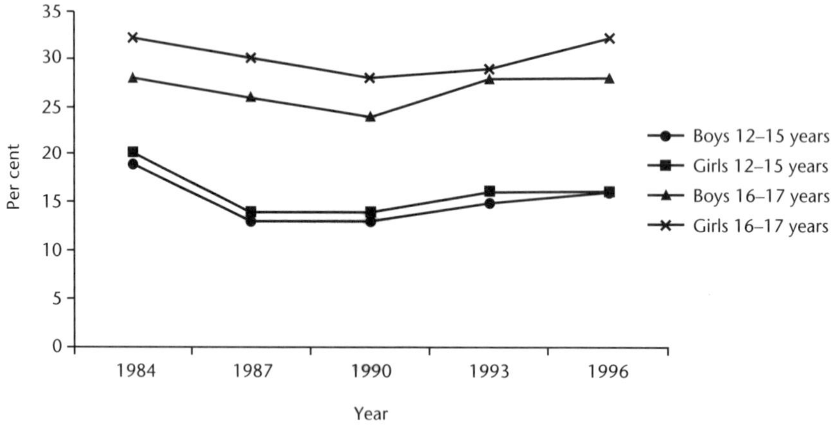

Source: AIHW 2001a

Alcohol consumption

Alcohol consumption is a risk factor for a large number of health conditions and injuries including stroke, liver cirrhosis, pancreatitis, diabetes, and some cancers, and is a significant factor in motor vehicle fatalities and injuries as well as falls, drowning, burns, suicide, and occupational injuries.

Nutrition

The Victorian Burden of Disease Study (DHS 1999) estimated that 2.8 per cent of total disease burden could be attributed to inadequate fruit and vegetable intake, exceeding the contribution made by alcohol (2.1 per cent), illicit drugs (1.9 per cent), unsafe sex (0.8 per cent) and occupational hazards (1.7 per cent). Dietary guidelines developed by the NHMRC (2001a, 2001b) recommend high intake of plant foods (e.g. cereals, fruit and vegetables, legumes, and nuts) and to limit fat intake to reduce the risk of coronary heart disease, several common cancers, obesity, and diabetes.

Information on the dietary intake of Australians is limited and the most recent National Nutrition Survey undertaken in 1995 (ABS and DHFS 1997) estimated that two in three persons were not consuming the recommended level of vegetables and four in five were not consuming enough fruit. More recent data from Victoria show that only 23.2 per cent of Victorians were consuming four or more serves of vegetables daily and 56 per cent were consuming two or more serves of fruit on a usual day (DHS 2002a). Overall, younger persons were less likely to be consuming adequate amounts of fruit and vegetables. This pattern is consistent with the increasing trend for young persons to consume large quantities of 'fast food' that is generally energy rich, fat laden and poor in nutritional content.

Physical inactivity

Participation in physical *activity* is an important protective factor for physical and mental health, significantly reducing the mortality and morbidity from cardiovascular disease, particularly coronary heart disease. Conversely, physical *inactivity*

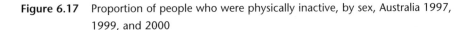

Figure 6.17 Proportion of people who were physically inactive, by sex, Australia 1997, 1999, and 2000

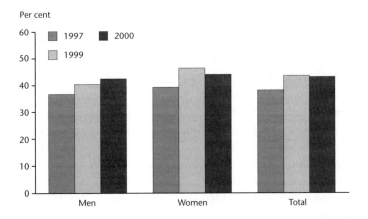

Source: AIHW 2002b

ranks second only to tobacco smoking in terms of its contribution to the BoD, accounting for around 6.5 per cent of the total BoD (DHS 1999; AIHW 1999b). In females, it is the most important risk factor for disease, contributing around 8 per cent of the total disease burden. Physical inactivity is strongly associated with other cardiovascular risk factors such as high blood pressure, high blood cholesterol levels, obesity, and diabetes. It also compounds the risks when associated with smoking, poor nutrition, and alcohol consumption.

Biomedical risk factors

A range of epidemiological and intervention studies have demonstrated that there are a number of biomedical or physiological factors that increase the risk of health problems. Some of the most important biomedical risk factors are blood pressure, blood cholesterol, and body weight. Information on the population distribution of these risk factors (prevalence) has to be collected from special surveys, which involve clinical examination and blood tests. Unfortunately, although this information is normally collected by general practitioners, there is no reliable or systematic data system available. Because of the difficulty and expense involved in the collection of representative data across the whole population, few good surveys have been conducted. The three important sources of data in Australia are:

- the National Risk Factor Prevalence Surveys 1980, 1983 and 1989 (NHFA and AIHW 1990)
- the 1995 National Nutrition Survey (ABS 1996; ABS and DHFS 1997)
- the 1999–2000 Australian Diabetes, Obesity and Lifestyle Study (AusDiab). (Dunstan et al. 2001)

Detailed information on biomedical factors is also comprehensively reported in *Australia's Health 2002* (AIHW 2002b).

High blood pressure

High blood pressure is a major risk factor for heart disease, stroke, peripheral vascular disease, and renal failure. This condition is more likely to develop in those who are overweight, physically inactive, have high dietary salt intake, and is also associated with emotional stress.

High blood pressure was the most commonly managed problem by Australian general practitioners in 2000–01, and in both the Victorian and National Burden of Disease studies accounted for more than 5 per cent of the total disease burden. Data from the 1999–2000 AusDiab study indicate that around 29 per cent or 3.6 million Australians over the age of 25 years had high blood pressure or were on medication for that condition. Data from the 1980, 1983, and 1989 Risk Factor Prevalence Surveys, the 1985 National Nutrition Survey and the AusDiab study show that the prevalence of high blood pressure has decreased significantly since 1980 for both males and females.

Figure 6.18 Proportion of people with high blood pressure, Australia 1980 to 1999–2000

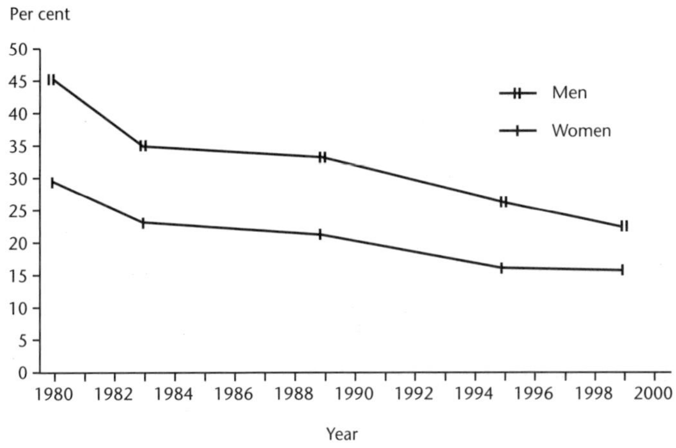

Source: AIHW 2002b

High blood cholesterol

High blood cholesterol is a risk factor for coronary heart disease and stroke, and causes almost 3 per cent of the total burden of disease. The AusDiab study estimated that around 50 per cent of both males and females aged over 25 years had elevated blood cholesterol levels (greater than or equal to 5.5 mmol/L). This equates to approximately six million people.

Since 1980 there has been no discernible change in the proportions of the population with high blood cholesterol; the proportion of males with elevated cholesterol levels has consistently exceeded the proportion of females with high levels.

Excess body weight

Excess body weight has an association with nearly all the risk factors discussed in this chapter, and is one of the most important public health problems in Australia. With the dramatic behavioural changes in modern society resulting in increases in dietary fat intake and physical inactivity, levels of excess body weight have reached epidemic proportions in all developed countries. Data from the USA provide the most striking example of this with a 61 per cent increase in obesity in US adults since 1991. In 2000, the prevalence of obesity was 19.8 per cent among US adults (Mokdad et al. 2001).

People who are overweight or obese have higher mortality and morbidity from a wide range of chronic diseases including the most common form of diabetes (type 2), coronary heart disease, respiratory disease, and some cancers. Other conditions associated with excess weight include gallbladder disease, osteoporosis, stroke, and a range of mental health disorders such as depression. Overweight accounts for around 5 per cent of the total burden of disease.

Excess weight is a condition of abnormal and excessive fat accumulation to the extent that a person's health and wellbeing may be adversely affected. The primary cause is a long-term imbalance in metabolism, with energy intake exceeding energy consumption. The measurement of excess weight as a risk factor for chronic diseases is not simple, as both the overall and regional distributions of fat in the body contribute to chronic disease development and progression. Two common measures of excess weight are body mass index (BMI) and waist circumference. Table 6.3 summarises the accepted approaches to the measurement and classification of excess weight.

The most recent data on overweight and obesity in Australia come from the AusDiab study. Using BMI as the index, 59.6 per cent of participants were overweight (67.4 per cent males and 52 per cent females) and 20.5 per cent were obese (19.1 per cent males and 21.8 per cent females). These data (obtained by physical measurement) are remarkably similar to the self-report data reported from the USA. While self-report data on BMI generally underestimate the extent of overweight and obesity, these data together with data from Canada (Joint Health Survey Unit 2001; Katzmarzyk 2002) show that Australians are among the most overweight in the world.

Table 6.3 Measurement of excess weight

MEASUREMENT OF EXCESS WEIGHT

Body mass index (BMI) is the ratio of weight (in kilograms) to height (in metres) squared. BMI classification consists of underweight, normal, overweight, and obese.

Body Mass Index (BMI):

Underweight:	< 18.5
Normal weight	18.5 and < 25
Overweight	25 and above, but < 30
Obese	30 and above

Waist circumference measures levels of abdominal fat mass and indicates an increased risk of metabolic complications associated with obesity. Two categories, overweight and obese, are identified.

Waist circumference:

Males:	Overweight	94 to 101 cm
	Obese	>/= 102 cm
Females:	Overweight	80 to 87 cm
	Obese	>/= 88cm

Source: AIHW 2001a

The data illustrated in figure 6.19 are derived from the 1980, 1983, and 1989 National Risk Factor Prevalence Studies (NHFA and AIHW 1990), the 1995 ABS National Nutrition Survey (ABS 1996) and the 1999–2000 AusDiab study (Dunstan et al. 2000), and show the national increase in prevalence of both overweight and obesity from 1980 to 2000 for both males and females.

Figure 6.19   Proportion of Australian adults (aged 25 to 64) overweight or obese, 1980–2000

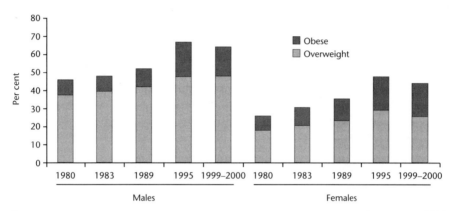

Source: AIHW 2001a

SUMMARY

- Health is measured through vast data collections but all information collected should have a practical purpose.
- Australia's population is slowly becoming proportionally older because of decline in births and longer life expectancy.
- Indigenous health inequalities are Australia's biggest challenge.
- Risk factor determinants of health include smoking, alcohol consumption, lack of physical activity, excess body weight, poor nutrition, use of illicit drugs, occupation, and sexual practices.

DISCUSSION TOPICS

1   What information can you find out from the LGA data about the health issues that impact on your community? What are the top ten BoD health issues? How does this list compare to the national data? What information can you glean about determinants that might contribute to the health issues of concern in your community? For instance, is access to transport limited? What implications

might this have for the community? Is social isolation likely to be a significant determinant? What causes you to draw this conclusion?

2   How might an understanding of the 'complex interrelationships of social, economic, cultural and political determinants…' influence key stakeholders and decision makers in planning strategies to address Indigenous health inequalities?

3   Apply your understanding of the determinants of health to suggest three actions that would improve the health of your community.

NOTES

1   Much of the material in this chapter has been derived from the Australian Institute of Health and Welfare (AIHW). *Australia's Health 2002* is the eighth in a series of biennial reports produced by AIHW that provides a comprehensive analysis of the health of Australians as well as aspects of performance of the Australian health system. Readers are encouraged to access this document through the AIHW web site (http://aihw.gov.au) for further detailed information.

2   A comprehensive description of the major causes of death is available in *Australia's Health 2002, The Burden of Disease and Injury in Australia, AIHW* and in *The Victorian Burden of Disease Study: Mortality, 1999.* These publications are accessible through the AIHW web site (www.aihw.gov.au) and the Victorian Department of Human Services web site (www.dhs.vic.gov.au/phd/bod).

3   The AIHW has kindly granted permission to use data and materials published in *Australia's Health 2002* and *Chronic diseases and associated risk factors in Australia, 2001,* for inclusion in this section of the chapter.

PUBLIC AND POPULATION HEALTH: STRATEGIC RESPONSES

Helen Keleher

Key concepts

- Population health
- Equity and inequity
- Evidence base
- Upstream–midstream–downstream intervention levels

Children, youth, young adults, new mothers, working age adults, newly retrenched, newly retired, and the elderly: what do they have in common? Any of these population groups is increasingly susceptible to the newest epidemic to affect the health of populations—that of mental illness. In the twenty-first century, it is expected that at some time in their life, one in five people is likely to suffer from a mental disorder or mental illness. Their families, friends, and colleagues too will experience its shadow.

In Australia, as in many other countries, this is a crisis of growing proportions—the prevalence and incidence of mental disorders and mental illness are creating enormous challenges for society. Many of us know someone who has suffered, or is suffering, from depression, anxiety, or perhaps a psychosis or bipolar disorder. We may know of someone who has self-harmed or attempted suicide. The extent of the problem is prompting not just major investment in individual treatment and support services but also in prevention and mental health promotion for the whole population, with a particular focus on those whose health is the most vulnerable. This is what is called a **population health** approach.

This chapter puts the case for population health to be modelled on a comprehensive approach, one that is solidly based on analysis of the determinants of health and statistical burden of disease data, rather than a selective evidence base that privileges statistical evidence or gives only token attention to the determinants evidence base. A comprehensive approach is critical because the kinds of evidence that are used to define problems also determine the responses that will be funded and sustained. In other words, if the goals of population health are comprehensive, then societal responses are likely to be more far-reaching. Thus, strategic population health has two goals: the first goal is to improve the health of the entire population; the second goal, simultaneous with the first, is to reduce health inequities among and between, specific population groups.

The concept of inequity is important for a comprehensive population health. In this chapter, various elements of a sound population health approach are discussed. These elements include the kinds of infrastructure needed for population health; some aspects of the evidence base on which to base decisions about priorities; and the importance of multifaceted, multidisciplinary programs with pathways into interventions, programs, collaborations, alliances and partnerships to develop effective upstream and downstream approaches. Using mental health and illness as a case study, approaches that are most likely to be effective in tackling population health problems are discussed.

DEFINING POPULATION HEALTH

Population health is an approach that turns the focus of attention on whole populations or subpopulations rather than on individuals, seeking sustainable changes to social and health systems in order to overcome inequities. Lilley (2000) argues that the expected outcomes from this approach go far beyond just health improvement:

Figure 7.1 The population health template

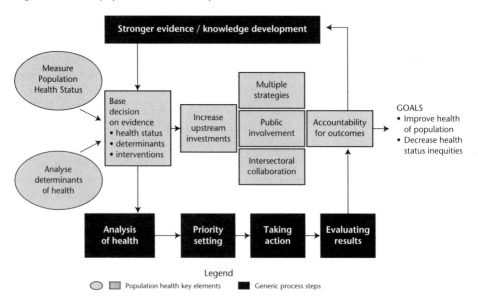

Source: Health Canada 2002

'the outcomes of benefits of a population health approach extend beyond improved population health outcomes to include a sustainable and integrated health system, increased national growth and productivity, and strengthened social cohesion and citizen engagement'. And further: 'The population health approach recognizes that health is a capacity or resource, rather than a state, a definition which corresponds more to the notion of being able to pursue one's goals, to acquire skills and education, and to grow. This broader notion of health recognizes the range of social, economic and physical environmental factors that contribute to health' (Health Canada 2002). Therefore, health is 'the capacity of people to adapt to, respond to, or control life's challenges and changes' (Frankish et al. 1996).

This definition encompasses understandings of the social, economic, cultural, and political factors and conditions that have an influence on health. It is essential to understand the shift in thinking that population health represents from the 1980s WHO definition of health. That definition—'that health is a state of physical, social and mental well-being'—confuses the actual state of health with what it is that determines health. It is a definition that masks the determinants by making the state of health itself the object of measurement, rather than focusing on the determinants as an object of measurement. Thus, a comprehensive population health model takes account of the effects of the determinants of health on the whole population as well as on particular population groups. This enables program/service delivery frameworks that address both the determinants of health and focus on the needs of those with disadvantaged health status, aiming to reduce health inequities.

There is a range of social determinants of health through which complex interactions occur and inequities arise. Some have been discussed in previous chapters. Table 7.1 lists the main categories of determinants, but it should not be

Table 7.1   Social determinants of health

1 Income, social status, and the social gradient	2 Social support networks
3 Early years of life	4 Unemployment, underemployment, and working conditions
5 Social environments, and social cohesion	6 Physical environments
7 Personal health practices and coping skills	8 Healthy child development
9 Transport	10 Education
11 Biology and genetic endowment	12 Social exclusion
13 Gender, racism, and all forms of discrimination	14 Culture
15 Food insecurity	16 Access to health services

Source: Wilkinson and Marmot 1998; Berkman and Kawachi 2000; Health Canada 2001

seen as definitive or unchanging because this is a dynamic field that is evolving as the research continues to emerge.

The sources for this list provide much more detail on the evidence base for each determinant than this chapter can provide, and together with the web sites at the end of this chapter, provide rich sources for further exploration.

EVIDENCE BASE FOR POPULATION HEALTH

Of the ten leading causes of disability world-wide, five are problems of mental disorders and mental illness, with an increase in the burden of illness expected to outstrip that for cardiovascular disease.

Hosman and Lopis 2000

Effective population health is modelled on an evidence base derived from two main sources of data: the measurement of health status and risk factors, such as burden of disease (BoD) studies; and by analysis of the determinants of health. The evidence base for mental health in Australia tells us that:

- the prevalence of depression at any one time among the population is about 6 per cent (DHAC 1999b) but that the lifetime prevalence is between 30 to 50 per cent (Hosman and Lopis 2000)
- women are twice as likely as men to have a depressive disorder
- rates for adolescent and younger women are particularly high
- in the utilisation of mental health services, people with depressive disorders are second only to people with schizophrenia (DHAC 1999b)
- costs to governments (for health services) and to society (loss of life to suicide, to productivity and for care) are intensifying (Hosman and Lopis 2000).

The field of mental illness exemplifies the importance of synthesising measurement of morbidity and mortality data with analysis of the determinants of health. If we were only to measure the incidence and prevalence of mental disorders or mental illness among the community, we would only be given a set of numbers. The BoD uses the DALY (Disability Adjusted Life Year) measure to account for the equivalent loss of healthy years of life through the existence of a disabling state or condition. It provides one form of evidence to assist with the setting of priorities for health planning. Yet, although such statistical measurement is useful to a point, it fails to help us understand people's social experiences of mental health problems, or the ways in which these problems affect people's daily quality of life, what difficulties they experience with treatment services, how stigma affects them, or the effect on their income or working life. Further, statistical measurement does not account for the flow-on effects that occur with respect to family, friends, and communities.

In Australia, governments have tended towards a selective population health model with a concentration on measurement, particularly through BoD studies and on disease states, rather than their underlying determinants. Significant investment has been made in BoD studies, into policy built around the disease priorities that emanate from those studies and with a strong focus on those diseases for which cost-effective interventions have been identified (Baum 2002, p. 104). Thus, a selective approach to health improvement is developed, one that is focused on diseases rather than determinants and inequities.

EQUITY AND INEQUITY

Definitional differences between inequality and inequity are critical for population health: 'Health inequality is a generic term used to designate the [measurable] differences, variations, and disparities in the health achievements of individuals and groups [whereas] health inequity refers to those inequalities in health that are deemed to be unfair or stemming from some form of injustice' (Kawachi et al. 2002, pp. 1–2).

In other words, inequality and equality are *dimensional* concepts meaning they are terms that simply refer to quantities or distributions that are measurable. Inequity and equity, on the other hand, are *relational* concepts, with political dimensions. Inequity and equity involve relations of equal and unequal power (political, social, and economic) as well as justice and injustice, and assert the need for public policy driven solutions. Kawachi et al. make the point that not only is it important to understand the essential differences between the concepts of inequality and inequity, but also appreciate that inequity is grounded in social justice. Social justice approaches to health are a necessary underpinning for health systems in order for priority to be put on the achievement of health as a resource and as a human right. Understanding inequity in moral terms provides the foundation for a population health model that seeks to tackle health inequities and injustices, while also seeking to improve the health of populations overall.

For example, inequalities in mental health relate to low socioeconomic status (Turrell et al. 1999) and to position in the social gradient (Marmot 1998). But in mental health, we need to know much more about pathways to good care and about client outcomes. For example, what is the relationship between mental illness, chronic illness, and low incomes? Given the stigma attached to mental health disorders, how are pathways to good care affected? To what extent do literacy and education affect people's mental illness experiences? To what extent is there a trickle-down effect for people with mental health disorders, of stigma, discrimination, and **social exclusion**; and what kinds of social support are available to them? What is the impact of violence, sexual assault, drug use or homelessness on their care? Too often, people with mental health disorders become isolated, and experience income decline and loss of social contacts, causing them to lack the kinds of social support that have such a profound influence on health. Thus, information about the mental health status of people is a much more complex story than that provided by morbidity and mortality measurements alone.

Levels of factors have a strategic importance not just for understanding health but also for policy and the design of interventions to tackle health issues such as mental health. There are three broad levels of factors:

Downstream factors. These are micro-level factors that include the effect of upstream and midstream factors on physiological and biological functioning. Proportionally, more investment is made in biological, physiological, and pharmaceutical research—in other words, in understanding interventions that will work on downstream factors. For example, the development of drug therapies for depression or psychiatric illness (or high blood pressure or to reduce blood cholesterol), or a focus on improving systems and the responsiveness of services such as community-based mental health services, is downstream investment.

Midstream factors. These are intermediate-level factors that include psychosocial factors, health-related behaviours and the role of the health system in health. Significant investment is also made at the midstream level, through lifestyle, behavioural, and individual prevention programs. Primary disease prevention is concerned with health risks and might include some form of opportunistic health education to encourage a client towards better health practices (Wass 2000). Disease prevention strategies are commonly framed as health education in primary care consultations, and target the individual for change rather than the social or environmental conditions that underlie the disease or condition (Keleher 2001). Social marketing and other behaviour change strategies are midstream interventions.

Upstream factors. These are macro-level factors that comprise organisational change and health development as well as global and structural influences on health and health systems, government policies designed to affect the social, physical, economic and environmental factors that determine health. In other words, upstream investments are directed at fundamental causes of poor health and inequities. One example of upstream investment in relation to depression is the investment by Australian governments in *beyondblue: the national depression initiative* to promote effective population health strategies.

Universal provision

An important foundation of any equity-driven approach to population health is a commitment to the **universal provision** of health care and health programs in order to make them accessible to all people on the basis of their need. Universally funded programs (e.g. QUIT, maternal and child health, drug and alcohol or health promotion) are most commonly provided through the community, primary and women's health sectors. Access to medical and hospital care and the Pharmaceutical Benefits Scheme (PBS) is funded through Medicare, Australia's national health insurance scheme. To date, access and equity to needed health services have been the foundations of Australia's health system but these fundamental principles are under threat from pressures exerted by the World Trade Organization (WTO) and its General Agreements on Tariffs and Trade in Services (GATTS) which do not identify goals of social equity (Schrader 2001). Through GATTS negotiations, multinational and predominantly US-based businesses are calling for majority foreign ownership of public health facilities, and thus, are seeking to gain a market share of public sector health system funding in Australia and other countries. The PBS is at the frontline of this battle. If the Commonwealth government allows the footprint of GATTS to be stamped on the PBS and/or Medicare, then community health, medical care and hospital care will be subject to increasing privatisation. Australia's health system will increasingly resemble that of the USA, with inevitable rationing of health programs and health care, as the principles of universalism are dismantled (Schrader 2001).

PUBLIC HEALTH: UPSTREAM INVESTMENTS FOR POPULATION HEALTH

Public health is a broad service system organised at the level of governments through government departments and agencies. It is primarily concerned with the prevention of disease and injury for whole populations and subpopulations. A popular definition of public health is that written by Professor John Last (1987) but is somewhat dated because of its lack of focus on inequities or the health of vulnerable groups:

> Public health is one of the efforts organised by society to protect, promote, and restore the people's health. It is the combination of sciences, skills and beliefs that is directed to the maintenance and improvement of the health of all the people through collective or social actions. The programmes, services, and institutions involved emphasize the prevention of disease and the health needs of the population as a whole. Public health activities change with changing technology and social values, but the goals remain the same: to reduce the amount of disease, premature death and disease-produced discomfort and disability in the population.

Last's definition tells us that public health is a field of both policy and practice that is necessary for population health. However, given that our societies in the twenty-first century are marked by increasing inequities and that we have a growing body of knowledge about the determinants of health, definitions of public health should be expanded to integrate social justice aims.

Public health in Australia has been conceptualised as traditional or 'old' public health and 'new' public health. The distinction between 'old' and 'new' illustrates the shift in thinking, since the 1970s, towards strategic ideas about how health can be supported and created, rather than the fairly singular focus on the treatment of disease that dominated previously. Traditional public health encompasses those services and approaches developed during the early public health movement of the nineteenth and early twentieth centuries. Clean accessible water supplies, sewerage systems, food safety including environmental controls over markets and food suppliers, and controls over air pollutants, are together vital foundations for public health. Today, with the advent of the new public health (see Baum 2002) with its closer integration of the new environmental health (discussed in Chapter 3), partnerships between sectors outside the health system, such as education, transport, agriculture, and social services, are critically important for health.

Public health is based on a foundation of evidence, programs, legislation, and regulation designed to safeguard our health. Put simply, public health can be thought of as large-scale problem solving. It involves identifying an actual or potential health problem, understanding the determinants and/or finding the cause, gathering and analysing data, devising and implementing solutions, and finally, checking the quality of the solution to be sure it is working. To be effective, public health needs well-planned strategic responses based on good-quality research. It also needs clear goals and policies and vision, with a coordinated planning for the future that addresses inequities and the needs of vulnerable groups, and those with the most disadvantaged health status.

Infrastructure

In order to respond to the determinants of health, government commitment is required at policy and program levels, as well as government investment in ongoing workforce training and development. Political and economic philosophies affect how governments will respond to the determinants of health agendas. Governments around the world are inexorably shifting to neoliberal philosophies with their focus on individualist marketplaces where everyone is encouraged to act in their own interests. Notions of social justice that call for interventionist government policies aimed at social and economic programs to reduce inequity are resisted by neoliberal governments. More extended discussion of political and economic policies in relation to public health can be found in Baum's *The New Public Health* (2002).

In relation to mental health, investment in infrastructure requires collaboration between sectors, research funding that is not just about clinical treatment but also about determinants of mental health and mental health promotion, effective dissemination strategies to enhance uptake of new knowledge, and the creation of a 'properly resourced policy platform on mental health' (Hosman and Lopis 2000, p. 37).

Resource allocation

Public health expenditure by governments, infrastructure within governments (rather than the private sector), and state funding for interventions are essential for good health. In Australia, public health expenditure is only about 2 per cent of the total health budget—the combined expenditure of Commonwealth and state governments on core public health activities in 1998–99 was $880 million (AIHW 2001). Eight major categories comprise this expenditure:
- communicable disease control
- selected health promotion activities
- immunisation
- environmental health
- food standards and hygiene

- breast cancer screening
- cervical screening
- all other core public health. (AIHW 2002b, p. xix)

With only 2 per cent of the total health budget, public health in Australia has a remarkable record of achievement and efficiency. The provision of state funding and intervention for public health is considered absolutely essential to prevent what Szreter describes as 'the four Ds'—disruption, deprivation, death, and disease (in Baum 2002, p. 102)—that comprise the major threats to the health of populations. Consider the state of health in countries and their communities where funding, infrastructure, and interventions to improve population health are not provided by the state. Those countries are characterised by lower life expectancy, high infant and maternal mortality, high childhood rates of infectious diseases and mortality, unstable social systems, and inequity. Redistributive policies that direct resources to underprivileged and vulnerable groups in society need to be managed by governments through policy and effective economic and social planning to ensure universal provision of services, to build social stability and to overcome gross inequities (Lowe 2002). The health of all people depends very much on commitment by ministers and departments of health to provide funding for, and drive, state interventions and systems that will create conditions that support and improve health.

Workforce development: new directions

Understanding a determinants approach means that the workforce, whether directly or indirectly involved in the delivery of health programs and services, requires additional competencies to those already mandated by the various professions. More specialised skills with a clearer sense of direction and purpose about population health are needed among the primary and community sectors, as well as in public health sectors.

The National Public Health Partnership (NPHP 2001) has researched the core skills for public health practice. In addition, practitioners engaged in practice directed at tackling inequities need to appreciate the depth of communication strategies required to work with culturally diverse, vulnerable, and disadvantaged groups. New skills for the twenty-first century include the ability to work collectively and in collaboration and partnerships for effective health program delivery that embraces consultation, citizen engagement, and the generation of upstream policy solutions (Baum and Keleher 2002).

COMMUNITY, PRIMARY, AND WOMEN'S HEALTH SECTORS

Community-based services are locally organised, and designed to deliver a range of programs and services in response to the needs for defined, local communities. They utilise downstream, midstream, and upstream strategies. Community-based services, together with general practitioners, are at the forefront of the delivery of services for people with mental health disorders.

Community health

At local levels, community-based health services are central to the delivery of primary health care, many personal services, health education, and local health promotion programs. There is a vast range of organisational and administrative patterns for community health services but they have some common features.

All had their genesis in the first government-funded program to definitively provide for community health services, which was the Community Health Program, established by the Commonwealth under the Whitlam government in 1973. Now the responsibility of the six states and two territories, Community Health Services (CHSs) are a model for the strategic organisation of a wide range of services and have a significant role in the organisation and provision of primary health care and health promotion. Community health services have in common a focus on a defined, local population. Staffing is purposely multidisciplinary including, for example, allied health staff from physiotherapy, podiatry, occupational health, speech therapy; community nursing; women's health clinics; maternal and child health nursing; health promotion programs including specific women's health and men's health programs; social work and family therapy; psychological and financial counselling; drug and alcohol workers; mental health services; and occasionally, general practitioners.

Community health services need to be responsive both to emerging population health data and to the needs of local communities. For example, in response to the evidence about the extent and burden of mental health disorders, Primary Mental Health Services are being established to work closely with general practitioners and community health services. Primary Mental Health Services encompass child and adolescent services, adult services, aged psychiatry, alcohol and drug programs, early intervention and crisis prevention, health education and health promotion programs. Community-based programs such as the Primary Mental Health Services, and organisations such as *beyond-blue* are able to plan strategically, direct research efforts, conduct health promotion, and raise levels of awareness about depression and its related disorders. Thus Australia is seeing multifaceted approaches, at a population health level, to the epidemic of mental illness and mental health disorders.

Strategies: primary health care and primary care

Primary health care (PHC) was first recognised through the Alma Ata Charter for Primary Health Care (WHO 1978). Its key principles were:
- *equity:* essential health care, universally accessible, and affordable
- *social justice:* achievement of health as a resource and a human right

- *reorienting health systems* towards raising the health status of individuals, families, and communities
- *enabling* people to lead socially and economically productive lives.

Primary health care is a health development model, a key strategy of public health derived from the **social model** of health specifically to deal with the determinants of health. Primary health care is more than a philosophy. It is also a system response to reducing health inequities and ameliorating the effects of disadvantage, to guide the delivery of primary health services (Keleher 2001). The model of PHC is for universal, community-based health promotion, prevention, and curative services, based on collaborative, multisectoral activities (e.g. education, transport, environmental health, agriculture) and authentic community involvement.

Primary health care is a different approach to primary care as it is practiced in medicine, nursing, and allied health therapies. In **primary care**, there is usually a single service or intermittent management of a condition with or without follow-up or interaction beyond that point. Primary care is focused on early diagnosis and timely, effective treatment, screening, surveillance, primary prevention, and disease management. Prevention in primary care is concerned with risk factors and risk conditions; secondary prevention, that is, early treatment to minimise complications; tertiary prevention, that is, concerned with rehabilitation; and often involves opportunistic health education and individualised, narrow forms of health education. Of course, primary care services may be delivered within a PHC service, but they must fulfil principles of equity, universal access, sustainability, cultural appropriateness, and health-worker accountability, and be provided at no cost to the consumer (Keleher 2001).

Primary health care has a broader vision to primary care and different intent with both bottom-up and top-down strategies. PHC practitioners work to change the social, political, environmental, and economic determinants of illness, in order to create better health in communities, regions, or cities. No one sector can deal with all determinants of health, so PHC is multisectoral and requires whole-of-government efforts, not just those of the health system. Primary health care practice requires the participation of those most affected by the problem and health-worker accountability for that participation. Practitioner focus is on the most urgent needs of communities, the priorities set by communities themselves, the equalisation of relationships between 'experts' and communities, health disadvantage and reducing health inequities, sustainability of the services provided, empowerment of people alongside efforts to help them be more self-determining, and the building of skills in individual clients and in communities to develop their capacity for self-determination.

Australia's Indigenous people have pioneered and championed both PHC philosophies and practices especially through the establishment of locally based Aboriginal Community Controlled Health Organisations. The Northern Territory is engaged in major reform of how programs and services are planned and delivered to local communities. In partnership with the Commonwealth Department of Health and Ageing, territory staff have worked with Indigenous people to develop the Primary Health Care Access Program (PHCAP) in remote areas of the Northern Territory. This is a system of funding to support comprehensive primary health care, and provides structures for partnerships between local communities and government for decision making and priority setting in planning and delivery of services and programs.

In mental health services, a primary health care approach is demonstrated in the case study presented in box 7.1.

Box 7.1 Community mental health nursing: A lifeline

The mental health workplace is most commonly out in the community where people live and work. Psychiatric nurses, Sarah and Joe, understand that while mental illness can be very debilitating, people can and do recover with appropriate professional help. Sarah explains that mental health nurses work with clients' basic needs, to help them regain their lives, and to reintegrate with work, family, and social networks. Joe will always remember being told that his work with a troubled teenage boy was critical to the boy's recovery: 'By talking through his interests, his family, his life, and getting to know him, I was able to use my skills to help him through what was a very difficult time in his life and get him into a treatment program. He is now back at school and doing well.'

The nurses whose work features in the case study incorporate many of the key features of PHC practice. Practitioners understand that people's basic needs must first be met before health advancement can occur. These basic needs are for shelter, social support, safety from violence, reliable and affordable food supplies, clean water, washing facilities, and waste disposal.

Primary health care also includes maternal and child health (reproductive health, contraception, breastfeeding); essential primary care (medicines, treatment, immunisation) at affordable cost; community engagement; working 'with' rather than 'on' communities; and health-worker accountability to communities. PHC is visionary, seeking solutions to problems that defy biological, genetic, or biochemical solutions, problems that demand new thinking, innovative approaches and values of universalism, accessibility, and affordability. Those most in need of PHC are least likely to access services for which cash payments might be requested.

Selective PHC has been developed by governments responding to Health Sector Reform agendas of the World Bank that advocate for user pays, cost recovery, private health insurance, and public–private partnerships (Hall and Taylor 2003). The focus is on individualised technologies, selected for the goal of reducing child mortality in developing countries. Comprehensive PHC was considered too expensive and therefore, idealistic. Selective PHC has little emphasis on equity or justice. At the beginning of the twenty-first century, it is more common to find health systems funding selective PHC rather than comprehensive PHC, which tackles determinants of health. Comprehensive PHC deals with basic needs in the context of a bigger vision including the desire for sustainable social and system changes. In this way, PHC has much in common with, for example, the provision of primary mental health programs in the community that seek to provide housing and employment assistance as well as case management and the development of personal skills through health education.

In Australia, as elsewhere, comprehensive PHC has not been well supported by governments despite the numbers of people living in poverty and disadvantaged circumstances who do not have access to basic services or to a healthy environment (Hall and Taylor 2003). The health of Indigenous people living in remote communities in Australia is strongly linked to these kinds of problems. Increasing numbers of Australians, including those with mental illness, and/or who are homeless, drug dependent, poor, refugees without access to Medicare or employment, prostitutes and street sex workers, are suffering from suboptimal access to basic services that they need.

Consumer engagement as a strategy

The Alma Ata Charter for Primary Health Care and the Ottawa Charter for Health Promotion both identify consumer participation as an essential, if not challenging, strategy. Since the creation of these charters, there has developed a body of literature about strategies designed to improve health services through consumer participation. In addition, there is a substantial body of literature about consumer partnerships and what they mean, and many excellent documents such as resource kits, fact sheets, and reviews to assist with community participation strategies and consultation processes. However, the central criticism of consumer participation is that its strategies are much more likely to give voice to people who are already empowered by education and likely to be in relatively comfortable circumstances.

Consumer engagement is a term somewhat more in its infancy (Bush 2002). Consumer engagement is emerging in relation to both health promotion and strategies to improve the use of, and access to, services. Specifically, consumer engagement seeks to increase the uptake of health services by a more diverse range of consumers, particularly vulnerable population groups including those experiencing disadvantage and/or social exclusion. 'By engaging citizens, population health approaches advance the health literacy of individuals and communities' (VicHealth 2002). The processes and philosophy of consumer engagement include the enhancement of services so that they are more likely to be used or taken up by those consumers. Issues of reach and uptake are important concepts in addition to a focus on extending the quality of health services provided through engagement with consumers, and enhancement of services through their participation. In effect, consumer engagement has the potential to be informed by social determinants of health evidence to improve access, especially of vulnerable population groups; improve the reach of programs; and increase the quality of information provided to consumers.

General practice and Divisions of General Practice

Under a program for reform of the general practice sector, Divisions of General Practice were established across the nation, and are funded by the Federal government. Divisional funding is intended to deliver outcomes in four to five quadrants of activity. These are:

- infrastructure to develop and maintain the capacity to provide Division services
- services to support general practitioners by the Division
- services provided by the Division to help general practitioners improve patient care
- selected population health programs including immunisation, and SNAP (smoking, nutrition, alcohol, and physical activity).

In 2000–01 for Divisions in rural and remote areas, More Allied Health Services (MAHS) was added to create a fifth sector of activity through the provision of allied health services for general practice clients (DHAC 1999c).

Population health activities (however defined) are only a part of Division activities. There is an argument that Divisions should be restructured and strengthened by the development of multidisciplinary population health teams. Divisions have managed to achieve a degree of engagement of many general practitioners in broader population health concepts, albeit a selective, primary care approach to population health. Maintenance of this engagement is important but should not be mistaken or seen as a substitute for comprehensive population health activities that are conducted from primary health care principles.

National Public Health Strategies

Since the 1980s, Australia has taken a national strategy approach to a range of domains of population health. Many have been revised since their first iteration. Governments in Australia have endorsed twenty-two National Health Strategies, with a number of new strategies under development. Public health strategies are intended to act on the determinants of health, but governments are typically more concerned with downstream and midstream approaches than with up-stream approaches. This means that National Health Strategies are more likely to involve a spectrum of interventions on prevention, early detection and screening, treatment and management, rehabilitation and palliation, than policy, legislation, and socioenvironmental approaches to population health improvement. There is certainly scope for National Health Strategy development to more deliberately incorporate upstream interventions that address the determinants of health including, for example, socioeconomic status, gender, socioecological issues, community capacity, and social support, and to conceptualise intersectoral issues, such as transport, that are key determinants of access to needed health services.

National Health Priorities

Australia's health ministers endorsed the establishment of National Health Priority Areas in 1996. This was a strategic initiative to provide planning and resources for improved continuity of care from treatment and rehabilitation through to primary prevention and health promotion in relation to conditions that represent the greatest burden of disease to the population. Seven National Health Priorities have now been endorsed: cardiovascular disease and stroke; cancer control; injury prevention and control; diabetes mellitus; mental health; asthma; and arthritis.

There is a clear social gradient in each of the National Health Priority Areas, related to a wide range of specific subpopulation groups and conditions including social isolation, social cohesion, social capital, marginalisation, and discrimination. It is widely understood that health inequalities need to be addressed by genuinely collaborative, multidisciplinary downstream, midstream, and upstream actions. While it is also recognised that upstream actions required are not the exclusive domain of the health sector, neither are they the domain of any one practitioner group within the health sector—multidisciplinary, intersectoral activities are required, as the population health template (figure 7.1) indicates.

National Public Health Partnership

The National Public Health Partnership (NPHP) is an intergovernmental partnership that was established in 1996 to provide a more strategic and systematic approach to planning and coordination of public health activities across Australia and to develop and implement major initiatives, new directions, and best practice. The NPHP has a broad focus on strengthening public health infrastructure in the areas of public health information, workforce, planning and practice, research and development and public health legislation.

SUMMARY

- Population health requires the incorporation of evidence about the determinants of health, which in turn requires commitment by governments to the genuine principles of primary health care, universal provision and consumer engagement that express a moral commitment to equity and social justice.

- Population health has the potential to be an effective model for the improvement of the health of populations and to tackle health inequities, but its effectiveness depends on the degree to which a comprehensive, rather than a selective, approach is taken.
- Definitions of public health need to recognise issues of inequity and the health of disadvantaged people.
- Mental health is a key health issue that requires strategic and comprehensive population health responses.
- Infrastructure and investment in upstream change are essential for the systemic change required for effective population health strategies to tackle inequities.

DISCUSSION TOPICS

1 Why is it that governments are '...typically more concerned with downstream and midstream approaches than with upstream approaches'?
2 In what ways might an understanding of the population health approach be used to highlight the limitations of strategies that are based exclusively on addressing the National Health Priority Areas?

USEFUL WEB SITES

Victoria's Primary Health Knowledge Base: www.dhs.vic.gov.au/phkb
beyondblue: the national depression initiative: www.beyondblue.org.au

Nongovernment organisations (NGOs) are at the forefront of advocacy to protect the principles of universal programs. The history and principles of Medicare and the PBS and current threats to them can be found on the following web sites:
Public Health Association of Australia (PHAA): www.phaa.net.au
Doctor's Reform Society (DRS): www.drs.org.au
National Medicare Alliance: www.nma.org.au
National Public Health Partnerships: www.nphp.gov.au (Follow the links to sites for Australia's National Health Strategies and National Health Priorities.)
National Aboriginal Community Controlled Health Organisations: www.naccho.org.au

HEALTH PROMOTION ACTION: RESPONDING TO THE DETERMINANTS

PART 2

MAJOR ACHIEVEMENTS IN PUBLIC HEALTH SINCE 1850

Damien Jolley

Key concepts

- Control of infectious diseases
- Sanitation, microbes, vaccines
- Control of noncommunicable diseases
- Cardiovascular diseases, tobacco, fluoridation, maternal health and babies, injury

'Public health' is one of the efforts organised by society to protect, promote, and restore the people's health (Last 2001). There is ample evidence to show that much has been happening over the last couple of centuries to improve the people's health. For example, life expectancy (the average length of life for the people in a community) of Australians increased steadily year-by-year through-out the twentieth century (figure 8.1). Australian women born in 2000 can expect to live twenty-three years longer than those born in 1900; for men, the gain is twenty-one years. How has our society managed to achieve this? In this chapter, we review some of the major achievements of public health, particularly over the last 200 years.

The very beginnings of humanity's efforts to improve its health can be found embedded within the rituals and rites of the many religions on the planet. For example, the Book of Leviticus (Leviticus 1954) contains explicit instructions for quarantine of 'plague' (used as a generic term for visible illness) and for destruction of infected clothing and possessions. In other religions, as well as in Judaism, consumption of foods more likely to harbour infection (e.g. pork) is explicitly forbidden.

Genetics, as part of evolution, has a role to play in protecting humans against disease. The genetic condition known as sickle cell mutation, for example, has been

Figure 8.1 The impact of public health on lifetimes in Australia: trends in life expectancy, Australia 1901–99

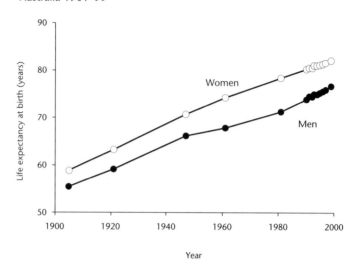

Source: AIHW 2002b

shown to be protective against malaria; thus, the mutation is very prevalent in countries where malaria is found, and it offers natural protection to the population living in those areas. (For further discussion of the sickle cell gene, see chapter 2.)

These are examples of innate, involuntary strategies to protect the health of our community. Public health is more than the automatic or natural response to disease, however; society's health strategies arise from the unique combination of the human mind, the human body and the natural world in which we find ourselves. The examples that follow demonstrate the breathtaking potential of this combination. In telling these brief stories, the names of individual players— the 'heroes' of public health, if you like—have been deliberately omitted. The real 'heroine' of all these tales is society itself, the community of people who together conspire to protect, promote, and restore their own health.

CONTROL OF INFECTIOUS DISEASES

Sanitation

Although there are many earlier examples of societies' attempts to control dis- ease, the first major inroads into population mortality and illness began in post- industrial Britain in the mid nineteenth century (Rosen 1993). That nation's Public Health Act of 1848 is the first formal use of the term.

Industrialisation saw a massive increase of population in the cities and towns of Europe; acute levels of morbidity and mortality in these areas followed. In 1842, a report into the 'Sanitary Conditions of the Labouring Population of Great Britain' revealed a critical problem of illness and death, particularly in the cities (HM Government 2003). Using data from this report, figure 8.2 shows that the life expectancy of labourers in English cities was as low as 15 years, while their counterparts in rural areas could expect to live to more than twice that age—compare these figures to our present Australian life expectancies (figure 8.1).

Figure 8.2   Average life expectancy by occupation in rural Rutland compared with cities in the north of England

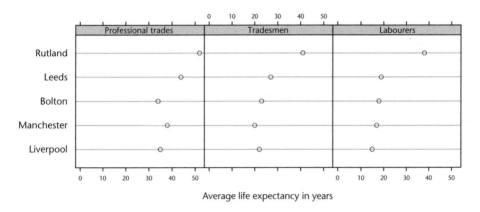

Source: HM Government 2003

Death rates are another part of this story of public health achievements. A death rate is the number of deaths per million people in each year; the lower the mortality rate, the healthier is the population—this is the opposite logic from life expectancy. The 1848 Public Health Act and its successors had a profound impact on mortality and illness in Great Britain. Table 8.1 displays the age-standardised death rates in England and Wales for 1848–54, 1901, and 1971, for a range of diseases attributable to micro-organisms and for all other conditions combined (McKeown 1976). The last half of the nineteenth century saw a 22 per cent reduction in overall mortality, and almost a 50 per cent reduction in water- and food-borne diseases.

Microbes and the germ theory of disease

The invention of the microscope in the seventeenth century revealed to humans the invisible enemies that were responsible for many of the diseases that had plagued the world since the beginning of time. Empirical observations of the late nineteenth century laid the foundations for an understanding of the underlying mechanisms of infection and disease. Bacterial culture techniques were developed, leading to postulates for proof of causation and to principles for isolation of people with disease and protection of others. In the last twenty-five years of the nineteenth century, a flood of discoveries led to immediate improvements in

Table 8.1 Death rates (per million per year) in England and Wales, for 1848–54, 1901, and 1971; rates have been standardised to the age and sex distribution of 1901

	1848–54	1901	1971	PERCENTAGE REDUCTION BEFORE 1901	PERCENTAGE OF OVERALL REDUCTION ATTRIBUTABLE TO EACH CATEGORY
Conditions attributable to micro-organisms	Death rates per million per year				
Airborne diseases	7259	5122	619	29%	40%
Water- and food-borne diseases	3562	1931	35	46%	21%
Other conditions	2144	1415	60	34%	13%
Total	12,965	8468	714	35%	74%
Conditions not attributable to micro-organisms	8891	8490	4670	5%	26%
All diseases	21,856	16,958	5384	22%	100%

Source: McKeown 1976

mortality and disease rates; the last column of table 8.1 shows that almost three-quarters of overall mortality reduction between 1850 and 1901 derived from conditions that were attributable to micro-organisms.

Vaccines and immunisation

Societies have exploited the body's natural defences against disease—immunity—since time immemorial, but it was not until the nineteenth century that safe vaccines against common virulent diseases were developed.

Perhaps the greatest success story of public health is the eradication of smallpox from the globe. In 1967, the World Health Organization (WHO) set out its plan of action in an Intensified Smallpox Eradication Programme; based principally on a vaccine derived from cows, but necessitating massive collaborative fieldwork and case-detection, this program succeeded, as the number of countries reporting wild cases of smallpox declined to zero over the next decade (figure 8.3) (Beaglehole and Bonita 1993).

Further disease eradication programs are presently under way, with poliomyelitis being the most advanced (in 2002). Figure 8.4 shows the global annual reported numbers of cases of polio to 2001 (WHO 2003b); although this graph is encouraging, it is likely that the number of wild-virus confirmed cases of polio will continue to ebb and flow at a low rate over the next decade.

Figure 8.3 Number of countries with smallpox reported, by year

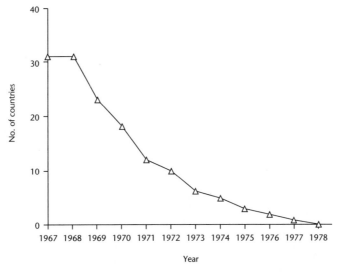

Source: Beaglehole and Bonita 1993

Figure 8.4 Global annual reported cases of polio, 1974–2001

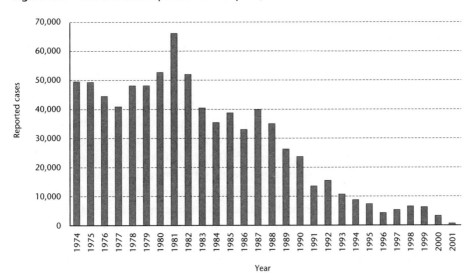

Source: WHO 2003b

Measles is another vaccine-preventable disease that was responsible for 30 million cases and 777,000 deaths (WHO 2003a) in 2001. Control of this disease (rather than eradication) is the strategic objective of WHO, with a target to reduce mortality by 50 per cent during 2001–05, compared with 1999 estimates. Figure 8.5 shows the dramatic impact of an effective measles vaccination program on the incidence of the disease (London School of Hygiene & Tropical Medicine 1990); if this pattern can be achieved in developing nations, then the WHO strategy may be successful.

Figure 8.5 Number of children born and number of measles notifications per four-week period, England and Wales 1950–89

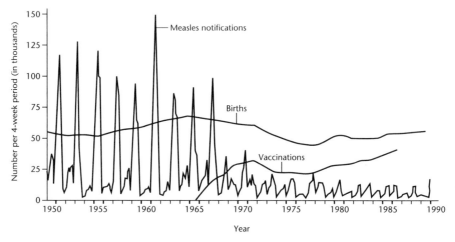

Source: London School of Hygiene & Tropical Medicine 1990

CONTROL OF NONCOMMUNICABLE DISEASES

Declines in deaths from heart disease and stroke

Public health achievements have occurred in diseases other than those caused by micro-organisms, of course. During the early part of the twentieth century, mortality levels from circulatory diseases climbed steadily, reaching annual peaks of over 750 per 100,000 males and 500 per 100,000 females during the 1960s and 1970s (figure 8.6). Since then, death rates from circulatory diseases, including coronary heart disease and stroke, have plummeted to levels less than one-third their respective peaks, and continue to decline into the twenty-first century.

Factors that have contributed to this decline include a reduction in cigarette smoking, particularly in men, decreases in population average blood pressure and blood cholesterol levels in both men and women, changes in dietary practices, and improvements in treatment for acute heart conditions.

Tobacco as a health hazard

The realisation that tobacco is responsible, at least in part, for the worldwide epidemic of coronary heart disease during the twentieth century came only after a series of studies aimed principally at a completely different epidemic. Lung cancer, a disease almost unknown until the early twentieth century, suddenly began

Figure 8.6 Age-standardised death rates in Australian men (closed circles) and women (open circles) by four leading cause-of-death groupings, 1921–2000

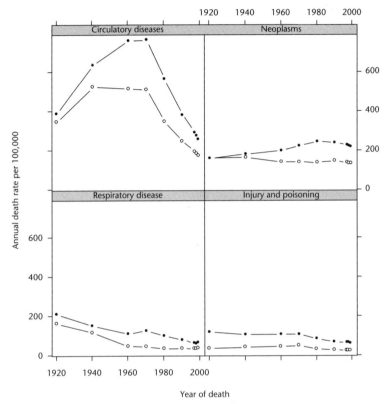

Source: AIHW 2002b

to account for more and more deaths, particularly among men, in the years following the Second World War. Public health investigators, in the USA and Great Britain, suspected that tobacco was responsible, but the convincing proof awaited lengthy follow-up studies (Doll and Hill 1964) in which individuals' smoking patterns and subsequent age and cause of death were related. These studies clearly showed the far-ranging mortal consequences of this single insidious exposure.

These and subsequent public health investigations have revealed a sobering portrait of the price the world community will have to pay if current tobacco smoking trends are not arrested. Table 8.2 displays data taken from the WHO Global Burden of Disease (GBD) Study (Murray and Lopez 1996), with estimates of total numbers of deaths attributable directly to tobacco for the year 2020, by global economic region. The table also shows the predicted loss of disability-adjusted life years (or DALYs) attributable to tobacco. By 2020, it is expected that tobacco will account for 12.3 per cent of deaths worldwide, and as much as 23 per cent of all deaths in the former socialist economies of Europe and 16 per cent of deaths in China. The GBD model also predicts that tobacco

Table 8.2 Estimated deaths and disability-adjusted life years (DALYs) attributable to tobacco use for 2020, by World Bank region

REGION	DEATHS ('000S)	% OF ALL DEATHS	DALYS ('000S)	% OF ALL DALYS
Established Market Economies	1286	14.9	16,499	17.0
Former Socialist Economies of Europe	1101	22.7	12,643	19.9
India	1523	13.3	24,024	10.2
China	2229	16.0	35,415	16.1
Other Asia and Islands	681	8.8	10,061	6.1
Sub-Saharan Africa	298	2.9	5457	1.7
Latin America and the Caribbean	447	9.4	7280	6.8
Middle Eastern Crescent	817	9.5	12,299	7.3
World	8383	12.3	123,678	8.9
Developed Regions	2387	17.7	29,141	18.2
Developing Regions	5996	10.9	94,537	7.7

Source: Murray and Lopez 1996

will be responsible for 8.9 per cent of all DALYs lost worldwide; in developed regions, tobacco will be responsible for more than 18 per cent of the total DALYs lost, and in the former socialist economies of Europe, 20 per cent of the total expected DALYs loss.

The task ahead for **public health is** to publicise these predictions as widely as possible, and to develop **behavioural**, structural, and legislative interventions to staunch the haemorrhage of **death and** disability attributable to tobacco use.

Fluoridation of drinking water

The achievements of public health are not limited to diseases that kill us. The prevalence of dental caries, or tooth decay, declined substantially during the twentieth century, and much of the reason for this decrease is the public health intervention of fluoridation of community drinking water. Figure 8.7 shows the average numbers of nonpermanent teeth with some history of caries among Australian children aged between five and 10 years old, over the decade from 1989 to 1998. Across all age groups, the caries prevalence has dropped by an average of 30 per cent; there is some evidence that the decline has tapered off since 1996, and public health investigations are under way to confirm this observation.

Figure 8.7 Impact of fluoridation on the oral health of Australia's children: the average number of primary teeth with caries experience (decayed, missing, or filled) by age and calendar year, Australia 1988–98

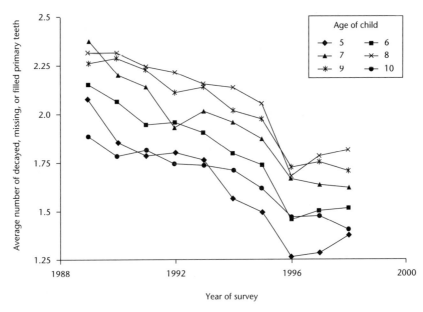

Source: AIHW 2002b

Healthier mothers and babies

Australia's infant mortality rate has dropped from over 100 per 1000 live births in 1901, to a low of 5.2 per 1000 live births in 2000, a dramatic decrease of over 95 per cent. Consistently, the infant mortality rate in Australia has decreased by about 3 per cent every year over the last hundred years.

At the start of the twentieth century, diarrhoea was a principal cause of death among infants, and much of the decline in infant mortality was brought about by the control of this one disease. Several factors contributed to diarrhoeal disease decreases; better nutrition and education of mothers were significant. One contributor was the Plunket Movement, started in Dunedin, New Zealand in 1907, which promoted a style of regimented infant care, with strict control over diet and an emphasis on education for mothers. This resulted in an immediate drop in the incidence of diarrhoea and a significant impact on overall infant mortality, which dropped from 88 per 1000 in 1907 to 32 per 1000 in 1937, the lowest in the world at the time (Royal New Zealand Plunket Society Inc. 2003). Similar Infant Welfare Societies developed in Australia from 1902 in the poorer suburbs of major cities (Keleher 2000). Such improvements did not happen uniformly across all echelons of society, however. The New Zealand Plunket Movement, for example, was in its early days a very middle-class organisation, with little influence on the lives of a significant minority of poor mothers and babies.

Pasteurisation of milk was introduced into the USA in 1908 and later into Australia. Education of women, family planning and contraception, improved economic conditions, and nutrition all contributed to the decline in infant death rates in developed countries. At the same time, maternal mortality has decreased, in Australia reaching 13 deaths per 100,000 confinements during the period between 1994 and 1996 (AIHW 2002b). Improved education of women, a decline in married fertility, and the control of septic deliveries were all important contributors to this decline.

Safe, legal abortion, still controversial in many states in the world, is an important contributor to the decline in maternal mortality. The risk of death from an unsafe abortion is more than 100 times that of a procedure conducted in safe conditions (Public Health Association of Australia 2003). Of the Australian jurisdictions, only one publishes its data on induced abortions; in 1999, there were 17.8 induced abortions per 1000 South Australian women aged 18 to 44 years, and almost one in four (23.4 per cent) of all pregnancies resulted in an abortion (AIHW 2002b). This rate is much higher than in other countries where data are available (e.g. Scandinavia, Netherlands, United Kingdom), which indicates the need for greater investment in family planning and reproductive health promotion (Public Health Association of Australia 2003).

Injury

Deaths on the road continue to take a toll among Australians aged between 15 and 30, particularly young men. In a series of public health initiatives since the mid-1960s, this road toll has more than halved; figure 8.8 shows the gradual increase in motor vehicle mortality since 1924, peaking in 1970, and then dropping sharply until the end of the century (AIHW 2002b). Improvements in

Figure 8.8   Injury mortality in Australian males, 1924–99

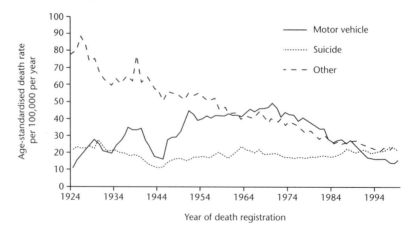

Source: AIHW 2002b

motor vehicle and road design have contributed to this decrease, as well as leg-islative initiatives such as seat-belt laws, random alcohol breath testing, red-light cameras, and speed restrictions. Australia's legislators and public health inter-ventionists have led the world in these initiatives.

Figure 8.8 shows not only the rise and fall of motor vehicle injury deaths, but also the dramatic decrease in 'other injuries' among males, consistently falling throughout the seventy-five-year interval. Workplace deaths are the main con-tributing factor to these other injuries; the graph shows that by 1999 these had dropped to less than half their 1925 rates, a testimony to the achievements of occupational public health and improvement in workplace safety.

CONCLUSION

Public health has made great advances since its beginnings in the early years of the nineteenth century. The examples above demonstrate our species' unique ability to organise itself to promote health and to improve the living conditions of its people. There have been many other wonderful achievements in public health which cannot be addressed in this short chapter. And, of course, there have been innumerable failures along the way, which have been deliberately overlooked. But perhaps even from a short list of triumphs, we can find some landmarks for the roads ahead.

We have mentioned sanitation, microbiology, vaccination, the decline in car-diovascular diseases, the fight against tobacco, fluoridation of water, healthier mothers and babies, and decreases in injuries on the roads and the workplace— are there any common threads? Is there a single idea, or just a couple of simple ideas, among these which can act as the signpost for the future?

SUMMARY

- Legislation is one common theme. From the original Public Health Act of 1848 in Great Britain, through to random breath testing and the banning of smoking in restaurants, successive governments in devel-oped countries around the world have found it necessary to enact their protective and preventive measures as laws, enforceable across all strata of society, often to protect the poor or the impotent.
- Of the eight measures described in this chapter, all but three (microbi-ology, cardiovascular disease declines, and healthy mothers and babies) have direct legislative enactment; even these three depend, at some level in their implementation, on legal intervention for their success.
- Education is another common characteristic of these achievements. Laws have little chance of existence, let alone success, if the majority of the population fail to understand their objectives. The decline of

cardiovascular diseases and the progress of healthy babies and mothers, the acceptance of the importance of sanitation and the war against tobacco, road and workplace safety changes were dependent upon concerted public education programs for their effectiveness.

- There remain many challenges ahead, however, particularly in the underdeveloped or developing world where achievements such as those we have described remain as objectives rather than trophies. We need to learn from our triumphs, and to avoid the pitfalls of our disasters, so that future objectives can be met.

DISCUSSION TOPICS

1 Compare and contrast the determinants of health throughout pre- and post-industrialised Britain.

2 Brainstorm examples of the behavioural, structural, and legislative interventions that have significantly contributed to a reduction in tobacco use in Australia. What might some of the barriers be to implementing such interventions in some developing countries that are currently experiencing a rapid increase in tobacco use?

3 What social determinants are likely to contribute to high rates of unwanted pregnancies in those countries discussed earlier under 'Healthier mothers and babies'?

4 Brainstorm a list of recent interventions that have contributed to a decline in injury rates, particularly for males.

5 Find out about the historical context of a public health challenge in a developing country of interest to you. What are the underlying determinants of this health concern? What lessons can we learn from history in seeking to overcome the adverse health outcomes linked to this health issue?

7 Find out about the protocols and processes currently utilised in Australia to address public health problems (e.g. an outbreak of Legionnaire's disease, severe acute respiratory syndrome, or other).

CRITICAL PERSPECTIVES ON PUBLIC HEALTH HISTORY

Judith Raftery

Key concepts

- Critical explanation and interpretation
- Contextualisation of public health stories

The history of public health is littered with good stories, and these stories are peopled with heroes. Some of these stories are so good, and their leading characters so heroic, that in some form or other they have emerged from the archives and become common knowledge. Thus, many people who have little interest in public health have heard of, say, Florence Nightingale, Joseph Lister, or Louis Pasteur and have some idea about their claims to fame. However, this process of reducing history to good stories and heroes frequently leads to distortion and the loss of any real insight that history might provide about what produces, protects, or threatens the health of the public. History is much more than stories about individuals: it is about ideas, movements, conditions and forces that shape societies and people's lives, that produce or inhibit change and that allow some people and some projects to flourish, while condemning others to wither or perish. Nevertheless, stories are part of history, and if we do tell them, we need to tell them well, in a way that situates them in the appropriate historical context and raises appropriate historical questions. Only then will they be a vehicle for worthwhile learning.

This chapter deals with three famous public health stories. It recalls the popular version of each story—versions that are heroic, truncated, decontextualised, and therefore not very instructive. It then demonstrates that if we extend the stories beyond these superficial versions, they can teach us much more about issues that it is important for students of public health to consider. The stories are about Edward Jenner and smallpox, Ignaz Semmelweis and puerperal, or childbed, fever, and John Snow and cholera.

PUBLIC HEALTH STORIES: THE POPULAR VERSIONS

Edward Jenner (1749–1823), was an English country doctor at a time when smallpox was a much-feared disease that appeared frequently in epidemic proportions and was associated with high mortality rates. Jenner had plenty of opportunity to observe the effects of smallpox in his medical practice, and he wondered why not all those exposed to this dreaded disease contracted it, why some got it only mildly, yet it killed others. By careful observation over a long period, collection of data on cases, deaths, and recoveries and, eventually, some judicious experimentation, he came to the conclusion that exposure to another much milder disease, cowpox, which could be transmitted from cows to people, conferred immunity against smallpox. Some country people had long been aware of this without understanding the process; they just knew that milkmaids who got cowpox did not seem to get smallpox. On the basis of his conclusions, Jenner published a scientific paper recommending a preventive intervention—inoculation with cowpox matter, which he called vaccination (after *vaccus*, Latin for cow), in order to produce immunity against smallpox.

Ignaz Semmelweis (1818–65) was a Hungarian doctor working in the obstetrics section of the General Hospital in Vienna in the 1840s. There were two obstetrics wards: in one the women were attended by midwives, and in the other by doctors and medical students. Semmelweis noticed that the rates of puerperal fever were far higher in the medical students' ward, and he wanted to find out why. He observed both situations carefully, made various changes to procedures, insisted on identical practices and treatment in each ward, kept careful records of the results, in terms of death rates, and compared them with death rates in the past, in order to gain a clearer picture of what was happening. Eventually, after pursuing various other hypotheses, he concluded that the problem was connected with the fact that the medical students regularly came straight from the morgue, where they dissected cadavers, to the obstetrics ward, without washing their hands, thus spreading fatal infection. He initiated a routine of thorough hand-washing with chloride of lime, and the mortality rates fell.

John Snow (1813–58) was a surgeon working in inner London. Like many doctors at that time he was perplexed by the periodic appearance of epidemics of infectious disease that cut a fearful swathe through the population. He was curious about the unproven theory that infections could be spread by particles that were transmitted through water. Through careful observation, counting of casualties and noting their geographical location, he became convinced that infected water from a particular source, the now-famous Broad Street pump, was the origin of a cholera outbreak in Soho in 1854. He demonstrated the validity of his data and his conclusions by having the handle removed from the pump and thus cutting off the supply of infected water, after which the outbreak quickly abated.

All of these famous stories seem to have both happy and healthy endings, which all depend on some basic descriptive epidemiology, a careful and coherent scientific methodology, and a single hero with some courage and imagination. But none of these popular versions is complete or entirely accurate, and all stand in need of some **exegesis**, that is, some critical explanation and interpretation.

PUBLIC HEALTH STORIES:SOME CRITICAL EXAMINATION

First let us consider the Jenner story. It reads as though Jenner was a lone thinker and observer, who happened on a wonderful new preventive strategy out of the blue. This is not usually the way great discoveries are made. The reality was that there was debate and experimentation about the process of inoculation with smallpox matter (variolation) in Britain and elsewhere throughout the eighteenth century. It did not provide complete protection against the disease but mortality rates from smallpox among the inoculated population were consistently and significantly lower than among the noninoculated. Jenner, like many of his medical colleagues, practised variolation, sometimes systematically inoculating entire communities when an outbreak of smallpox occurred. Thus his 1796 cowpox experiment occurred in a context of widespread faith in the concept and practice of inoculation (Miller 1981). His great contribution was to discover a method of inoculation that was safer and more effective than the existing methods. Jenner now enjoys hero status as the great pioneer of vaccination, but that status was not immediately bestowed on him, as the popular story might suggest. In fact, the scientific establishment of his day jeered Jenner. He was told by members of the Royal Society that he had come to audacious conclusions on the basis of slim evidence and suggested that if he valued his reputation he should keep quiet about using infective material from cowpox to provide immunity against smallpox. Although vaccination was quickly adopted as standard protection against smallpox, and to great effect, for the next hundred years debate continued about it in medical and scientific communities. Jenner, far from being a universal hero, was vilified by some as 'little better than a criminal and money grabber', and his method as 'mythical' and 'a foul poisoning of the blood' (Porter and Porter 1988).

Why was this the case? Given the degree to which inoculation was accepted it seems unlikely that Jenner's idea seemed too new, or too revolutionary, although since it required the use of animal rather than human matter it may have been considered too risky as well as distasteful. Conservatism played a part, however. There were people who clung to older disease theories that were at odds with the theory underlying the practice of vaccination, and who, for various reasons, remained unconvinced by the evidence of the success of vaccination. Professional jealousy may also have been involved. Jenner was outside the social and scientific establishment and his insights were developed through respect for traditional, 'country knowledge' that did not cut much ice with modern, city-based scholars. There is a happy ending to Jenner's story. Vaccination became a respected medical procedure, with broad application, and in the case of smallpox has enabled us to defeat the disease. But we can learn much about what helps or hinders advances in the public's health by thinking about why this acceptance did not come easily.

Now let us revisit the Semmelweis story. The story is a moving one, on several levels. The women who gave birth in the Vienna Hospital came overwhelmingly from the poorer sections of society, since in Vienna, as elsewhere at that time, better-off women were able to choose the more expensive, but safer, option of giving birth at home, attended by their own doctor. The deaths that so concerned Semmelweis were thus a result of social inequalities as well as of what now appear as careless and cavalier hospital practices. However, at the time, neither of these things caused widespread concern. In fact, some doctors and students at the Vienna Hospital were greatly offended by Semmelweis's ideas and tried to sabotage his efforts. Not only did his discoveries fail to make him a hero, but they led to his dismissal from the obstetrics department and subsequent failure to obtain other appointments at the hospital.[1]

As with Jenner, professional jealousy, leading to defensiveness, seems to have been part of this reaction. Semmelweis's experimentation and the resulting reduction in puerperal fever mortality highlighted the greater loss of life that had occurred when others had been in charge of the obstetrics wards. Some of his colleagues took offence at this, and thought his ideas were a slur on their competence and reputation. Prejudice of several kinds was involved. Semmelweis was a Hungarian, and in Vienna that made him a foreigner and an outsider. And since he was young and not very well established professionally, it was easy for him to be snubbed and for his ideas to be disregarded by those who were older and better established. Resistance to new ideas was also part of it. Not much was understood about processes of infection in the 1840s, and although the other doctors and students at the Vienna Hospital had no more-convincing explanations, they did not take kindly to an explanation that implicated their own behaviour and practices. As with the smallpox story, there was a happy ending, eventually. In time, sanitary reform and antiseptic and aseptic practices in hospitals lessened the risks of puerperal fever and other hospital-induced fevers—but not in Semmelweis's time, and not without other doctors and scientists confirming and extending his theories, putting them to the clinical test and talking and writing about them in places that counted. In the meantime, people continued to die from hospital-induced infections. The Semmelweis story teaches us that these deaths were the result of the inertia exerted by tradition, of professional jealousy and protection of territory, and of social inequalities, and not just of incomplete understanding and the deadly work of some invisible pathogen. It alerts us to the likelihood that such factors still result in preventable suffering and death today.

Finally, let us engage in some historical exegesis of the John Snow story. Some ill-informed popular versions of the story have Snow removing the handle from the Broad Street pump himself. Of course he did not. As a doctor, Snow had no authority to interfere with the public water supply, but he knew that the local government body, acting under powers given to them by the 1848 Health Act, did have the authority to act to avert a threat to the public's health when mortality rates rose above the expected level. And so he went to the local authority and argued that the pump handle be removed. They were 'incredulous but had the good sense to carry out his advice' (Frost 1936). Why was Snow so confident? Part of the answer is his own careful local case-finding and communication with other doctors in the area in order to establish the geographical distribution of cholera deaths.[2] And, in fact, it was this investigatory work, rather than the removal of the pump handle, that was Snow's real contribution to insight into and control of the cholera epidemic. But Snow had other sources of information as well. Due to when he was working (and *timing* remains important in history even though memorising dates has fallen into disfavour), he was able to rely on central government data that were available to him through two sources: the General Register Office, established in the 1830s, and the national census, held in 1851. He had much more to go on from these sources—about population numbers, house occupancy, death rates, *and which water companies serviced particular streets*—than he could learn from just knocking on doors, as some of the stories have it. Despite all this, not everyone was convinced by Snow's argument, or by the results of the removal of the pump handle, and he certainly was not accorded hero status.

As in the case of Semmelweis, Snow's ideas seemed too new and his solution bizarre. Various disease theories competed for scholarly status and many of his medical and scientific contemporaries were happy to dismiss his arguments because they did not positively identify 'the cholera poison'.[3] Almost four decades after Snow's demonstration of the role of impure water in the dissemination of cholera, and nine years after the identification of the infective agent, *vibrio cholerae*, the prestigious Royal College of Physicians was giving the following advice about preventing cholera. It made no mention at all of water or water quality.

Advice on Preventing Cholera (1892)

The house must be clean, light, thoroughly dry and well-ventilated.

Inhabitants must eat three or four nourishing and ample meals each day, but not soup or cheese which are indigestible. Alcohol may be taken in moderation, but sparkling wines are to be shunned, as well as over-fatigue, emotional excitement and undue mental strain.

Regular exercise, plenty of sleep, and the pursuit of an occupied and tranquil life are recommended.

Smith 1979

In addition—and this is probably the most significant point of all—Snow's ideas were not readily embraced by his colleagues and other influential groups, because they indicated the need for reform that was outside the doctor's sphere of operation. It was not clinical reform that was needed. The problem was not to do with how doctors treated patients. Snow's work pointed to the need for much more thorough social and economic reform, implying enlarged roles for government and enlarged notions of civic responsibility. At least partly for that reason, this story does not have a happy ending. Probably, the Soho epidemic of 1854 would have been worse if Snow had not had the pump handle removed. But what he was able to do in Soho did not make the world safe from cholera. Cholera struck again in England within a few years and is still a major killer, even though we now know a great deal more about it than Snow did. We still give advice about it, and although it is now usually good advice, like boiling water before using it, it is nevertheless ineffectual advice if people cannot afford the fuel needed to boil the water, as is the case in some parts of the world where cholera epidemics still occur.[4]

The key lesson that emerges from the Snow story is that we cannot protect people from preventable suffering and death just by identifying pathogens and providing advice on how to avoid them. Protection of the health of the public depends on ensuring the extension of the basic prerequisites of health—such as safe and adequate water, access to a reliable food supply, appropriate shelter—to all. And that takes a comprehensive commitment on the part of society and government, not just the discoveries of inventive, individual heroes.

Thus we can see that these classic public health stories—and there are many others—when contextualised and subjected to some historical exegesis encourage us to think about those forces that act as either constraints on or enablers of what we can achieve in public health.

SUMMARY

- We can see that these classic public health stories (and there are many others) benefit from being contextualised and subjected to some historical exegesis.
- Critical thinking about public health stories encourages us to think about those forces that act as either constraints on or enablers of what we can achieve in public health.
- We can learn much when we look beneath the simplified, surface versions of the past and ask critical questions.

DISCUSSION TOPICS

1 Find out more about one of these and other public health stories. How might your knowledge of the social, biological, and environmental determinants of health help you to better understand the contexts in which these stories occur?

2 Develop a conceptual diagram to illustrate the interrelationship between the underlying determinants of health for one of these stories.

3 To what extent might a focus on public health heroes or champions be considered unhelpful when reflecting on significant public health actions that have led to improved health outcomes?

NOTES

1   For futher insights into the Semmelweiss story, see Semmelweis, I. 1983, *The Etiology, concept and prophylaxis of childbed fever*, trans. K. C. Carter, The University of Wisconsin Press, Madison, [1860].

2   The stories here are fascinating. For example, Snow observed that inmates of the local workhouse were protected because the workhouse had its own pump-well, and that the Broad Street brewery workers who were given a daily ration of beer while at work were also less at risk. Not so fortunate was a widow from the cholera-free area of Hampstead, who had water brought to her from the Broad Street pump daily, because she liked the taste!

3   Reluctance to embrace the thinking behind Snow's theory was apparent even in high places. See, for example, Eyler, John M. 1973, 'William Farr on the cholera: the sanitarian's disease theory and the statistician's method', *Journal of the History of Medicine and Allied Sciences*, vol. xxviii, no. 2, pp. 79–100.

4   See, for example, Jeffrey, P. 1992, 'Cholera: disease of the poor', *Christian Century*, 29 January, pp. 84–5.

HEALTH PROMOTION: ORIGINS, OBSTACLES, AND OPPORTUNITIES

John Catford

Key concepts

- The new public health and the Alma Ata Declaration
- Ottawa Charter for Health Promotion
- Adelaide Recommendations on Healthy Public Policy
- Sundsvall Statement on Supportive Environments for Health
- Jakarta Declaration on Health Promotion into the 21st Century
- Mexico Ministerial Statement for the Promotion of Health: From Ideas to Action
- WHO leadership and future challenges

The last twenty years has seen an exponential growth in a new movement for health known as 'health promotion'. Across the world there are government health promotion strategies and reviews, statutory authorities and foundations, consumer interest groups, professional associations, and journals. University departments and professors proudly bear the name, Masters and Bachelor degrees are in abundance, and a new textbook seems to appear every few months. The International Union of Health Education, for example, included health promotion in its title in 1994, thus formally recognising the broader base of its activities. Millions and millions of dollars are now increasingly being invested in health promotion programs by governments and international organisations, e.g. the World Bank, as well as through voluntary contributions from individuals. It is quite remarkable that this has all happened in just two decades.

This chapter reviews the development of health promotion, outlines some of the important milestones, and looks to the future for new opportunities and challenges.

THE NEW PUBLIC HEALTH

Public health improvements in the nineteenth century were largely the result of a few individuals taking action centrally to improve living and working conditions. Through regulation and legislation the major determinants of ill health could be tackled. For example, infectious diseases could be controlled through cleaner water, safer sanitation, and purer air, and malnourishment through income support and better food supply. However, with the ascendancy of noncommunicable diseases, such as heart disease and cancer, health behaviours and lifestyle become all important.

During the 1980s public health leaders became aware of these radical changes. Epidemiological assessments needed to be balanced against the felt needs of populations. Individuals should be viewed not as health consumers, as if health services were the source of health, but rather as health creators, recognising that health is won by people themselves. Increasingly there was a shift to an ecological, holistic view of health from a medical, reductionist one. Some health service workers found this loss of power and status threatening. One way to overcome this was to improve understanding of the issues and provide practical examples of successful initiatives. As a response the World Health Organization (WHO) set up *Health Promotion International* in 1986, a quarterly journal published by Oxford University Press, to provide a vehicle for describing progress in health promotion and the positive benefits of such an approach.

As a result of these developments health has become an agenda item for a much wider group of sectors than before. The requirement is not so much for

---

Box 10.1   What is health promotion?

Health promotion is the process of enabling people to increase control over and to improve their health. This perspective is derived from a concept of 'health' as the extent to which an individual or group is able, on the one hand, to realise aspirations and satisfy needs, and on the other hand, to change or cope with the environment. Health is seen therefore, as a resource for everyday life, not the objective of living; it is a positive concept emphasising social and personal resources, as well as physical capacities.

Health promotion represents a comprehensive social and political process, not only embracing actions directed at strengthening the skills and capabilities of individuals, but also action directed towards changing social, environmental, and economic conditions so as to alleviate their impact on public and individual health. Community participation is essential to sustain health promotion action.

Source: WHO 1984, 1998b

more public health policy but rather more **healthy public policy**, ensuring that all policies—be they fiscal, environmental, agricultural, industrial—promote health rather than weaken it. For example, the health benefits of cycling should be considered when formulating transport policy; food policy should take into account the health advantages of supporting the fishing and fruit industries. This is not to suggest that specific health legislation, such as banning tobacco advertising, is not important. Rather it recognises that all policies at both local and national level have the potential to influence health and that their health impact should be considered.

In addition to recognising the importance of intersectoral action for health, the active participation of the public is also essential. Merely 'instructing' people on hygienic practices is ineffective when complex health behaviours are involved such as eating, smoking, exercise, drinking alcohol, and sexual behaviour. There needs to be a shift from experts telling people 'what they should do', to an approach that equips people with the knowledge and skills to make their own decisions. This empowerment process is fundamental to the concept of health promotion, that is, helping people to take control of their own health. This paradigm shift has been fostered by WHO, particularly the regional office in Europe (WHO EURO), which since the early 1980s has been encouraging member states to move away from doctrinaire, authoritarian, and medically dominated approaches to more participative ones.

During this period the term 'health promotion' was becoming increasingly used by a new wave of public health activists who were dissatisfied with the rather traditional and top-down approaches of health education and disease prevention. It signalled a positive, creative, and outcome-oriented approach. However, in some contexts and languages the term 'promotion' was considered synonymous with 'marketing' and 'selling' rather than 'enhancement' and 'empowerment'. This led to WHO calling a special meeting in 1984 at the WHO EURO headquarters in Copenhagen to provide some clarity and direction. This in turn led to the first substantive document on health promotion, the Concepts and Principles of Health Promotion (WHO 1984).[1] In addition to proposing a series of principles (see box 10.2), a number of subject areas, priorities, and dilemmas were also presented.

The origins of the health promotion movement are complex and no single driver is responsible. However, most commentators would agree that the shift in thinking began to occur around an important Global meeting of WHO at Alma Ata in the state of Kazak in the former Soviet Union in 1978. The declaration that resulted crucially recognised that health improvements would not occur just by developing and financing health services, which had been the focus for investment since World War II (WHO 1978). It provided the seedbed for the development of health promotion in the following decade to reach out to other sectors (box 10.3).

In addition, the Declaration of Alma Ata formally adopted Primary Health Care (PHC) as the principal mechanism for health care delivery. This was a vital

Box 10.2   The principles of health promotion

First proposed by a WHO working group in 1984

1   *Health promotion involves the population as a whole in the context of their everyday life, rather than focusing on people at risk for specific diseases.* It enables people to take control over, and responsibility for, their health as an important component of everyday life—both as spontaneous and organized action for health. This requires full and continuing access to information about health and how it might be sought for by all the population, using, therefore, all dissemination methods available.

2   *Health promotion is directed towards action on the determinants or causes of health.* Health promotion, therefore, requires a close cooperation of sectors beyond health services, reflecting the diversity of conditions which influence health. Government, at both local and national levels, has a unique responsibility to act appropriately in a timely way to ensure that the 'total' environment, which is beyond the control of individuals and groups, is conducive to health.

3   *Health promotion combines diverse, but complementary, methods or approaches,* including communication, education, legislation, fiscal measures, organizational change, community development and spontaneous local activities against health hazards.

4   *Health promotion aims particularly at effective and concrete public participation.* This focus requires further development of problem-defining and decision-making life skills both individually and collectively.

5   While health promotion is basically an activity in the health and social fields, and not a medical service, *health professionals—particularly in primary health care—have an important role in nurturing and enabling health promotion.* Health professionals should work outwards developing their special contributions in education and health advocacy.

Source: WHO 1984

signal to developing countries that were increasingly investing in high-cost hospital systems that were only available to a limited few, namely, those in urban centres who could pay. Alma Ata heralded the shift in power, which is fundamental to health promotion, from the providers of health services (the doctors, nurses, health administrators) to the consumers of those health services and the wider community who ultimately pay for them.

The consequence of the declaration was that the majority of countries, particularly in the developing world, adopted PHC as their principal health response. This led WHO to prepare a global strategy 'Health for All by the Year 2000' with a series of measurable targets and goals (WHO 1981). Health for All

> **Box 10.3   The Declaration of Alma Ata**
>
> **Extracts from the International Conference on Primary Health Care**
>
> The Conference strongly affirms that health, which is a complete state of physical, mental and social well being, and not merely the absence of disease or infirmity, is a fundamental human right and that the attainment of the highest possible level of health is a most important world-wide social goal whose realization requires the action of many other social and economic sectors in addition to the health sector.
>
> Governments have a responsibility for the health of their people, which can be fulfilled only by the provision of adequate health and social measures. A main social target of governments, international organizations and the whole world community in the coming decades should be the attainment by all peoples of the world by the year 2000 of a level of health that will permit them to lead a socially and economically productive life. Primary health care is the key to attaining this target as part of development in the spirit of social justice.
>
> Primary health care is essential health care based on practical, scientifically sound and socially acceptable methods and technology made universally accessible to individuals and families in the community through their full participation and at a cost the community and country can afford to maintain at every stage of their development in the spirit of self reliance and self determination.
>
> *Source*: WHO 1978

fast became the driving force for comprehensive health development over the following two decades and provided the right environment for the concept of health promotion to foster and grow.

THE OTTAWA CHARTER FOR HEALTH PROMOTION

In 1986 the first of a series of global health promotion conferences was organised by WHO to provide impetus and profile to the newly emerging concept of health promotion. Held in Ottawa, Canada during November snow blizzards, it brought together 212 representatives from thirty-eight countries and was organised in partnership with the Canadian government and the Public Health Association (WHO 1986a). Ottawa is seen as the formal birthplace of health promotion; not only did this conference endorse and legitimise some of the work that had been going on behind the scenes through WHO, but it cascaded action into a number of countries. The charter that emerged is now considered the bedrock of the health promotion movement (WHO 1986b) and the logo has

Figure 10.1 Logo of the Ottawa Charter for Health Promotion

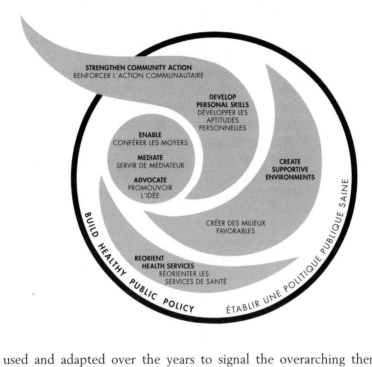

been used and adapted over the years to signal the overarching themes and approaches of health promotion (WHO 1986c) (figure 10.1).

The Ottawa Charter for Health Promotion set out three complementary ways to foster health. Health promoters were encouraged to advocate, to mediate, and to enable rather than to dictate, to rule, and 'to blame the victim'. Through **advocacy**, health promotion action aims at making the underlying determinants of health as favourable as possible. These include political, economic, social, cultural, environmental, behavioural, and biological conditions.

Health promotion action also aims at reducing the differences in current health status and ensuring equal opportunities and resources to *enable* all people to achieve their fullest health potential. This includes a secure foundation in a supportive environment, access to information, life skills, and opportunities for making healthy choices. Finally it is recognised that the prerequisites and prospects for health cannot be ensured by the health sector alone; coordinated effort is needed across all sectors—government, public, private, and community. Health promoters therefore have a major responsibility to *mediate* between different interest groups in society for the pursuit of health.

Specific challenges were also identified at Ottawa—to build healthy public policy, develop personal skills, strengthen **community action**, create supportive environments, and reorient health services (box 10.4). These have commonly become the framework for many health promotion strategies at local, regional, and national levels as they simply and clearly set out the mix of action that is required.

Box 10.4   The Ottawa Charter for Health Promotion

Extracts from the First International Conference on Health Promotion in Ottawa, Canada

Health Promotion Action means:

Build Healthy Public Policy
Health promotion policy combines diverse but complementary approaches including legislation, fiscal measures, taxation, and organizational change. It requires the identification of obstacles to the adoption of healthy public policy in non-health sectors, and ways of removing them. The aim must be to make the healthier choices the easier choices for policy makers as well.

Create Supportive Environments
Systematic assessment of the health impact of a rapidly changing environment—particularly in areas of technology, work, energy production and urbanization—is essential and must be followed by action to ensure positive benefit to the health of the public. The protection of the natural and built environment and the conservation of natural resources must be addressed in any health promotion strategy.

Strengthen Community Action
At the heart of this process is the empowerment of communities, their ownership and control of their own endeavours and destinies. Community development draws on existing human and material resources to enhance self-help and social support, and to develop flexible systems for strengthening public participation and direction of health matters.

Develop Personal Skills
Health promotion supports personal and social development through providing information, education for health and enhancing life skills. Enabling people to learn throughout life, to prepare themselves for all its stages and to cope with chronic illness and injuries is essential. This has to be facilitated in school, home, work and community settings.

Reorient Health Services
Health services need to embrace an expanded mandate, which is sensitive and respects cultural needs. This should support the needs of individuals and communities for a healthier life, and open channels with other sectors. This must lead to a change of attitude and organization of health services, which refocuses on the total needs of the individual as a whole person.

Source: WHO 1986b

Looking back twenty years later, the key achievements of Ottawa were to legitimise the vision of health promotion by clarifying the key concepts, highlighting the conditions and resources required for health, and identifying key actions and basic strategies to pursue the WHO policy of Health for All. Importantly, the charter also identified the prerequisites for health including peace, a stable ecosystem, social justice and equity, and resources such as education, food, and income. It highlighted the role of organisations, systems, and communities, as well as individual behaviours and capacities, in creating choices and opportunities for better health.

THE ADELAIDE AND SUNDSVALL CONFERENCES: BUILDING THE BASE

Since the 1986 Ottawa conference, WHO has organised, in partnership with national governments and associations, a series of follow-up conferences that have focused on each of the five health promotion action themes, as outlined in

---

Box 10.5   Adelaide Recommendations on Healthy Public Policy

Extracts from the Second International Conference on Health Promotion in Adelaide, Australia

Healthy public policy is characterized by an explicit concern for health and equity in all areas of policy and by an accountability for health impact. The main aim of health public policy is to create a supportive environment to enable people to lead healthy lives. Such a policy makes health choices possible or easier for citizens. It makes social and physical environments health enhancing. In the pursuit of healthy public policy, government sectors concerned with agriculture, trade, education, industry, and communications need to take into account health as an essential factor when formulating policy. These sectors should be accountable for the health consequences of their policy decisions. They should pay as much attention to health as to economic considerations.

Government plays an important role in health, but health is also influenced greatly by corporate and business interests, nongovernmental bodies and community organizations. Their potential for preserving and promoting people's health should be encouraged. Trade unions, commerce and industry, academic associations and religious leaders have many opportunities to act in the health interests of the whole community. New alliances must be forged to provide the impetus for health action.

Source: WHO 1988

box 10.4. This initiative has also provided the opportunity to track how health promotion is being interpreted and developed over time and across the world.

Building healthy public policy was explored in greater depth at the Second International Conference on Health Promotion in Adelaide, Australia in 1988. Organised to coincide with Australia's bicentenary, an invited audience of 240 participants from forty-two, mainly developed, countries attended. The conference confirmed that equity and accountability were key issues (Svensson 1988). Public policies in all sectors influence the determinants of health and are a major vehicle for actions to reduce social and economic inequities, for example by ensuring equitable access to goods and services as well as health care. The Adelaide Recommendations on Healthy Public Policy called for a political commitment to health by all sectors (see box 10.5). Policy makers in diverse agencies working at various levels (international, national, regional, and local) were urged to increase investments in health and to consider the impact of their decisions on health. Four priority areas for action were identified—supporting the health of

---

Box 10.6   Sundsvall Statement on Supportive Environments for Health

Extracts from the Third International Conference on Health Promotion in Sundsvall, Sweden

In a health context the term supportive environments refers to both the physical and the social aspects of our surroundings. It encompasses where people live, their local community, their home, where they work and play. It also embraces the framework, which determines access to resources for living, and opportunities for empowerment. Thus action to create supportive environments has many dimensions: physical, social, spiritual, economic and political. Each of these dimensions is inextricably linked to the others in a dynamic interaction. Action must be coordinated at local, regional, national and global levels to achieve solutions that are truly sustainable.

Key strategies at a community level are:

1 Strengthening advocacy through community action, particularly through groups organized by women.

2 Enabling communities and individuals to take control over their health and environment through education and empowerment.

3 Building alliances for health and supportive environments in order to strengthen the cooperation between health and environmental campaigns and strategies.

4 Mediating between conflicting interests in society in order to ensure equitable access to supportive environments for health.

Source: WHO 1991

> **Box 10.7   The ten vital signs of quality in health promotion**
>
> 1   Understanding and responding to people's needs fairly
> 2   Building on sound theoretical principles and understanding
> 3   Demonstrating a sense of direction and coherence
> 4   Collecting, analysing, and using information
> 5   Reorienting key decision makers
> 6   Connecting with all sectors and settings
> 7   Using complementary approaches at both individual and
>   environmental levels
> 8   Encouraging participation and ownership
> 9   Providing technical and managerial training and support
> 10 Undertaking specific actions and programs
>
> Catford 1993

women; improving food security, safety, and nutrition; reducing tobacco and alcohol use; and creating supportive environments for health (WHO 1988).

The focus of the Third International Conference on Health Promotion in Sundsvall, Sweden, in 1991 was on creating supportive environments. It came at a critical time as it provided the first opportunity for health professionals from all over the world to consider how environments—whether physical, social, economic, or political—can be made more supportive for health (Catford 1991). Armed conflict, rapid population growth, inadequate food, lack of means of self-determination and degradation of natural resources were among the environmental influences identified at the conference as being damaging to health. The Sundsvall Statement on Supportive Environments for Health stressed the importance of sustainable development and urged social action at the community level, with people as the driving force of development (WHO 1991) (box 10.6). This statement and the report from the meeting were presented at the Rio Earth Summit in 1992 and contributed to the development of Agenda 21. A set of briefing books together with the conference report, handbook, and a simple practical 'how to do it' manual were other useful products from the conference (see WHO 2003c). Over time Sundsvall spawned a number of other developments such as the ten 'vital signs' of quality in health promotion (Catford 1993) (box 10.7).

THE JAKARTA AND MEXICO CONFERENCES: EXTENDING THE REACH

The Fourth International Conference on Health Promotion held in Jakarta, Indonesia in 1997 reviewed the impact of the Ottawa Charter and engaged new players to meet global challenges. It was the first of the four International Conferences on Health Promotion to be held in a developing country and the

Box 10.8   Jakarta Declaration on Health Promotion into the 21st Century

Extracts from the Fourth International Conference on Health Promotion in Jakarta, Indonesia

Priorities for Health Promotion in the 21st Century

1   Promote social responsibility for health

Policies and practices should be pursued that: avoid harming the health of other individuals; protect the environment and ensure sustainable use of resources; restrict production and trade in inherently harmful goods and substances; safeguard both the citizen in the marketplace and the individual in the workplace; and include equity-focused health impact assessments as an integral part of policy development.

2   Increase investments for health development

Increasing investment for health development requires a truly multisectoral approach, including, for example, additional resources to education and housing as well as for the health sector. Investments for health should reflect the needs of certain groups such as women, children, older people, indigenous, poor, and marginalised populations.

3   Consolidate and expand partnerships for health

Health promotion requires partnerships for health and social development between the different sectors at all levels of governance and society. Existing partnerships need to be strengthened and the potential for new partnerships must be explored. Partnerships offer mutual benefit for health through the sharing of expertise, skills, and resources.

4   Increase community capacity and empower the individual

Improving the capacity of communities for health promotion requires practical education, leadership training, and access to resources. Empowering individuals demands more consistent, reliable access to the decision-making process and the skills and knowledge essential to effect change.

5   Secure an infrastructure for health promotion

'Settings for health' represent the organisational base of the infrastructure required for health promotion. New health challenges mean that new and diverse networks need to be created to achieve intersectoral collaboration. Training in and practice of local leadership skills should be encouraged to support health promotion activities.

Source: WHO 1997a

first to involve the private sector in an active way (WHO 1997a). The evidence presented at the conference and experiences of the previous decade (e.g. Kickbusch 1997; Gilles 1998; Nutbeam 1998) showed that health promotion strategies contribute to the improvement of health and the prevention of diseases in developing and developed countries alike. These findings helped to shape renewed commitment to the key strategies and led to further refinement of the approaches in order to ensure their continuing relevance. Five priorities were identified in the Jakarta Declaration on Health Promotion into the 21st Century (box 10.8). These were confirmed in the following year in the

---

Box 10.9   Mexico Ministerial Statement for the Promotion of Health: From Ideas to Action

Extracts from the Statement signed by 87 Ministers of Health or their representatives on 5 June 2000 in Mexico City

Gathered in Mexico City on the occasion of the Fifth Global Conference on Health Promotion, the Ministers of Health who sign this Statement subscribe to the following actions:

A To position the promotion of health as a fundamental priority in local, regional, national and international policies and programmes.

B To take the leading role in ensuring the active participation of all sectors and civil society, in the implementation of health promoting actions, which strengthen and expand partnerships for health.

C To support the preparation of country-wide plans of action for promoting health, if necessary drawing on the expertise in this area of WHO and its partners. These plans will vary according to the national context, but will follow a basic framework agreed upon during the Fifth Global Conference on Health Promotion, and may include among others:

- The identification of health priorities and the establishment of healthy public policies and programmes to address these.
- The support of research which advances knowledge on selected priorities.
- The mobilization of financial and operational resources to build human and institutional capacity for the development, implementation, monitoring and evaluation of country-wide plans of action.

D To establish or strengthen national and international networks which promote health.

E To advocate that UN agencies be accountable for the health impact of their development agenda.

F To inform the Director General of the World Health Organization, for the purpose of her report to the 107th session of the Executive Board, of the progress made in the performance of the above actions.

Source: WHO 2000

Resolution on Health Promotion adopted by the World Health Assembly in May 1998 (WHO 1998b).

Despite the progress and developments in health promotion over the previous decade, two important challenges still remained. The first was to demonstrate and communicate more widely, particularly to developing countries, that health promotion policies and practices can make a difference to health and quality of life. The second was even more important—that health promotion action can achieve greater equity in health and can close the health gap between population groups.

Although equity is at the core of health promotion and was the thread that ran through the previous conferences and their declarations, there was still a general concern that health promotion was more effective for the privileged groups in society and for the richer developed world. Yet inequities in social and economic circumstances continued to increase and to erode the underlying conditions for health. For these reasons, the Fifth Global Conference on Health Promotion in Mexico: Bridging the Equity Gap focused on health inequalities both within and between countries. The joint organisers were WHO, the Pan American Health Organization (PAHO/AMRO), and the Ministry of Health of Mexico. The three main conference objectives were to show how health promotion makes a difference to health and quality of life, especially for people living in adverse circumstances; to place health high on the development agenda of international, national, and local agencies; and to stimulate partnerships for health between different sectors and at all levels of society. The products of the conference included six technical reports, case studies, the Mexico Ministerial Statement for the Promotion of Health: from Ideas to Action, the Framework for Countrywide Plans of Action for Health Promotion, and a conference report (WHO 2000).

The ministerial statement affirms the contribution of health promotion strategies to the sustainability of local, national, and international actions in health. It also pledges to draw up country-wide plans of action to monitor progress made in incorporating strategies that promote health into national and local policy and planning (box 10.9).

WHO LEADERSHIP: FUNDAMENTAL FOR SUCCESS

Although the Mexico conference helped to put health promotion on a wider political agenda and spread the concept to Central and South America, there was some controversy about whether the leadership of health promotion through WHO was losing its way. There was robust discussion in *Health Promotion International* (see vol. 16, no. 1, 2001) together with a strong rebuttal by the then Director General, Dr Gro Harlem Brundtland.

Much credit for this truly pioneering work goes to Dr Ilona Kickbusch. She has been the key instigator of WHO's approach to health promotion and has been extremely successful in placing it high on international, national, and local health agendas. For example, at international level, the 51st World Health Assembly adopted the first global health promotion resolution and urged all member states to implement the five priorities set out in the Jakarta Declaration (WHO 1998b). While at a national level in the United Kingdom, the Royal College of Physicians used the Ottawa Charter as the platform for policy development concerning alcohol and smoking control (RCP 1992, 1995). At operational levels the Ottawa Charter and latterly the Jakarta Declaration have also been used as the basis for planning by literally thousands of health projects across the world.

Until September 1998, Ilona Kickbusch was Director of the Division of Health Promotion, Education and Communication in Geneva and was previously in a similar position at WHO EURO. She has since taken up an appointment as Professor of Public Health at Yale University in the USA, where she is leading a major new initiative on international health. She was one of the founders of *Health Promotion International* (now in its eighteenth volume) in 1986 and currently still chairs the editorial board.

Many other individuals have, of course, contributed to the development of health promotion, and their work is documented in *Health Promotion International*. While WHO has been at the centre of developments, its influence has waxed and waned according to budget, individuals, and political opportunities. Currently the responsibility is sited within the Department of Non-Communicable Disease Prevention and Health Promotion under the directorship of Professor Pekka Puska. He is well known for his leadership of the North Karelia project, a long-term community-based heart disease prevention program in Finland that was set up in the 1970s.

One of the compelling reasons for the continued involvement of WHO is that public health issues have national and international dimensions as well as local ones. Community-based strategies are vital if appropriate services and environments are to be offered to people. But increasingly these are shaped by larger forces. For example, HIV, acid rain, and refugees do not recognise national or local boundaries. Satellite television will make targeted public education more difficult as well as providing opportunities for unhealthy commercial pressures. The tobacco, alcohol, and food industries have well-funded international marketing strategies that are hard to combat without collective action. Strong international cooperation is therefore essential to ensure environmental protection, access to adequate resources for healthy living, and high-quality health care.

Periodically there are calls for reform within WHO. With the appointment of the new Director General, Dr Jong Wook Lee from Korea in 2003, improvements are likely to continue. Despite the concerns about the inefficiency, remoteness, and lack of focus of large bureaucracies, we can state with confidence that WHO is likely to continue to 'make a difference' in health promotion development. It is undeniable that under WHO's leadership over two decades, a new health and social movement has been conceived, birthed, and nurtured with far-reaching effects (see for example Catford 1996, 2002). The contributions of WHO's health promotion program delivered through its Geneva headquarters and regional offices, including in the Western Pacific region (WHO 2003c), are now legion.

FUTURE CHALLENGES: KEEPING UP THE MOMENTUM

One of the great attractions of health promotion is that it is strong on innovative approaches (e.g. empowerment) but silent on health topics (e.g. tobacco). This is not a deficiency but a strength because as a proven 'technology' it can be applied to new or existing health issues in novel and creative ways. The themes that a health promotion perspective brings include:

- person focused—with a strong consumer/citizen orientation
- holistic health—incorporating mental and spiritual aspects
- values dominant—particularly regarding health disparities
- determinants based—with a socioecological perspective
- social capital—with emphasis on partnerships and alliances
- reaching out—by engaging, connecting, and horizontal networking
- cutting edge—through innovation, risk taking, and boundary riding
- capacity building—with communities, organisations, and workers.

Health promotion utilises a series of strategies that seek to foster conditions that allow populations to be healthy and to make healthy choices. The range of strategies now draw on a wide number of disciplines including anthropology, epidemiology, sociology, psychology and other behavioural sciences, public health, political science, education and communication. However, in broadening its base and becoming part of the main stream—which are all good developments—it runs the risk of being less innovative and radical.

Indeed to some, health promotion has now become part of 'establishment speak'. Unfortunately this has resulted in the term sometimes being misused, its values becoming distorted, and its meaning being lost. A further danger is that its cutting edge could easily become blunted. When faced with such challenges the best strategy is to look forward and then to move forward. Surely we need to rise to the new opportunities and threats of the next millennium and in so doing inject new energy and passion. But how could we act differently and better? Where should we be spending our efforts? Is there a new dimension of thinking and action that we should be moving into?

If we look at the development of the contemporary health promotion movement over three decades we see some interesting themes emerging. In the 1970s we started by tackling preventable diseases and risk behaviours primarily through information and simple education (e.g. heart disease, cancer, tobacco, nutrition). We could call this the first dimension of health promotion. In the 1980s we emphasised the importance of complementary intervention approaches (e.g. Ottawa's healthy public policy, personal skills, supportive environments, community action, health services); this was the second dimension of health promotion. In the 1990s we learnt the value of reaching people through the settings and sectors where they live and meet (e.g. schools, cities, health care settings, workplaces); and this was the third dimension of health promotion.

In the 2000s we need to sustain the momentum and add a fourth dimension of health promotion. But what is this? Does it exist? The answer is that it has always been there, but we have not been sufficiently confident or skilled to respond to it. We need to move—not just in our words but also in our actions—from the narrow entry point of disease prevention and control to the wider agenda of social determinants. The challenge now is to respond to the global trends of massive social change that impact on health, welfare and the environment. This fourth dimension is the most demanding, but it may be mastered if we use the tried and tested tool-kits derived from the first three dimensions together with new concepts, approaches, and theories. (See chapter 11 for an in-depth discussion on this fourth dimension of health promotion.)

What then are the social trends that we should be concerned about from a health promotion perspective? Seven are important:

- habitats—unrelenting increases in urbanisation and rural deprivation
- families—massive shifts in structures, responsibilities, and roles
- work—major new patterns, pitfalls, and potentials
- ageing—progressive lengthening of life span and dependency
- violence—rising aggression, conflicts, victims, and refugees
- markets—sharp movements towards consumerism and privatisation of services
- communication—revolutionary changes in information transfer and learning.

How can we 'surf' these seven major social trends to improve health? Country after country in the industrialised world is recognising that major and sustainable improvements in health status can only be won through a health promotion approach. This realisation also applies to developing nations, as the seminal 1993 World Bank report emphasised: 'If the right policy choices are made, the payoff will be high'. But here lies the stumbling block, for the science of 'delivery' has not kept pace with the science of 'discovery'. Although the necessary information to take action is available, often the right decisions are not made, not implemented, or not sustained. Leadership, together with better intelligence on 'how' to act effectively, can bridge this gulf, but our investment in this area to date has been poor (Catford 1997).

Effective leaders in health promotion are particularly important, not least because of the uncertain and demanding future that lies ahead. For example, some of the challenges facing the health promotion sector include:

- How to respond to the changing burden of disease.
- How to address increasing environmental health problems due to degradation of the environment and rapid urbanisation.
- How to secure better equity and access of health promotion services.
- What balance to strike between health promotion investments in population versus personal health care services.
- How to resist demands for inappropriate technology and high-cost services of low return.
- What new financing sources and mechanisms to introduce.

- What sort of health promotion workforce to provide and develop.
- What health promotion sector reforms and strategies to adopt.
- What planning, management and evaluation methods to use.

As we look into the twenty-first century the picture is getting bigger and the terrain more hazardous. Although we have much to celebrate about the development of health promotion knowledge and practice over the last two decades, we dare not be complacent—as Mark Twain said, 'Even if you are on the right track, you will get run over if you just sit there'.

SUMMARY

- Health promotion is a dynamic, far-reaching field with a strong record of strategic thinking and planning to cope with challenges and change.
- Health promotion workers and advocates will need to be well equipped to deal with social trends and unhealthy influences that threaten the health of people.
- Leadership development coupled with a focus on the social determinants of health is a key dimension for the continued growth and well-being of health promotion beyond 2003.

DISCUSSION TOPICS

1 How might the principles of the Ottawa Charter be utilised when planning an integrated intersectoral approach to mental health promotion at national and community level? In what ways might your discipline contribute to this approach?

2 Can you identify examples of the ten vital signs (box 10.7) having been implemented in your local community?

3 Develop a case study to illustrate the tension between community-based healthy public policies and the broader influences of unhealthy international pressures.

4 Why is it that health promotion strategies in years gone by were often described as being aimed at the 'middle class worried well', but less effective in reaching marginalised and disadvantaged groups?

5 Create a conceptual diagram of the evolution of health promotion from the Alma Ata to the Mexico conference, highlighting the key achievements of each conference.

6 In your opinion, what are the main health challenges facing your community now and in the future? How might documents such as the Ottawa Charter and the Jakarta Declaration influence decision makers in seeking to address these existing and emerging health trends?

7 What are the obstacles and opportunities for your discipline to contribute to promoting health at local, national, and global levels?

USEFUL WEB SITES

A wider range of **WHO health promotion publications** is available at: www.who.int/dsa/cat98/healthpro8.htm

Articles published in **Health Promotion International** can be accessed through: www.heapro.oupjournals.org

NOTES

1   The *Concepts and Principles of Health Promotion* is available through the WHO archiving service and is also reproduced in **Health Promotion International** 1986 1:1 pp. 73–6.

IN SEARCH OF THE FOURTH DIMENSION OF HEALTH PROMOTION: GUIDING PRINCIPLES FOR ACTION

Berni Murphy

Key concepts

- A determinants approach to promoting health
- Evidence-based health promotion
- Building collaborative partnerships
- Strengthening community and workforce capacity
- Leadership in promoting health
- A framework for health promotion action

dev.

'HEALTH PROMOTION MUST BE EVERYONE'S BUSINESS RATHER THAN SOMEONE'S JOB DESCRIPTION'

This chapter will take a practical approach, in that the 'how to' aspects of health promotion action will be considered, and a set of *guiding principles* for that action constructed. Let us first begin by revisiting the appraisal in chapter 10 of the evolutionary phases of health promotion, the so-called three dimensions. John Catford describes the first dimension of health promotion in the 1970s as focusing on tackling preventable diseases and risk behaviours. The second dimension during the 1980s focused on the importance of implementing complementary approaches, shaped largely by the Ottawa Charter for Health Promotion (WHO 1986a). The third dimension evolved during the 1990s and was concerned with reaching out to people in the contexts in which they live their lives through focusing on settings and sectors. While each of these phases or dimensions has steadily improved the efficacy of health promotion action, a more sophisticated approach is now required if we are to address emerging social and environmental global trends and their health implications. New horizons call for a new stratagem: the fourth dimension of health promotion. What then might the fourth dimension of health promotion look like? And how might we, as health professionals, contribute to this new paradigm? This brings us to the first of the *five guiding principles for health promotion action*.

A DETERMINANTS APPROACH: THE FIRST GUIDING PRINCIPLE FOR ACTION

Before we can hope to create healthier and supportive environments, and develop strategic responses to identified health problems, we must first understand the underlying social, economic, environmental, and political determinants of health as they impact on individuals, communities, and populations. We can no longer be satisfied that genetics or individual lifestyle choice are entirely responsible for health outcomes. A growing body of evidence now recognises that international factors such as globalisation, environmental degradation, and political instability significantly impact on health, with those who are most disadvantaged experiencing the worst outcomes. One need only look to regional conflicts, the refugee crises, poverty, food insecurity (i.e. not having enough food or money to buy food), and the suffering they create to realise the impact that macro-level determinants can have on health.

Keleher and Murphy (2002) theorise that in a rapidly changing social milieu, the complex nature of the social determinants, their interrelationships and their influence on health, necessitates a particular focus for those charged with setting priorities, planning strategic responses and implementing interventions. Health promoters have opportunities to take leadership roles in sharing their knowledge and understanding of the underlying determinants of health within the health sector, and across other sectors that have the capacity to influence health outcomes. Turrell et al. (1999) argue that health leadership must 'fund, develop and sustain the critical mass of R & D activity that will be required to make a difference' to health inequalities as we move into the new millennium (p. xii). Much of this research should focus on better deepening our understanding about the determinants of existing and emerging health issues, particularly as they impact on vulnerable groups, and will be crucial to informing effective and socially just responses.

EVIDENCE-BASED HEALTH PROMOTION: THE SECOND GUIDING PRINCIPLE FOR ACTION

Central to the quest for new approaches must be a commitment to building a comprehensive body of evidence upon which to base strategic responses. Chapter 6 introduced some of the ways that Australia currently measures population health, including morbidity and mortality data, life expectancy, perinatal birth rates, and specific disease registers such as those monitoring cancers and infectious diseases. The epidemiological data is clearly crucial in contributing to decision-making processes about setting priorities for health policy and practice.

Qualitative studies help to interpret the epidemiological data, giving meaning to the statistics, particularly with respect to nonfatal outcomes that nevertheless contribute to the burden of disease (e.g. mental health conditions such as depression, anxiety, and phobias). But what else do we need to know? Where are the gaps in knowledge? What health promotion responses have worked, with which groups, and in what contexts? Conversely, what has been evaluated as ineffective, and would therefore be a waste of precious dollars in future strategic planning? And what is the significance and meaning of the evidence emerging about the impact of the social determinants on health?

The second guiding principle for health promotion action is that strategic responses must be based on a sophisticated body of evidence, one that has accumulated through the gathering and analysis of accurate and comprehensive health data, together with intervention impact and outcome evaluation findings. Further, health research must continue to stretch beyond a narrow disease focus if we are to better understand the implications for health of social and economic trends such as urbanisation, the transformation of communities and social capital, widening economic disparities, shifting work patterns, increasing gender equality, migration, and an Australian population that is ageing. But what are we to do when the evidence is not yet available to us? Must we wait for the evidence to catch up before we commit resources, even though we can be reasonably confident that particular interventions are likely to be successful? The answer, of course, is that effective leadership must dictate when it is timely for interventions to be implemented *ahead* of the evidence, as has been the case with several mental health interventions that have specifically sought to address underlying social determinants. For instance, VicHealth's 'Together We Do Better Campaign' focuses on raising awareness among decision makers as well as the community about the psychosocial environments that promote mental health and wellbeing.

BUILDING COLLABORATIVE PARTNERSHIPS: THE THIRD GUIDING PRINCIPLE FOR ACTION

The fourth dimension of health promotion calls for collaborative partnerships to promote health in ways that might otherwise be beyond the scope of agencies and sectors working in isolation. Collaboration within the health sector can deliver more integrated services that have been reoriented to better fit the changing needs of individuals and communities. However, it is at the intersectoral level that the potential to address underlying determinants of social and health outcomes can clearly be recognised. This requires a shift in thinking at the macro level regarding infrastructure and systems, particularly with respect to policy, funding, and service delivery. The benefits of collaborative endeavours are various, and include:

- an increased capacity to respond to existing and emerging health problems, and their determinants

- improved resource allocation and utilisation
- opportunities to strengthen the community's capacity to identify and respond to factors promoting and inhibiting health in the local context
- opportunities to implement innovative upstream approaches leading to infrastructure and systems changes that are likely to have a broad and sustained impact.

In many instances, partnership arrangements determine the extent of their health promoting influence. For example, *informal networks* might offer referral services, commission research, raise awareness, and advocate for change. The health promoter can be pivotal in conceptualising, establishing, and facilitating such networks. Alternatively, *collaborative alliances* involve contractual obligations and must be built on trust and mutually beneficial relationships. As such, these alliances are more likely to exert significant upstream influence through systemic and process changes.

The phases in the collaborative process will obviously vary depending on the nature of the partnership, but are likely to include the development of a shared understanding by stakeholders of the goals and planning logic; and the development of an agreement with respect to roles, responsibilities, and resourcing. It is during the latter phase that the tensions that can threaten collaborative endeavours often surface, particularly when shared understandings, roles, and responsibilities have been assumed rather than implicitly stated and documented.

The following case study (box 11.1) describes an innovative approach to addressing the underlying determinants of health for Victorian youth that involved building intersectoral collaborative partnerships. Stakeholders recognise that this investment will of necessity stretch into years and possibly even decades before socioecological changes are likely to be embedded in the state's infrastructure and systems.

Box 11.1 Case study 1

'Common solutions to common problems': intersectoral partnerships in focus

VicHealth joined other key stakeholders (including the Royal Automobile Club of Victoria and the Transport Accident Commission) in conceptualising an intersectoral approach to addressing the underlying determinants of health for young people. This initiative was founded on research indicating that many of the same social determinants leading to adverse health outcomes were evident for a range of risky behaviours (e.g. drug and alcohol misuse) and conditions (e.g. homelessness). Further, VicHealth recognised that over forty different silo programs with a health focus, instigated by a diversity of stakeholders, were at that time competing for curriculum space in Victorian schools. Examples included harm minimisation drug and alcohol programs, road safety programs, and mental health promotion programs. VicHealth took a leadership role in brokering initial meetings between key stakeholders from sectors and services, including education, welfare, mental health, drug and alcohol services, gambling, criminal justice, transport, housing, and employment. The intent was to raise awareness of the common underlying determinants of health for young people, and to build capacity for collaborative action, while reducing the number of silo programs operating. VicHealth fostered opportunities for intersectoral partnerships and created a climate conducive to strategic innovation. Some two years after its inception, the initiative has metamorphosed through several conceptual phases and is still in train. At times it appears to lose momentum, as is often the case with initiatives requiring both long-term commitment and investment, and a relinquishing by stakeholders of long-held attitudes, beliefs, and territory. Nevertheless, project leaders and many of the stakeholders remain committed to this socioecological approach, and are optimistic that such collaborative partnerships are, in fact, the way of the future.

Source: VicHealth project worker 2003

ADVOCACY, ENGAGEMENT, AND EMPOWERMENT: THE FOURTH GUIDING PRINCIPLE FOR ACTION

The fourth guiding principle for action focuses on a commitment to strengthening the capacity of individuals, communities, and the workforce to recognise and respond to factors influencing health in their local contexts. Social movements that lead to better health outcomes are likely to emerge when communities are engaged, supported, empowered, and motivated to challenge the status quo. However, effective engagement and empowerment can only happen when skilled communicators are attentive to the issues, the context, and the stakeholders, as well as to their needs and concerns. *Community engagement* requires patience and a commitment to the process. It assumes a more collaborative and mutual relationship than *community participation*, which can be quite *top-down* in practice, despite the best intentions to promote empowerment and independence.

Within the fourth dimension, health professionals will focus more on working *with* individuals and communities rather than *on* them. The skilled health promoter will recognise the importance of genuinely engaging with communities around health issues, and will demonstrate a range of skills to facilitate this important process. Some of these professional skills, strategies, and values are presented in box 11.2.

Advocacy and community engagement are effective health promotion tools, particularly when the aim is to build the capacity of marginalised and vulnerable groups to address social and health inequities most relevant to them. Collaborative partnerships with health and other workers enhance effectiveness.

Box 11.2   Skills, strategies, and values for effective community engagement

- Leadership, political acumen, and respect for community members, their values, attitudes, and beliefs.
- Understanding of the community and their needs, the issues, determinants, and the context.
- Willingness to consult from top echelons of government, INGOs, NGOs, down to grass roots. Commitment to engaging the community in every step of the process.
- Ability to plan, organise, implement, review, and modify.
- Willingness to establish transparent processes.
- Commitment to establishing networks, building capacity, supporting, and empowering.
- Ability to mediate, advocate, create, negotiate, and resolve conflicts with integrity.
- Communication skills including engaging, listening, persuading, encouraging, and feeding back.
- Ability to conduct effective meetings, and to present verbal and written reports.
- Patience, persistence, resilience, and commitment.

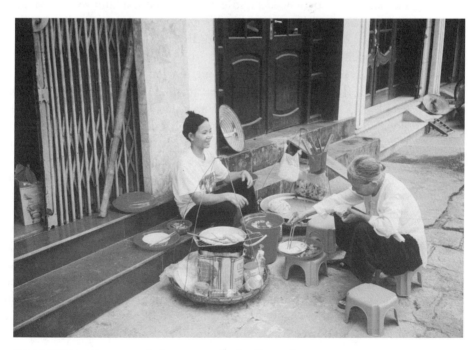

Young Vietnamese woman helps prepare the family meal

The following case study (box 11.3) about youth in Vietnam demonstrates the role that leading health agencies can play in *advocating* for change, as well as the difficulties encountered when trying to *engage* and *empower* young people to be more actively involved in decisions that impact on them.

Empowerment must happen at a number of levels in order to effect the social changes likely to address health inequities while promoting health for all. Empowerment at the individual and community levels can be about developing knowledge and understanding of issues, determinants, and contexts, as well as building the personal skills and confidence to take action. Implicit in this scenario, however, is the need for people to have opportunities to exercise greater control over social and other conditions impacting on their lives. In this regard, the work of health and other sectors is pivotal to creating supportive environments conducive to social change. In the fourth dimension, we will hopefully see workforce development prioritised to better equip health professionals and other sectors to collaborate in respectful partnerships with individuals and communities to assess needs, and to plan and implement multilevel actions that are targeted at sustainable enhancement of health.

Box 11.3   Case study 2

Advocacy, community engagement, and empowerment: Youth in Vietnam

Vietnam has experienced rapid economic, cultural, and social change in recent years. Approximately 40 per cent of the population of 80 million are under 25 years of age, and more than 1.2 million young people are now flooding the job market each year. While education is valued in Vietnam, access to vocational training remains limited and illegal migration from regional and remote areas to the cities is increasing as young people seek opportunities for economic participation. Youth now access global information through the Internet, billboards, and other media. Vietnam's social fabric is changing, with traditional family structures and values being challenged. Research suggests that family breakdown, frustration at limited job opportunities, emerging mental health issues, drug use, and crime are all of growing concern in relation to young people. United Nations agencies have recently begun to *advocate* on behalf of youth by lobbying the Vietnamese government, INGOs, NGOs, and other key stakeholders involved in research, funding, policy, and practice. The UN agencies *mediate* to broker partnerships that will improve the situation for youth, and recognise the need to involve youth in the process. *Youth forums* have been conducted across the country to *engage* young people in identifying and discussing issues most pertinent to them, and to ultimately empower youth to participate in decision-making processes.

However, young people in Vietnam do not have a tradition of speaking out, and community elders do not traditionally invite the contribution of youth. Some observers have applauded the spirit fostered at the forums of collaboration between youth and decision makers, with young people gradually developing the skills and confidence to voice opinions, and elders learning to listen and to better understand their perspectives. Others, however, have been less effusive, and have contended that *participation* in such forums is not necessarily testament to genuine *engagement*, with tokenism being evident in some instances. Incidents of social desirability bias were also reported, whereby some youth felt pressured to express opinions that they believed their elders wanted to hear. Even the critics, however, acknowledge the potential of these forums to *engage* and *empower* youth, and argue that adults must now genuinely invest in the process and gain the skills to facilitate the voices of youth. In so doing, these adults will be working *with* youth as agents of change.

Adapted from Ridge and Murphy 2002

LEADERSHIP IN HEALTH PROMOTION: THE FIFTH GUIDING PRINCIPLE FOR ACTION

The fourth dimension of health promotion is unquestionably the most challenging for health professionals. No longer can we simply respond to adverse health data with interventions that work predominantly midstream and downstream. The challenge now is to be much more proactive in recognising the conditions that compromise health, and to then work upstream in pre-empting the impact of these determinants with timely, innovative, and strategic responses. Effective leadership will of necessity comprise many facets and provide many opportunities. Those in health leadership roles must, in particular, demonstrate a profound understanding of the social determinants of health, and conceptualise and share a vision for collaborative action to address these determinants, as well as a commitment to social justice and equity.

The health leader must be cognisant of the existing and emerging evidence around issues, determinants, and approaches, and seek to *mediate* between communities, health providers, and other sectors (e.g. education, transport, housing, welfare) in strengthening existing partnerships and in building new ones. The health leader should *advocate* for change, while being sensitive to the needs of the community and respectful of individual values where they differ from the collective goals. Finally, the health leader should *enable* others to share the vision, by spreading the word about the determinants of health within the health workforce, other sectors, and the community. Communities and workforces that better understand the contexts that promote and inhibit health are more likely to foster movements for socioecological change. The fifth and final guiding principle for action, then, is about leadership that understands health and its determinants, that shares a vision for improving health for all, and that acts to build the capacity of communities, the health workforce, and other sectors to enact timely and efficacious evidence-based policies, practice, and social change.

PUTTING THEORY INTO PRACTICE: A FRAMEWORK FOR HEALTH PROMOTION ACTION

We have explored the guiding principles for action, but how can we as health professionals best *implement* these principles? What are the approaches and interventions that contribute to health promotion action in the fourth dimension? Figure 11.1 provides a useful tool for conceptualising and operationalising a range of approaches and interventions.

This framework sets out the three main approaches for health promotion action: the downstream *primary care approach*, the midstream *lifestyle/behaviourist approach*, and the upstream *socioecological approach*. (See chapters 2 and 7 for a more detailed explanation of the downstream, midstream, and upstream metaphor.) It is important to recognise that all of these approaches make a valuable contribution to enhancing health, and that health promotion is at its most effective when it involves multilevel, integrated, and complementary interventions that are supported by health and other sectors working in collaborative partnerships with the community.

Figure 11.1 Framework for Health Promotion Action

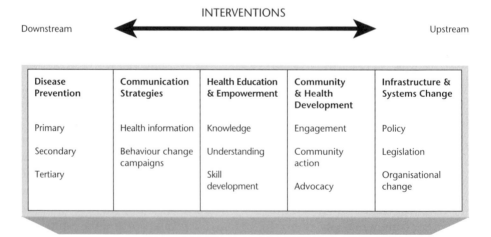

INTERVENTIONS

Downstream ⬅——————————————➤ Upstream

Disease Prevention	Communication Strategies	Health Education & Empowerment	Community & Health Development	Infrastructure & Systems Change
Primary	Health information	Knowledge	Engagement	Policy
Secondary	Behaviour change campaigns	Understanding	Community action	Legislation
Tertiary		Skill development	Advocacy	Organisational change

Primary Care Approaches   *Lifestyle/Behaviourist* Approaches   *Socioecological* Approaches

Source: Murphy, B. and Keleher, H. 2003

The primary care approach: starting downstream, moving upstream

Depending on the focus of your particular health discipline, you might concentrate your efforts in one or more of the intervention categories. For instance, a community health nurse might currently be primarily involved in primary disease prevention (e.g. conducting screening and risk assessment programs). However, the opportunity for this health professional to do so much more than primary disease prevention becomes apparent as we scan the Framework for Health Promotion Action. Community health nurses who develop further skills then have the scope within their work practice to incorporate a range of other activities consistent with contemporary health promotion and primary health development approaches. These activities might include provision of health information, development of locally targeted communication strategies, the facilitation of health education and

Table 11.1 Primary care approach: heart health in focus

PRIMARY CARE CLINIC A	PRIMARY CARE CLINIC B
• Primary care clinic introduces a 'healthy heart' program to proactively address the risk of heart disease in male clients aged 40–70 years.	• Clinic convinces health network partners to fund a heart health project worker.
• Clinic invites all clients in target group to a 30-minute interview with clinic nurse via personalised letter.	• Network successfully lobbies several donors to boost funding (e.g. local government, state government, Heart Foundation). Project funding now secure for five rather than two years.
• Clinic raises awareness of issue in local newspaper and through displays at local pharmacy.	• Project worker uses community engagement skills to invite community to be actively involved in process.
• Sixty-eight per cent of clients take up invitation to attend.	• Aims are established as: (i) building community knowledge and understanding about heart health and its determinants; (ii) building community capacity and resources to identify issues and develop effective responses; (iii) advocating for infrastructure changes to support heart health.
• Nurse checks blood pressure, weight, and cholesterol, and completes questionnaire about risk behaviours (e.g. diet, physical activity, smoking, alcohol, stress).	
• Ten per cent of clients are referred to specialists for further screening/treatment.	
• Nurse provides brochures and personal advice tailored to meet the needs of the client about eliminating unhealthy behaviours.	• Community members and health professionals work collaboratively to identify needs and to plan multilevel complementary interventions.

cont.

Table 11.1   Primary care approach: heart health in focus (continued)

PRIMARY CARE CLINIC A	PRIMARY CARE CLINIC B
• Client evaluation sheets find that 86 per cent describe the session as 'worthwhile and informative'. • Clinic annual report commends the 'healthy heart' initiative as successful and worth the investment. • Follow-up phone survey 12 months after consultation finds that less than 7 per cent have made lifestyle changes to improve their heart health. Primary care clinic decides to adopt a primary health development approach to promoting heart health in response to local burden-of-disease data.	• Clinic conducts heart health screening after an awareness campaign focusing on positive ways to improve heart health rather than focusing only on risk factors. • Education programs are planned and facilitated to meet the needs of the participants, and to build their knowledge, skills, confidence, and motivation to take actions that support healthy living. • Partnerships are developed with over twenty-five community groups (e.g. sporting organisations, seniors groups, gardening groups, parent groups, support networks). • 'Men's shed' initiative deemed a success. This invites men to work together to build toys, furniture, etc. for the community and also reduces social isolation among these men (social isolation is a risk factor for heart disease). • After three years, the project worker reports on policy and infrastructure changes that provide supportive environments for healthy living. These include smoke-free venues; increased availability of affordable healthy food options; a vegetable garden planted and maintained at the seniors community centre; increased active living options due to more safe public spaces and walking tracks; and increased opportunities for social connection through the arts and recreation programs.

skill development programs, contribution to community action groups, as well as membership of committees that develop policies and practices in support of local municipal health plans. In this way, people working predominantly 'downstream' in the primary care domain also have the capacity to influence midstream and upstream action. Table 11.1 provides an interesting contrast between two *primary care* clinics seeking to address heart health concerns in their locality. The core business for both clinics might once have been positioned downstream, but we can see that clinic A has attempted to expand its work into the midstream domain, while clinic B has attempted to exert influence both midstream and upstream.

The lifestyle/behaviourist approach: starting midstream, moving upstream

This approach recognises that lifestyles, behaviours, and personal choices influence health outcomes. For instance, social isolation, stress, poor nutrition, smoking, alcohol misuse, and physical inactivity have all been identified as risk factors for a range of diseases. In its simplest form, this approach seeks to better inform people about these risks and consequences through provision of information and targeted behaviour change campaigns, as well as to increase personal knowledge and skills through health education programs. The theory here is that if we can increase knowledge, understanding, and personal skills, individuals will be more likely to make healthier choices. However, the extent to which this occurs depends on a range of factors, including the effectiveness of interventions in reaching the target audience; the degree to which the individual feels motivated and empowered to make lifestyle changes; the individual's locus of control; and the extent to which external influences support or compromise attempts to adopt healthier behaviours (see chapter 13 for further discussion of these issues).

Table 11.2 provides a contrast between health providers in two different towns conducting diabetes information and education programs. The Town A health providers tend to work midstream by adopting a traditional lifestyle behaviourist approach. However, the Town B health providers also seek to collaborate with their community and work towards infrastructure and systems changes. In so doing, the Town B health providers can be said to be operating both midstream and upstream.

Table 11.2 Lifestyle/behaviourist approach: diabetes education in focus

TOWN A HEALTH PROVIDERS	TOWN B HEALTH PROVIDERS
• Doctor diagnoses condition.	• Doctor diagnoses condition.
• Doctor refers client to diabetes educator.	• Doctor refers client to diabetes educator.
• Additional referral to hospital dietitian.	• Additional referral to hospital dietitian.
• Doctor referral to diabetes educator and dietitian is the result of a long-standing informal network arrangement.	• Doctor, diabetes educator, and dietitian collaborate to optimise treatment and future health plan for client.
• The three health professionals do not talk to each other about this client.	• This is a consequence of deliberate effort to improve effectiveness of the network.

cont.

Table 11.2 Lifestyle/behaviourist approach: diabetes education in focus (continued)

TOWN A HEALTH PROVIDERS	TOWN B HEALTH PROVIDERS
• Diabetes educator is described as 'practical and supportive' by client. • Diabetes educator links client into Diabetes Australia register to access cheaper products required to manage condition. • Diabetes educator tells client where to buy blood-testing kit. • Diabetes educator teaches client how to monitor blood sugar. • Diabetes educator sees client on three occasions to monitor progress and offer support, in keeping with standard procedures.	• Diabetes educator encourages client to bring partner to consultations, recognising the importance of social support in dealing with condition. • Diabetes educator links client into Diabetes Australia register to access cheaper products required to manage condition, and to access support groups. • Diabetes educator tells client where to buy blood-testing kit. • Diabetes educator teaches client how to monitor blood sugar. • Diabetes educator seeks to enable client to self-manage condition. Sees client when necessary to monitor progress and offer support. • Diabetes educator encourages client to attend diabetes education workshop. Client reports the session was 'engaging, empowering and very motivating'. Client attends a later workshop to share experiences with others.
• Dietitian provides general advice about diet. • Dietitian does not consult client about dietary preferences, attitudes, and beliefs. • Dietitian sends client home with two pages of general advice regarding 'do's' and 'don'ts'. • Dietitian suggests client purchase certain recipe books for diabetics. • Client comments that the dietitian does not 'share the knowledge'.	• Dietitian is positive and supportive. • Dietitian encourages client to bring partner to consultations, in keeping with network philosophy to encourage supportive environments. • Dietitian consults client and partner on dietary preferences, attitudes, and beliefs. • Dietitian provides client with general information, plus recipes suited to the clients' preferences. Suggests recipe books to purchase and web sites to check. • Dietitian shares knowledge, and seeks to enable client to make healthier choices.

cont.

Table 11.2 Lifestyle/behaviourist approach: diabetes education in focus (continued)

TOWN A HEALTH PROVIDERS	TOWN B HEALTH PROVIDERS
• Dietitian pencils in several forward appointments but client never returns.	• Client volunteers to return for further consultations when required and complies with advice given by dietitian.
• Dietitian and diabetes educator collaborate once a year to run 'diabetes week' in the town. • They organise a diabetes information display in the shopping mall to raise awareness of the high incidence of diabetes in the population, and to encourage those in high-risk groups to be screened for the disease. • They jointly write an article for the local newspaper about risk factors for diabetes.	• The network recognises that poor diet, physical inactivity, and social isolation are determinants of several illnesses (including diabetes) highlighted in recent local burden-of-disease data. • The network lobbies local food outlets to offer healthy choices, and to promote these options. • The network lobbies state and local government for funding to increase parklands, and walking and cycling paths to encourage people of all ages to be more active.

The socioecological approach: working upstream

The term 'socioecology' refers to the complexity of interactions between people, and their social and physical environments. The *socioecological approach* acknowledges the influence that infrastructure and systems can exert on these interactions, particularly with respect to social and health outcomes. The Framework for Health Promotion Action identifies community engagement and development, as well as infrastructure and systems change, as key interventions that support a socioecological approach. The social movements that can grow from community engagement and empowerment were discussed earlier in this chapter (see 'Advocacy, engagement, and empowerment'). It is important to realise, however, that community action takes time, and is therefore often at odds with current government funding models that demand more immediate and tangible returns. Investment in **community development** approaches by governments must be consistent with a genuine commitment to a social model of health, rather than an excuse to defer or avoid essential infrastructure and systems changes and their associated costs. *Infrastructure* usually refers to policies and resources (e.g. money, people, time, transport, education, welfare, childcare), while *systems* refers to processes to manage the infrastructure, which include feedback, promotion and grievance mechanisms, induction and mentoring systems, and funding arrangements, as well as processes to effect change. It is at this macro level that significant improvements in

Table 11.3   Socioecological approach: organisation responses to workplace conflict and stress

Scenario: Workplace conflict is reported in three different organisations, with the conflict impacting on the productivity and stress levels of the workers and their colleagues. The organisations report their responses to the situation, and the workers involved describe the outcomes.

ORGANISATION A	ORGANISATION B	ORGANISATION C
• This organisation is concerned that the conflict is impacting on productivity and stress levels, and therefore acknowledges that it should support the workers in dealing with this issue. • The organisation offers counselling to the workers with an emphasis on cognitive techniques, including learning how to reframe unpleasant experiences. The counsellor also suggests the workers consider relaxation strategies (e.g. massage). • The manager offers to pay for the workers to attend a workshop on developing personal coping strategies. • The manager suggests that the workers attend a tai chi class offered by the organisation once a week at lunchtime to help manage stress.	• The organisation recognises that it has an important role to play in addressing workplace conflict. • It acts quickly to eliminate the conflict by moving one worker to another area. • The manager then puts processes in place to uncover the source of the conflict. A mediator is brought in to speak independently to each worker. The mediator then works towards a resolution satisfactory to the workers. • This organisation encourages workers to be active and healthy, and to therefore be more productive and able to cope with workplace and life stressors. To this end, it subsidises gym memberships for its workers. This organisation is committed to providing a safe and supportive environment for its workers.	• The organisation is working towards more collaborative management styles and transparent processes. • The organisation subsidises the social club and gym memberships as part of its commitment to being a health promoting setting for all employees. • The organisation offers workforce training in antidiscrimination, effective negotiation, and resolving conflicts. • The organisation's equal opportunity officer, who is trained in counselling, mediation, and conflict resolution, consults the workers to uncover the cause of the conflict. • The organisation has clearly documented grievance procedures. After due consideration one of the workers decides to go through formal proceedings.

cont.

Table 11.3 Socioecological approach: organisation responses to workplace conflict and stress (continued)

ORGANISATION A	ORGANISATION B	ORGANISATION C
• The workers report that while they have undertaken counselling, the coping strategies course and the relaxation classes, the cause of the conflict remains. The workers are unsatisfied with the outcome and one worker is now on stress leave.	• The workers report satisfaction with the mediation process, but are frustrated with the organisation's systems, management styles, and lack of consultation with workers. They feel grievance issues are dealt with ad hoc rather than in accordance with formal policies and procedures.	• The workers and management say that the conflict has been resolved satisfactorily. The workers report that they felt empowered to address the issue due to their skills, management support, and effective processes. The cause of the conflict and all grievance proceedings remain confidential.

health outcomes can be made, particularly with respect to vulnerable groups and those suffering health inequities. Collaborative intersectoral partnerships, therefore, underpin much of the upstream work now being undertaken to improve the health of groups and to create healthier settings.

Originally a 'setting' was viewed as a place to *do* health promotion to people. Here was a captive audience for our midstream behaviour change health messages, education programs, and targeted interventions, with typical settings including workplaces, hospitals, communities, and schools. However, during the 1990s, the *settings approach* became more sophisticated, and involved, first, studying the ways in which the setting impacted on the health of those within, and, second, working towards change within the setting to make it more health promoting. In this sense, the settings approach can now operate more upstream than was originally the case. Kickbusch (1997) contended that the settings approach must now be expanded to include social development and social spaces such as childhood and being female, as well as marginalised and excluded populations (e.g. those living in remote regions and slum dwellings).

In some instances, significant *organisational change* is required to create workplace settings that promote the health of employees, visitors to the workplace, and the wider community. The extent to which organisations can influence the health and wellbeing of employees is becoming more apparent as research uncovers the interrelationship between workplace factors, such as stress, and health outcomes. Table 11.3 provides a contrast between three different organisations faced with a dilemma: in this instance, it is workplace conflict. The strategies adopted by each organisation highlight very different approaches, with one organisation (A) attributing responsibility to individuals to change their behaviour; the second (B) supporting the individuals and attempting to address the immediate *causes* of the behaviour; and the third (C) taking a more socio-ecological approach to the organisation–worker interface by seeking to create organisational structures and systems that are health promoting, while also empowering the individuals to exercise greater control within their own contexts. Analysis of the differing strategies offers insight into downstream, mid-stream, and upstream organisational approaches, while also flagging the debate around 'who is responsible for health?' Is it the responsibility of the individual, or of society, or a measure of both?

A final word on the downstream, midstream, and upstream metaphor...

Imagine you are a skilled swimmer standing in the middle of a stream, able to manoeuvre comfortably in your immediate vicinity. The current is flowing swiftly downstream, so you could also easily choose to go with the current. But you gaze upstream and realise that the real rewards lie in that direction. You face upstream and feel the current working against you. While it will be hard work, you recognise that the rewards will be worth it, and you strike out with power-ful strokes upstream.

In this scenario, the skilled swimmer is a health worker with professional skills. *Midstream* is where you focus behaviour change approaches, and *down-stream* is where you focus the primary care approaches. Both of these approaches will continue to make valuable contributions to the spectrum of health promo-tion action. But as we begin the fourth dimension of health promotion, it is the *upstream* socioecological approaches that have the potential to reap new rewards. Do we have the skills and the courage to turn and face upstream?

SUMMARY

- This chapter has considered the guiding principles for health promo-tion action in the new millennium.
- Health promotion action must be underpinned by a knowledge and understanding of the determinants of health.
- Strategic responses must be evidence-based, but effective leadership must determine when the interventions should occur ahead of the evidence.
- Collaborative partnerships within the health sector and intersectorally can promote health more effectively than organisations operating in isolation.
- Community and workforce capacity must be strengthened to promote health, and to respond to health concerns and their determinants.

- Effective leadership requires leaders who are willing to share a vision for collaborative action to address the determinants of health, underpinned by a commitment to social justice and equity.
- The Framework for Health Promotion Action is a useful tool for conceptualising and operationalising the range of health promotion approaches and interventions.

DISCUSSION TOPICS

1 If you were working as a health professional at a refugee mandatory detention centre, how might you *mediate, advocate,* and *enable* on behalf of young children and youth being detained there? Who might you *engage* in the process? What skills would you need to *advocate* and *engage*? What processes would you undertake?

2 In what ways does the fourth dimension of health promotion differ from previous dimensions? How might your profession contribute to this fourth dimension?

3 Which stakeholders could contribute to an intersectoral collaboration for a disadvantaged group in your local context? What might the key objectives be, and what skills would you need to facilitate this process?

4 What skills would you need to develop in order to increase your professional capacity to enhance the health of communities through socioecological approaches? Write a personal action plan for your professional development.

USEFUL WEB SITES

Ottawa Charter for Health Promotion:
www.who.int/hpr/archive/docs/ottawa.html
Jakarta Declaration on Health Promotion into the 21st century:
www.who.int/hpr/archive/docs/jakarta/english.html

HEALTH PROMOTION IN ACTION: CASE STUDIES FROM AUSTRALIA

Bernie Marshall

Key concepts

- Unpacking the determinants of health
- Taking action on the determinants of health
- Case study 1: Road trauma
- Settings approaches to health
- Case study 2: Health promoting schools

You have already been introduced to the field of health promotion in chapter 10. There you examined the Ottawa Charter for Health Promotion (WHO 1986a), one of the key documents in public health. It defines health promotion as 'the process of enabling people to increase control over, and to improve, their health', or the process of individuals and communities taking control over the determinants of their health. In order to do this, people must be able to 'identify and realise aspirations, satisfy needs, and to change or cope with the environment'. In this chapter, two case studies are used to examine ways in which the determinants of health and key documents such as the Ottawa Charter are used to inform, organise, and practise health promotion in Australia.

In health promotion, our task clearly is to provide what people need in order to be able to change the factors (determinants) that impact on their health. Sometimes this means we work to change attitudes and beliefs, and to increase people's health knowledge, skills, and motivation. But often people need access to resources or opportunities in order to have healthier lives, and many times we need even bigger changes in community attitudes and social norms, and in the policies and practices of governments and social institutions such as workplaces and schools, in order to make a difference. This range of health promotion work is summarised in the five action areas of the Ottawa Charter.

If health promotion involves increasing people's control over the determinants of their health, two questions arise:
- What are the determinants of a particular aspect of health?
- What do people need in order to be able to take action on these determinants? It is these two questions that will guide this chapter.

UNPACKING THE DETERMINANTS OF HEALTH

The causes or determinants of health are very wide ranging—just try to identify all the factors that influence your own health, both positively and negatively. To help in identifying such determinants, models or frameworks are often used. One of the most straightforward models is the 'iceberg model' (Ryan and Travis 1988); this model identifies the connections between a particular state of health and its determinants. In figure 12.1, you will notice that only the smallest section of an iceberg is seen above the waterline—this represents the identified and visible state of health. The invisible expanse below the waterline represents the underlying hidden determinants (or causes) of this visible state of health.

The section immediately below the waterline is directly connected to the visible state of health and can be identified and described without too much difficulty. This layer represents the factors that directly contribute to the state of

Figure 12.1 The health iceberg

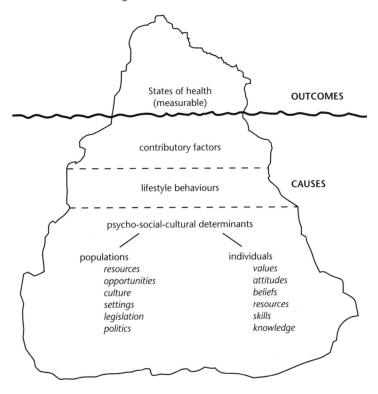

health, either positively or negatively. For states of negative health, we usually refer to this layer as 'risk factors'. Good examples are the links between obesity and heart disease, between smoking and lung cancer, and between extended exposure to loud noise and deafness.

Underlying these contributing factors are the less well-defined lifestyle behaviours—the accumulated behaviours that 'create' the risk/contributing factors in the layer above; we can imagine that these are what we would observe if we spent a week or two with the person concerned. Sometimes these links to contributing factors and states of ill health are clear, as in the case of the links between a poor diet and obesity leading to heart disease, between a lifestyle that involves extended periods of sunbaking, or working outdoors without adequate protection, leading to excessive UV exposure which in turn is the major risk factor for skin cancer. Sometimes the links are tenuous and circumstantial, as in the case of links between asthma attacks and allergies associated with a person's way of life.

Below these, well below the surface and hard to observe without further investigation, are the determinants that structure and impact on the way people live their lives, the determinants of their lifestyles and behaviours. These hidden determinants include psychological, social, cultural, environmental, economic, and political factors. We may not even be aware of how these factors influence our actions, the sorts of lives we live, the social and economic conditions we strive for, or our eventual health status. In figure 12.1 separate lists are given for factors at population levels (such as cultural norms, health-related opportunities available to people, and access to community resources) and at the level of individuals (such as an individual's resources, beliefs, values, attitudes, knowledge, and skills).

It is this underlying level of the iceberg that we generally need to focus on if we are to take effective action to promote health—it contains the 'real' determinants of people's health, often termed the 'upstream' determinants (box 12.1). We will return to this point after looking at an example of analysing a

Box 12.1 'Upstream' determinants

'There I am standing by the shore of a swiftly flowing river and I hear the cry of a drowning man. So I jump into the river, put my arms around him, pull him to shore and apply artificial respiration. Just when he begins to breathe, there is another cry for help. So I jump into the river, reach him, pull him to shore, apply artificial respiration, and then just as he begins to breathe, there is another cry for help. So back into the river again, without end, goes the sequence. You know I am too busy jumping in, pulling them to shore, applying artificial respiration, that I have no time to see who the hell is upstream pushing them all in.'

McKinlay 1979

health issue using the iceberg (figure 12.2). While not necessarily comprehensive in this example, it gives you an idea of how the levels of the iceberg can be used to identify determinants of health and illness.

Three things become obvious in looking at figure 12.2. First, the lists grow longer as we go to lower levels of the iceberg, down to the psycho-socio-cultural determinants of health. There are clearly many factors that influence how people live their lives and there are many social factors that directly affect people's health. Second, we can advance from one layer of the iceberg down to the next by asking the question 'Why'? Why is someone at risk of heart disease? Because they are overweight? Why is he or she overweight? Because they do little exercise? Why so

Figure 12.2   The determinants of heart health

State of Health: Heart disease

Contributing Factors: High blood pressure
>   Elevated cholesterol
>   Overweight/obese
>   Smoking
>   Family history of heart disease

Lifestyle Behaviours: Lack of exercise: busy life with little time for exercise; uses the car for all local and distant travel
>   Works long hours
>   Lots of takeaway foods/eating out
>   Going to pubs and clubs where smoking is the norm
>   Unemployed and spends much of the time at home watching TV

Psycho-socio-cultural Determinants:
>   No interest in participating in physical activity—boring, not for me, too hard
>   Grew up in a family where physical activity was not valued
>   Employer expectations/requirements to work long hours
>   Poor experiences of competitive sport at school
>   Lack of a comprehensive physical education program at school
>   Fear of looking silly/incompetent during physical activity
>   No convenient, safe or affordable facilities for activity
>   Smoking is normal behaviour/valued among friends and family
>   Smoking is affordable in comparison to other activities
>   Low income so cannot afford a range of healthy foods
>   Lack of knowledge of healthy diet
>   Poor food preparation skills
>   Belief that it won't happen to me or that if anything does happen doctors will be able to fix it
>   No one to exercise with
>   Can't afford to join a gym
>   Poor body image prevents them joining others in public physical activity
>   Watches lots of TV and so sees many commercials for unhealthy products
>   Unemployed and so little money and poor self image
>   In a job where there is quite a bit of stress and little opportunity to make decisions about work

little exercise? Because they have no time, or because they are embarrassed about body shape, or because there are few facilities available in the local community for safe participation in activity, or … Third, many of the determinants we have identified for heart disease are common to a number of other health conditions, such as diabetes and a number of cancers. This contrasts with the way much of our health system is organised and funded around priority health issues and risk behaviours, such as smoking, leading to 'silos' of health sector funding and activity, where there is little linkage between programs that need to address the same powerful upstream determinants of health.

In figure 12.2, you can start to see the intervention points that heart health promotion programs might target. We could concentrate on the 'risk/contributing factor' level and put out lots of brochures and posters telling people that for the sake of their heart health they should reduce their weight or their blood pressure. Or we could go to the next level, and have materials promoting a healthy diet or being physically active. And we do all of this in health promotion—you will all have seen such materials in your local area and at health services. But health promotion has often been criticised for leaving the 'job' there, as if the determinant of people's health behaviour is simply a lack of awareness. When we move to the bottom layer of the iceberg, however, we begin to find the factors that we need to target if we want to make a difference. So to plan an effective health promotion initiative to address heart health, we would need to identify and target the factors at the level of the individuals in a specific population (e.g. their knowledge, skills, beliefs, attitudes) and at the population level (e.g. resources and opportunities in the community for people to be physically active, cultural norms around eating, the settings in which people live, work and play, and policy at government and organisational level). Developing an integrated heart health program to address a bank of these factors is certain to be more effective than simply targeting the knowledge and skills of individuals.

This leads us to some important points about health promotion:

- In order to address the broad range of determinants of health, health promotion needs to involve combinations of strategies and approaches, not just one-off programs.
- People will only take action about the determinants of their health if they have an active role in decisions and self-determining action. Community participation is a key element of health promotion. Thus health promotion works *with* and *for* people, not *on* them.
- Since many of the determinants of health lie outside the responsibility of the health sector, effective health promotion relies on collaborations and partnerships between different sectors of the community and workforce.

The iceberg provides a useful model of the determinants of health, particularly for aspects of health that are linked to our lifestyles. But it is a simple model, and you will recognise that it does not readily lead us to the complexity of determinants of health.

Table 12.1 The five action areas of the Ottawa Charter for Health Promotion

1 BUILD HEALTHY PUBLIC POLICY	2 CREATE SUPPORTIVE ENVIRONMENTS	3 STRENGTHEN COMMUNITY ACTION	4 DEVELOP PERSONAL SKILLS	5 REORIENT HEALTH SERVICES
Smoke-free workplace policies	More bike paths	Peer education in the gay community	Safe sex education in schools	Incidental counselling by general practitioners about smoking or physical activity
Pool-fencing laws	Syringe disposal bins in public places	Women's health groups	Pre-driver education	
No hat, no play policies in schools	Safe water supply	Local environmental action groups	Diabetes management education	Breast cancer screening programs
Bicycle-helmet laws	Shaded areas in schools for play and sport	Alcoholics anonymous groups	Cooking skills classes for older men	Brochures and information sheets available on a range of health issues
Improved safety requirements for cars	Greater availability of low-fat, low-salt foods	Breast cancer support groups	Physical education classes	
Requirements for nutrition labelling on food products	Alcohol-free dances for under 18s	Community setting up walking groups	Community education on 'slip, slop, slap'	Multidisciplinary teams in health services
Reducing taxes on low-alcohol beer	Access ramps for people in wheelchairs	Patient rights and consumer groups	Stress management programs	Medicare
Drink-drive laws	OK to talk about sexual activity publicly	Youth groups organising alcohol-free events	Parenting courses	Divisions of General Practice contributing to community health education and promotion
Environmental protection laws and regulations	Making smoking socially unacceptable	Local action to establish alcohol-free Indigenous communities	QUIT courses	
Occupational health and safety laws	Establishing a community attitude that if you drink and drive, you're a bloody idiot	Young mothers' groups	Teaching IDUs safe injecting techniques	Health promoting hospitals
Antibullying policies in schools and workplaces				

TAKING ACTION ON THE DETERMINANTS OF HEALTH

Now that we have investigated the determinants of health, we can consider what people need in order to be able to take action on these determinants. This is the work of health promotion.

The Ottawa Charter for Heath Promotion presents five domains for health promotion action that will help people to be able to have greater control over their health. Examples of actions in each of these domains are given in table 12.1. You could add more examples from your own knowledge and experience. See also chapter 10 for more details on these five domains.

In working to achieve its five action areas, the Ottawa Charter identifies three key roles for health promotion workers: *enabling*, *mediating*, and *advocating*, which are covered in detail in chapter 10. Box 12.2 presents a case study about the actions that can arise within a community when people work together to address conditions adverse to healthy living.

Box 12.2   Community action: people power

A new subdivision on the outer fringe of the city had a delightful bush feel, with tree-lined streets and public spaces. What it did not have, however, were footpaths, since the Council had not required the developer to include hard surface pavements in their plans. Young mums with prams and toddlers, children walking to school, young children on bicycles, and people exercising their dogs, were all forced to walk on the unsealed verges of the local streets. After several reported near misses between vehicles and pedestrians, a group of parents from the local primary school decided it was time to take action. They formed a Resident's Action Group, and co-opted the school principal, local maternal and childcare nurse, church representatives, bicycle user's group, and the senior citizen's management committee. They held a meeting, and strategically planned their course of action. They wrote letters to the local newspaper, mayor, and parliamentary representative. They held a public meeting to raise awareness and invite support. A petition was organised as a result of that meeting, and was presented to the Council. A carefully worded letter accompanied this petition, drawing attention to the Council's own Municipal Health Plan, which proclaimed a commitment to creating supportive environments. The letter pointed out that the Council was clearly failing to do so with respect to pedestrian safety, and it was also failing to provide opportunities for people to be physically active near where they lived. The Council eventually agreed to build hard-surface shared footways for pedestrians and cyclists on one side of each road and street in the subdivision.

Health promotion practice thus spans a broad range of actions with an even broader ranger of players. We will explore health promotion practice further by examining two case studies in areas where Australia is a world leader: road trauma and health promoting schools.

CASE STUDY 1: ROAD TRAUMA

Figure 12.3 Injury mortality in Australian males, 1924–99

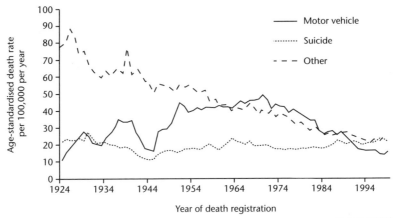

Source: AIHW 2002b

Figure 12.3 shows a clear increase in road deaths in Australia for most of the twentieth century as car ownership rapidly grew. At that time, motor vehicle accidents (MVA) accounted for a large proportion of all death due to injury. But it is clear that since the 1970s, there has been a significant decrease in MVA deaths in Australia, even though both the total number of vehicles on our roads and the total distance they cover have continued to rise (AIHW 2002b). To set figure 12.3 in some context, the decrease in MVA deaths since the 1970s in just one state, Victoria, translates to an additional 650 people alive every year, and over 6000 people not suffering serious injury.

What has caused this amazing and rapid decline in our road toll? How did it come about, and was it planned or did it just happen? If we were to construct an iceberg around this health issue, we would list many determinants of motor ve-hicle accidents in the bottom layer, both in relation to individuals and the com-munity. People's attitudes and behaviours in relation to speed, drink driving, road behaviour, and risk taking are clearly important. So are the knowledge and skills of drivers. And of course the design of our roads and cars can have a major impact on road safety, as does the availability of public transport as an alterna-tive to driving. Figure 12.4 (see p. 178) gives an indication of the impact of some of the actions that have been taken to lower the road toll.

To think about this in health promotion terms, it is useful to categorise some of these initiatives under the five action areas of the Ottawa Charter. Box 2.3

Figure 12.4   Victorian road toll 1970 to 2000⁺

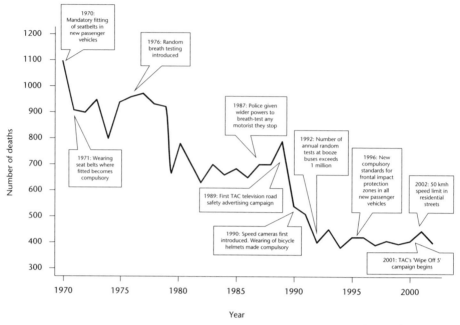

Source: The *Age* 2002

provides an insight into the applications of the Ottawa Charter action areas to the road safety context.

The public health actions taken in Australia to reduce the road toll give us a clear picture of the nature of contemporary health promotion:

- It is based on a sophisticated system of data collection to learn more about the issue and the impact of action that has been taken. In the case of road trauma, there are comprehensive data collections on aspects such as mortality and morbidity, accident black spots, data from speed cameras, data on breathalyser testing, surveys of driver attitudes and behaviours, crash testing of new vehicles, and the characteristics of drivers involved in motor accidents. These are all determinants of road accidents.
- Australia has adopted multilevel, multicomponent strategies that target a broad range of the determinants of this health issue.
- There has been active engagement with communities, and collaborations and partnerships across sectors. In this case, intersectoral action has brought together the police, the court system, local government, road authorities, education systems, employers and unions, the alcohol industry, and car designers and manufacturers.
- There has been a deliberate effort to keep the community well informed about the health issue and the actions taken to address it.
- The action taken to address the health issue has been sustained over a number of years. One-off interventions are seldom likely to be effective.

Box 12.3 Road safety measures: the action areas of the Ottawa Charter

Building healthy public policy
- Collaboration between key stakeholders including road-traffic authorities, insurers, police, car manufacturers, local government, and other sectors, to continually seek ways to enhance road safety through new laws and policies.
- Drink-driving and speeding legislation (penalties include fines, loss of license and demerit points for transgression).
- Enforcement mechanisms to deter unsafe road user behaviour, including speed cameras, red-light cameras, and random breath-testing.
- Legislation to make it compulsory to wear seat belts in cars (Australia was the first country in the world to use this action).
- Annual road-worthiness certification for certain vehicles (e.g. tourism transport buses).
- Policies in sporting clubs, hotels, and bars concerning responsible serving of alcohol.

Creating supportive environments (this refers to both social and physical environments)
- Improvement to road design and construction (e.g. accident blackspot identification).
- Improved lighting and traffic management systems.
- Improved car safety design (e.g. crumple zones, airbags, ABS braking systems).
- Mass media campaigns to gradually create a shift in societal attitudes (e.g. towards drink driving, risk taking and driver fatigue).
- Having a range of low-alcohol alternatives available in licensed premises and encouraging their consumption.
- Gathering data that informs the development of road safety policies and programs.

Strengthening community action (i.e. actions taken by community members rather than campaigns or interventions that target the community)
- Creation of Community Road Safety Councils. This involves building partnerships between local government, police, road traffic authorities, parent groups, cycling groups, and other sectors. These councils have addressed local road safety and traffic management issues.
- Lobbying for improved public transport, safer transport, and bicycle lanes.

- Creation of Walking Bus programs. This involves adults/parents escorting children to school on foot via a designated route. They collect children along the way, as a bus would. This enhances the safety of participants, is physically active, and socially connecting.

Developing personal skills
- Programs to improve driver skills (e.g. more comprehensive learner driver guidelines, pre-driver education, improved licensed testing procedures) and mass media campaigns to promote safer practices on the road.
- Bike Ed and Cycle On cycling programs in primary and secondary schools.
- Computer interactive simulated driver programs to improve decision-making skills.
- Alcohol education programs in schools and other community settings.

Reorienting health services
- Development of quicker and more effective responses from road trauma teams resulting in many lives being saved.
- Medical associations and doctors advocating for road safety measures.
- Road trauma teams participating in media awareness-raising efforts regarding the dangers of drink driving and speeding.

SETTINGS APPROACHES TO HEALTH

Now that we have established some of the characteristics of health promotion practice, it is clear that health promotion is quite different from curative medical services in the way it is practised—people don't go along to a 'health promotion centre' for a health promotion treatment. Rather, health promotion practitioners seek to work with people in the contexts of their everyday lives. Health promotion recognises the idea that people live in social, cultural, political, economic, and environmental contexts. Ilona Kickbusch, former Director of Health Promotion for WHO, summed up this important characteristic of health promotion:

An ecological approach (to public health) ... starts with the basic and simple question: where is health created? The ecological answer—in the language of everyday—is health is created where people live, love, work and play. It is created by human beings in their interactions with each other and with their physical environments. The consequence for a public health strategy is to commence from the settings of everyday life within which health is created (rather than start with disease categories) and to begin with strengthening the health potential of the respective settings.

Kickbusch 1989a

Kickbusch points out the importance for health of the settings in which people live their lives: schools, workplaces, hospitals, communities, parks and gardens, prisons, and sporting organisations, to name just some. The health world has used such settings for a long time, seeing them as a geographical area or an organisation containing a captive audience to which health messages and programs can be delivered effectively: schools are good places to educate children; and shopping centres are good places to deliver health information to the general public.

Kickbusch, however, makes an important point—settings themselves can have a direct impact on health. Many aspects of workplaces and work can impact considerably on the health of workers, either positively or negatively: for example, work-related stress; job satisfaction; work-based harassment; hazardous equipment and chemicals; feedback and involvement in decision making; shift work; passive smoke inhalation in the office; feelings of being appreciated and of belonging; and policies on flexible work hours and family leave to care for sick children.

An important aspect of 'settings' is that most of them lie outside the formal health sector. They are the responsibilities of many different organisations and groups, who are unlikely to have health as their prime concern. This has two important implications:

- Health promotion in these settings must be intersectoral in nature, bringing together the major stakeholders.
- In working in and with these organisations, we need to take account of the priorities, structures, and dynamics of the setting.

The earliest examples of a purposeful settings approach to health promotion are the Healthy Cities projects that developed from the late 1980s under the auspices of WHO EURO. The network of WHO 'healthy cities' has grown to include a number in Australia, including Canberra and Noarlunga in South Australia. But other formal settings approaches have also developed, with health promoting schools being the most prominent.

CASE STUDY 2: HEALTH PROMOTING SCHOOLS

The 'health promoting school' (HPS) has emerged during the 1990s as a promising and cost-effective framework for enhancing the health of students and their families (Jones et al. 1995; St Leger 1998). Schools represent the only public institution that reaches nearly every young person in Australia and they often have considerable and extended contact with students' families. Over the last decade, we have seen shifts from simple health teaching and school linkages to specific child health care services (e.g. immunisation) towards health promotion programs run in, with, and by schools. More recently, schools are considering how their day-to-day operations can change to create a more health promoting setting (Rowling 1996).

At an international level, WHO has provided considerable leadership in the development of HPSs. WHO EURO has been responsible for the establishment of networks of HPSs in thirty-seven countries to provide a framework for innovations in health promotion and mechanisms for dissemination of good practice (St Leger 1998; Thomas et al. 1998). The WHO Western Pacific Regional Office has developed comprehensive guidelines to support its thirty-two member countries develop the health promoting capacity of their schools (WHO 1996).

Within Australia, the National Health and Medical Research Council has developed a rationale and direction for HPSs (NHMRC 1997) and a significant number of school-based health promotion initiatives have been funded by most states. Formal and informal networks of HPSs can be identified both at state and national levels. The Australian Health Promoting Schools Association (AHPSA) operates nationally to support, and advocate for, HPSs and to increase intersectoral collaboration around school health. In contrast to the European networks, school membership of Australian HPS networks or AHPSA does not involve selection based around meeting formal criteria. Rather, Australia has developed a more open approach, encouraging all schools to see themselves as being on the path towards operating as a HPS.

In Australia, Rowling has defined health promoting schools broadly as having 'an organised set of policies, procedures, activities and structures designed to protect and promote the health and wellbeing of students, staff and wider school community members' (Rowling 1996). A number of frameworks have been developed in Australia to operationalise this definition of a HPS, and these can be simplified to three major aspects of school operations (Marshall et al. 2000) as shown in figure 12.5:

- the school's health curriculum, and the nature of the teaching and learning processes occurring in classrooms
- the ethos and organisation of the school, including its social and physical environments and its policy framework
- the links and interactions between the school and its families and community, including partnerships with health-related services and agencies.

Figure 12.5 The health promoting schools framework

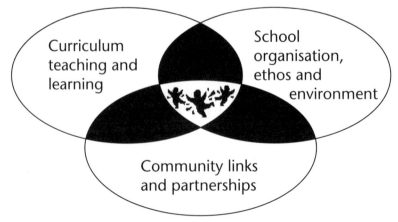

Source: Deakin University and Department of Education Employment and Training 2000

It is clear that these three aspects encourage a far broader approach than the health education role that used to underpin the work of schools in respect of student health. Interventions that combine classroom activities with changes to the school's environment, and with work in the school community (including parents and health services) have been shown to be more effective than educational

Table 12.2 Health promoting schools in action

CURRICULUM TEACHING AND LEARNING	COMMUNITY LINKS AND PARTNERSHIPS	SCHOOL ORGANISATION, ETHOS AND ENVIRONMENT
• Include study of antidiscrimination and harassment in curriculum.	• Build partnerships with parents.	• Implement effective welfare support and management strategies.
• Include resilience and coping strategies in curriculum.	• Build partnerships with health and other services in the locality.	• Implement effective behaviour management policies.
• Include understanding mental illness, stigma, grief, and loss in curriculum.	• Foster links with sporting, creative arts, performing arts, and leisure groups in the community.	• Offer opportunities for peer support, leadership. and citizenship.
• Encourage positive, caring, and supportive teacher–student relationships.	• Forge links with community groups and organisations (e.g. support meals on wheels for seniors, collect for charitable organisations such as the Red Cross, participate in peer support programs with feeder primary schools).	• Celebrate the diversity of the school community population.
• Build collaborative approaches to teaching and learning.		• Work to create safe, attractive, and functional physical spaces that promote the social, intellectual, physical, and mental wellbeing of the school population.
• Create positive class-room environments where students can learn in a safe yet challenging climate.	• Implement effective transition programs from primary to secondary, and from secondary to post-school education, training and workplaces.	• Recognise that the well-being of the staff will impact on that of the students (e.g. offer professional development in resilience, leadership, and conflict resolution).
• Include student initiatives and interests in the teaching program.		• Commit to transparent and collaborative decision-making processes.

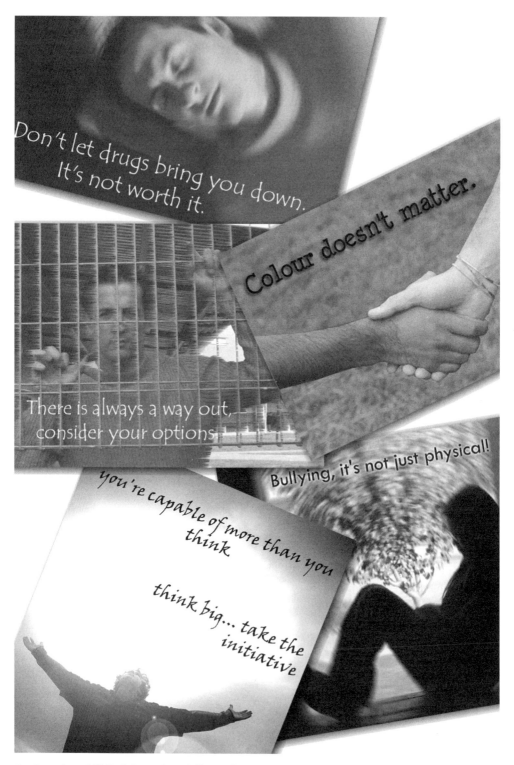

Students from Mill Park Secondary College take action to creatively promote positive mental health interventions alone (NHMRC 1997; Lister-Sharp et al. 1999; Ridge et al. 2000; Wagner 2002). Some of the many ways in which schools have implemented the HPS initiative are listed in table 12.2.

An example of this comprehensive approach to school health is the MindMatters project, a national mental health promotion in secondary schools program funded by the Commonwealth Department of Health and Ageing under the National Mental Health Strategy and the National Youth Suicide Prevention Strategy. The case study shown in box 12.4 exemplifies how one school actively involved the students in promoting positive mental health within the school community.

Box 12.4   Promoting mental health in a school setting

After attending a MindMatters Conference, the student welfare coordinator decided to more actively promote positive mental health around the senior campus. However, commercial posters and other resource materials were either too expensive or not necessarily relevant to the issues confronting her students. She approached the school's media department about getting the students actively involved in developing more appropriate posters for their context. The Year 11 media studies class embraced the project and worked as a collaborative team in identifying the mental health promotion issues of concern to their peers. They then worked to create images and key messages in poster format that they believed would really speak to the school community. Their work is currently displayed at both the senior and junior campuses, with one poster also being selected to promote the school's caring social environment in the wider community. Students have observed that they are now more aware of underlying issues around mental health promotion, and that they are proud of their work and feel empowered from their involvement in this initiative.

Source: Verbal report from Janine Pike, Student Welfare Coordinator, Mill Park Secondary College. A sample of the work produced can be seen on p. 184.

SUMMARY

- Health promotion is a broad field of activity, ranging from actions that are essentially medically focused and individual (such as individual risk-factor assessment and counselling) to actions aimed at helping people to change their behaviour, and further along to actions that seek to create supportive environments and settings that address a broad range of social and environmental determinants of health.

- There is a fundamental requirement for health promotion to address inequalities in health, to address the social determinants of health, and to promote community engagement.
- This is a challenging agenda, but essential if health promotion is to move beyond preaching to the converted and working with those members of the community whose health needs and interests are already well catered for.

DISCUSSION TOPICS

1 Select a setting such as a tertiary institution, your local community or workplace. Within this setting, whose health needs are most likely to be met and whose needs are likely *not* to be met? Who are the *most* vulnerable?

2 How might you *enable, mediate,* and *advocate* with respect to vulnerable groups in the setting you have just identified? In what ways did people use the skills of enabling, mediating, and advocating in the community action outlined in the case study described in box 12.2?

3 What upstream strategies should now be considered in the continuous fight to reduce the impact of road trauma on the community?

4 Consider the examples presented in table 12.2. Can you think of other initiatives that demonstrate a holistic approach to health in the school setting? Now categorise the examples given according to the Jakarta Declaration (see box 10.8).

USEFUL WEB SITE

MindMatters: www.curriculum.edu.au/mindmatters

HEALTH EDUCATION AND COMMUNICATION STRATEGIES

Berni Murphy

Key concepts

- Health literacy: a determinant of health
- Health literacy and empowerment
- Developing effective health education programs
- Behaviour-change health communication strategies

The Framework for Health Promotion Action presented in chapter 11 identified a range of interventions that seek to improve the health of individuals, communities, and populations. This chapter reviews midstream interventions from that framework, being *health education* and *communication strategies*, and examines the contribution of these interventions to the five action areas of the Ottawa Charter (WHO 1986a), and to the Jakarta Declaration (WHO 1997a).

HEALTH LITERACY: A DETERMINANT OF HEALTH

Access to information and education has long been recognised as a powerful determinant of health. Communication strategies have been utilised to raise awareness of health issues and to persuade individuals to make healthier choices. Health education programs attempt to go further, in that they aim to develop the knowledge, understanding, and personal skills of program participants to enable them to make informed decisions to enhance their health. However, the extent to which individuals attend to the health information presented, understand it, and can apply it to their own contexts is largely dependent on their health literacy.

Fundamentally, **health literacy** is about being sufficiently educated to access and use information that can impact on health status. This can manifest in a range of ways at the individual level, including being able to read labels on food packaging and medicines, being able to understand health information presented in posters, brochures and on medical forms, and being able to follow written and verbal instructions. It is also about having the personal skills to know what to ask and where to find the answers. Further, it is about making informed choices based on a capacity to integrate health information with personal values. In this sense, health literacy provides individuals with options that would otherwise not be available to them. With health information becoming more available through the Internet, the ability to search for and filter credible health web sites now introduces a new dimension to the concept of health literacy.

HEALTH LITERACY AND EMPOWERMENT

Higher levels of health literacy within communities are likely to lead to a collective deeper understanding of social, environmental, organisational and political factors that impact on health. Community members are likely to be more *empowered* to engage in debates around local health issues, and more *enabled* to collaborate with others in *advocating* for change at community and government level, thus supporting the original intent of the Ottawa Charter. Targeting health communication and education interventions at decision makers rather than just at individuals can provide the impetus to challenge existing policies and practices deleterious to the health of communities and populations. For instance, such interventions targeted at the organisational level through professional development short courses, can build the collective health literacy and capacity of the workforce across sectors to address social and health issues. Such has been the case with workforce development strategies implemented by the Department of Human Services (DHS) across Victoria since 2000. A key element of this strategy has been to create environments through these short courses that foster workforce networks and partnerships conducive to more collaborative intersectoral responses to community health concerns.

Striving for high levels of health literacy within communities is therefore also consistent with the Jakarta Declaration's Third and Fourth Priorities for Health Promotion: 'to consolidate and expand partnerships for health', and 'to increase community capacity and empower the individual' (WHO 1997a). Conversely, low levels of health literacy serve to reinforce existing social and health inequities, by excluding disadvantaged and marginalised individuals and groups from information and services that could enhance their social and health outcomes across the life span.

HEALTH EDUCATION

Health education and health promotion are sometimes incorrectly used as interchangeable terms. However, a review of the Framework for Health Promotion Action in chapter 11 clearly positions health education as a subset of health promotion, and therefore *one* of several interventions available to the health promoter.

Health education is a particularly valuable tool in the clinical setting, where health professionals are often required to work one-to-one, or in small groups with clients, around prevention and rehabilitation issues.

Health education programs can be very effective in assisting people to develop the knowledge, understanding and personal skills that can enhance their health. Further, the sense of empowerment that participants experience from appropriate and sensitively planned programs, can have a ripple effect beyond the health domain to other facets of their lives. For instance, Keleher and Murphy (2002) contend that 'the gaining of new social skills can lead to increased social competence, confidence and income generation' (p. 24).

Health education programs must therefore do more than simply tell people what they need to *know*, and what they must *do* in order to be healthier. Such programs have the potential to be patronising, can be driven by the values of the health educator, and can inadvertently lead in victim blaming. Programs that focus on a single health issue such as diabetes, or a risk behaviour such as poor nutrition, are particularly prone to being expert driven, less inclusive, and less respectful of the participant's context. Though the facilitators might feel confident that they have successfully delivered the 'must know' content in such programs, evaluations routinely indicate that participants do not necessarily feel empowered or motivated to make healthier choices, even though they are now more knowledgeable. Whenever participant investment and a sense of ownership is absent from a program, the evidence points to disappointing outcomes.

Principles of effective health education programs

If we are to conduct health education programs that are consistent with the Ottawa Charter's intent to develop personal skills and to enable participants to make healthier choices (WHO 1986a), and with the Jakarta Declaration's priority to increase community capacity and empower the individual (WHO 1997a), then the principles listed in box 13.1 should apply.

Box 13.1   Principles of effective health education programs

- The program is carefully planned to incorporate and attend to the needs of the group.
- The program is culturally sensitive and appropriate.
- The planning process incorporates recognition of the social contexts in which people live their lives.
- The planning process incorporates recognition of the impact of determinants on participants' attitudes, behaviours, and capacity to make healthier choices.

- The facilitators recognise that the entry-level knowledge base will vary across the group.
- The facilitators work to engage, empower, and enable the participants.
- The facilitators recognise and respect the different values, attitudes, and beliefs that participants will bring to the health education program.
- The facilitators do not preach or chastise participants for their beliefs or choices.
- The facilitators encourage and value the input of participants throughout the program, and recognise their life experiences as being relevant.
- The key messages are explained in plain language, illustrated with visual support (e.g. diagrams, graphs, photos), and reinforced with exemplars relevant to the audience.
- The program increases the knowledge and understanding of participants around broad and specific issues impacting on their health.
- The program increases the skills of the group to make healthier choices and to take actions at both the individual and community level that are likely to improve social and health outcomes.

Planning effective health education programs

The planning process is clearly vital in developing and implementing effective health education programs. Further, the concept of program planning must not merely be confined to such issues as the number of participants invited to attend the program, the venue, the duration of the program, the materials required, and so forth. These administrative elements must of course be spot on. But health education planning must involve much more than just attention to program administration. The planning cycle must attend to three key elements: *administration*, *content*, and *process*, with *content* referring to the knowledge base to be included in the program, and *process* referring to how it is to be delivered.

The program designers must be clear about the actual purpose of the program. What are the objectives, and how can they best be achieved? What do they hope to accomplish by the end of the program? The Framework for Developing Effective Health Education Programs presented in figure 13.1 provides a useful tool for guiding the development of health education programs.

This framework highlights the importance of undertaking a series of discrete yet interrelated steps in the planning process. The program designers must first analyse and understand the health issue/s from a determinants of health perspective. They must then consider the question: What is realistically possible with respect to the scope of the program? Next, the planning process must involve developing an understanding of the target group, its needs, expectations, and learning preferences. During this stage of planning, several questions must be answered, such as: What style of delivery would best suit this group and this issue? Is a lecture delivery style appropriate in this instance, or would a more

Figure 13.1   Framework for developing effective health education programs

Framework for Developing Effective Health Education Programs

WHY

Why is this health issue a problem?
Analyse the health issue/s within the context of a determinants of health model. What are the underlying causes of the problem/s? Can the health education program improve personal skills and also impact in some way on the underlying determinants? Consider what is realistically possible.

WHO

Consider the target group
What are the needs and expectations of the group?
What are their values, attitudes, and beliefs?
What are their learning preferences?

WHAT

What do you hope to achieve?
What will be different for this group at the end of the program?
Establish aims and learning objectives for the program.

HOW

How will you implement an effective education program?
What delivery methods best suit the issues and the group (e.g. lecture, peer education, experiential learning, group process, reflection)?
What content? What must the participants know at the conclusion of the session?
What activities are suited to the learning objectives, the participants, and the venue?
What resources do you need to run the program?

EFFECTIVE?

How will you know your program has been successful?
Have you met your aims and objectives?
What criteria will you use to measure success?
What went well and what would you do differently next time?

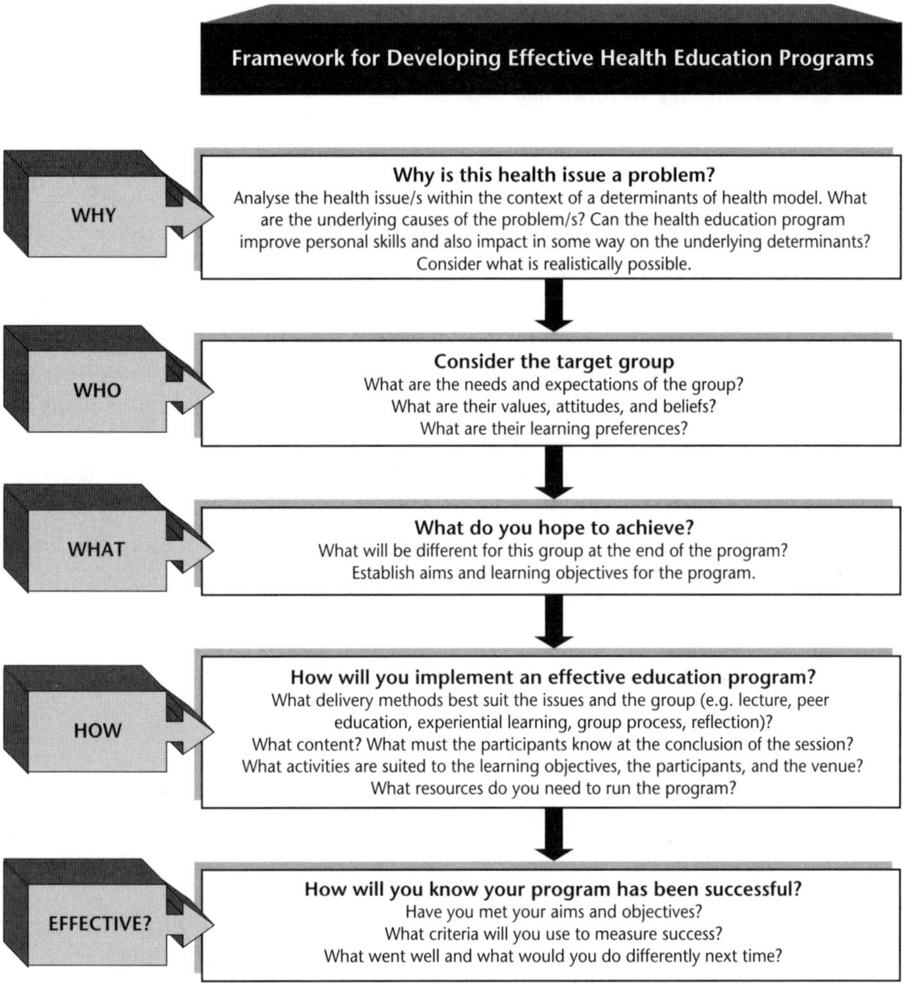

Source: Murphy, B. 2002

relaxed and interactive approach create an atmosphere conducive to facilitating learning? What content *must* be included? What activities and resources would best support the selected delivery style?

It is important to note that most people learn best by *doing*, in challenging yet safe learning environments. Why is it then that so many health educators resort to noninteractive, didactic, delivery modes? The answer is that this mode often suits the expert who is delivering the program. But expert-driven lectures are not necessarily the most effective or appropriate means of getting a message across. The needs and preferences of the group should be paramount in deciding on the most appropriate approach in this regard. While attending to administration and content goes partway to delivering the message, the skilled health educator will recognise that it is the decisions about process issues that will determine whether the message is heard. Finally, health educators intent on delivering effective programs will also recognise the value of building an evaluation strategy into their planning cycle, and in so doing, will commit to an ongoing review of the program and its capacity to influence change.

Measuring the effectiveness of health education programs

Health education program evaluation must be more than a token review of the basic aspects involved in conducting the program. Such evaluations routinely seek to report on the fundamentals. How many attended? Were they satisfied with the program? Did they take resource materials away with them? Much of this information is often gathered by a so-called 'happy sheet' or evaluation form, completed by participants at the end of the program. But what does this information really tell us? While this information is critical to ensuring the program reaches the target group and is pitched at the right level, the evaluation must not end there.

The evaluation strategy needs also to measure whether the learner has achieved the impacts we are seeking. This question encourages us to consider changes the learner experiences with respect to the following:
- knowledge
- ideas/thoughts/decisions
- thinking processes/perceptions
- feelings and values
- actions/behaviours
- performance, competence, or skill. (adapted from Kirkpatrick 1994)

Some of the methods commonly utilised to measure these changes include observation, and pre- and post-testing. Focus group interviews are useful in exploring changes in knowledge and attitudes, as well as *intent* to change behaviour. Alternatively, participants might be asked to record their behaviour changes and/or reflections in a personal diary. This is often the case with respect to nutrition and weight management programs.

Regardless of the methodology employed, the purpose of the evaluation process is twofold: to measure the *effectiveness* of the program in meeting its objectives; and to measure the *impact* of the program on the participants in the short, medium and longer term. In addition, uncovering the prevailing barriers to sustained impact can serve to further inform planning and enhance program effectiveness. Experienced health educators often chant the mantra 'what went well and what would I do differently next time?' While this statement is simplistic, the message is nevertheless important: health educators must continually seek to improve the administration, content, and processes of their programs, and in so doing strive to deliver effective health education programs that can genuinely make a difference to social and health inequities.

BEHAVIOUR-CHANGE HEALTH COMMUNICATION STRATEGIES

Lifestyles and health behaviours that contribute to adverse health outcomes first became the target for health promotion interventions during the later part of the twentieth century. Health messages were delivered with a scattergun approach through various mass media channels, under a social marketing banner. These messages were designed to raise awareness of the consequences of sedentary lifestyles and unhealthy risk behaviours such as smoking cigarettes, sunbaking,

Table 13.1   Strengths and limitations of behaviour change communication strategies

STRENGTHS	LIMITATIONS
Can raise awareness of unhealthy lifestyles and behaviours.	Awareness raising can further marginalise those in the target group.
Can discourage unhealthy behaviours while offering alternative healthier options.	Can be unappealing to those living *in the moment*, in that the campaign expects people to give up behaviours they enjoy now, in order to avoid adverse health outcomes in years to come.
Has the potential to reach mass audiences.	Capacity to reach marginalised and disadvantaged groups is often less evident.
Has the potential to affect behaviour change among literate individuals, with supportive networks and reasonable locus of control.	Has limited impact on more vulnerable individuals and groups, particularly those of lower socioeconomic status, with less education, weaker support networks, and less control over their lives.
Is a cost-effective prevention strategy when incorporated with complementary and integrated interventions.	Can be a pretext for noninvestment in infrastructure and systems changes that are likely to have the greatest impact on health.
Well-designed programs can be very persuasive.	Ill-conceived campaigns can be driven by the values of health promoters, and can be coercive rather than persuasive.
Can create a climate conducive to societal and infrastructure/systems change, particularly when determinants of health are incorporated into intervention planning processes.	Can ignore the underlying determinants of health and attribute responsibility for health outcomes entirely to the individual choice.

and drink driving. Many of these campaigns were based on the assumption that simply raising awareness of the risks of unhealthy behaviours would influence miscreants to adopt healthier practices. The role of underlying determinants and contexts in these health communication campaigns were either not well understood or ignored. Instead, the health behaviour-change messages were kept simple: stop doing what you are doing, even though you might enjoy it!

In order to understand the role that behaviour-change communication can play in contemporary health promotion, it is important to first acknowledge the strengths and inherent limitations of this type of intervention. Table 13.1 presents a summary of some of these strengths and limitations.

It would appear that the *impetus* for conducting a campaign, in many instances, shapes the format the campaign takes, and is a key indicator of its potential impact. For example, if the purpose is to address a single risk factor or multiple risk factors that are recognised as contributing to the burden of disease, then the campaign is more likely to be a **silo** or stand-alone intervention, exclusively focused on persuading individuals to change their behaviours. The role of the underlying determinants of health, or the contexts in which people live their lives, is not considered or incorporated into these intervention strategies. The evidence suggests that the impact of such approaches is often limited to more literate individuals, who exhibit reasonable locus of control, have access to supportive networks, and are motivated to adopt healthier practices in the first place. However, research further indicates that people from lower socioeconomic backgrounds, who have weaker support networks, and less control over their lives, are in fact less likely to be influenced to either adopt behaviour changes, or to sustain any attempts to modify unhealthy practices. This is particularly the case when the individual habitually relies upon the behaviour as a coping mechanism (e.g. smoking cigarettes or drinking alcohol).

If, however, the initial motivation for conducting a health communication campaign is to address social and health inequities, the shape the campaign takes is likely to be very different. In this instance the health behaviour-change message is likely to be one of several complementary and integrated strategies drawn from the breadth of the health promotion action spectrum. An example of how such an integrated approach might take shape is:

- The behaviour-change communication strategy is developed to raise awareness of adverse health outcomes associated with risky or unhealthy choices.
- Follow-up phases of the campaign propose healthier options, while continuing to discourage unhealthy choices.
- The campaign is sensitively planned and will *not* create an atmosphere of victim blaming.
- The campaign is supported by constructive health education programs.
- Opportunities are specifically created for community engagement and empowerment.
- The campaign incorporates communication strategies targeting decision makers rather than individuals. In this sense, communication strategies are used as an effective tool to advocate for upstream change.

- A climate conducive to infrastructure and systems change is promoted, understanding that this might take years or even decades, as was the case with tobacco control in Australia.

MODELS FOR HEALTH BEHAVIOUR CHANGE

With table 13.1 in mind, let us now examine some of the more popular models for health behaviour change communication. Brief case studies from local and global contexts have been included to illustrate key points.

KAB: knowledge, attitude, behaviour change

The belief that increased *knowledge* will lead to an *attitudinal change*, which will in turn lead to a *behaviour change*, has underpinned many behaviour change interventions over the years. Figure 13.2 is a diagrammatic representation of the KAB model.

Figure 13.2   KAB model for behaviour change

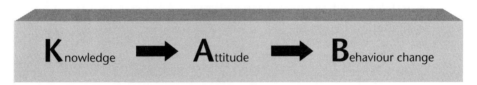

This model does have merit, in that some individuals are likely to be motivated by access to new information, leading to some attitudinal shift, and, as a consequence, the adoption of healthier practices. However, the extent to which people can attempt to modify their behaviours, or are able to sustain changes, is dependent on a range of factors, most notably the contexts in which they live their lives. If they have support at the micro level, say from family, friends, and neighbours, then the changes might be maintained in the short term. However, if macro level structures and systems (e.g. access to sufficient income, supportive childcare policies, inclusive community services) do not support the change, then

Figure 13.3   Reverse KAB model for behaviour change

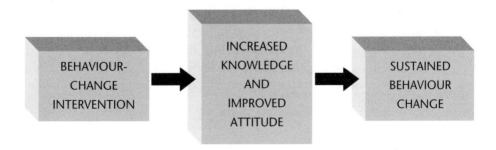

the likelihood of sustaining healthier practices in the longer term is less certain.

Another variation on the KAB model is the reverse KAB model. Figure 13.3 (see p. 195) is a diagrammatic representation of this model.

In this instance, the intervention first attempts to break the habit of unhealthy practices by introducing opportunities to experience new behaviours and their inherent benefits. The theory here is that breaking the unhealthy cycle and encouraging healthier choices will be very motivating for those involved in the program. Other aspects of the program then work to gradually shift attitudes and build more knowledge pertinent to the targeted health issues. Once again, this strategy can be effective in the short term, but if the infrastructures and support systems at the micro and macro level are not conducive to change, then sustainability beyond the lifespan of the program becomes problematic. The case study described in box 13.2 involving a women's participation program illustrates some of the difficulties associated with KAB and reverse KAB models for behaviour change.

Box 13.2 Case study 1

Behaviour change and infrastructure support: The Women's Participation Program

A 10-week program for socially isolated teenage single mothers was conducted in a low socioeconomic outer Melbourne area. These women were identified as being extremely marginalised and disadvantaged, with low income and poor access to support networks. The program involved facilitator-led discussions around personal development themes such as goal setting, managing stress, financial planning and healthy eating. In addition, the participants were introduced to a different physical activity each week, such as walking in the natural environment, weight resistance training, tai chi, yoga, rock climbing, belly dancing, picnics, bus trips, and swimming. The program was heavily subsidised, but participants were asked to contribute $5 each week towards costs. While some initially found the social interaction with the group intimidating, they were all excited by the prospect of new experiences, and reported a new 'zest for life'. And yet, after just four weeks the program had to be abandoned. Typical of suburban fringe developments, the area is poorly serviced by public transport, so one participant walked 5 km to the venue, pushing a pram. She gave up when it rained during the third week. Another had to rely on neighbours for childcare, but after being let down at the last minute on two occasions, she lost motivation. A third woman simply could not afford the $5 each week but was too embarrassed to admit it. She stopped going after three weeks.

> The take-home message here is clear: an intervention that aims to effect behaviour change is only sustainable with adequate infrastructure support. This program offered hope for a better future, but ultimately only served to reinforce the reality of life as a single mum without access to sufficient income, transport, or affordable childcare.
>
> Adapted from Murphy 2003

Stages of Change model for behaviour change

Prochaska, DiClemente, and Norcross (1992) developed a Stages of Change model for behaviour change that is commonly used in clinical practice, particularly with respect to nutrition programs, smoking cessation programs, and overcoming physical inactivity and sedentary lifestyles. Many health professionals attest to the strengths of this model, in that it accurately reflects the various stages that individuals experience in attempting to change behaviours that impact on their health. These stages are identified as *pre-contemplation, contemplation, preparation, action,* and *maintenance.* Further, this model identifies opportunities for the health professional to intervene at crucial times by offering support, encouragement, and additional resources. However, some commentators believe that incorporating recognition of external factors that act on the individual, whether in supportive or unhelpful ways, could further strengthen the model. For instance, support from family and friends for a person who is trying to give up smoking cigarettes can be very important during the *action* stage of behaviour change. Conversely, a work environment that condones smoking on the job, or working with colleagues who are mostly cigarette smokers, is counterproductive to *maintaining* the behaviour change, and might contribute to a relapse.

Table 13.2 Prerequisites for behaviour change

1	The change must be self-initiated
2	The behaviour must become salient
3	The salience of the behaviour must occur over time
4	The behaviour is not a coping strategy
5	The individual's life must not be chaotic or problematic
6	The individual has access to social support networks

Source: Pill and Stott 1990

Pill and Stott (1990) contend that models such as that developed by Prochaska et al. assume that the decision-making processes undertaken by individuals are rational, and that attempts to change behaviour further assume a reasonably high locus of control. As a result of a five-year study, they developed six prerequisites for behaviour change (table 13.2, p. 197).

IEC: Information Education Communication

A more integrated approach to health behaviour-change communication that has emerged in recent years is the IEC model, which links information, education, and communication in a midstream response to health concerns. Figure 13.4 is a diagrammatic representation of this model.

Figure 13.4 IEC behaviour change model

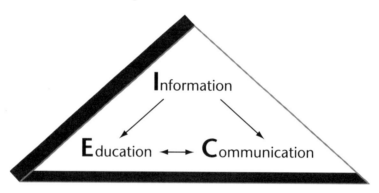

The *information* aspect of the IEC model calls for the gathering of baseline data to inform the development of health enhancement approaches. This data might include morbidity and mortality statistics, life expectancy, and factors contributing to the burden of disease. Health *education* programs are central to the IEC response, and specifically work to address health concerns highlighted in the data. Finally, the *communication* aspect of the approach incorporates mass media behaviour change communication to persuade individuals to adopt healthier practices. The IEC model clearly links responsibility for health outcomes with the individual's capacity to change unhealthy practices, though recognition of contexts and the underlying determinants of health are ordinarily not implicit in intervention responses.

The IEC approach can be effective if it is supported by opportunities for communities to engage in the debates around the issues and their determinants, and by significant infrastructure and systems change. However, without the support of these more upstream socioecological approaches, IEC is likely to have limited impact. It is interesting to note that some developing countries are embracing IEC as a solution to their considerable health problems, but until sufficient investment is made in infrastructure and systems change, the real potential of IEC is unlikely to be realised. The case study described in box 13.3 illustrates some of

> **Box 13.3   Case Study 2**
>
> ### IEC: Getting the healthy eating message across
>
> Baseline data indicated that particular groups of refugees who had settled in Australia from Africa and Asia were not adopting healthy diets. It was thought that this was about a range of factors including cultural differences, cost, and access to food supplies. A campaign was conducted to raise awareness of the importance of healthy eating. This involved the social marketing of health messages, and education workshops to increase knowledge, understanding, and skills, with respect to making healthy food choices. A follow-up evaluation found that when asked what healthy eating meant to them, study participants universally replied that it was about eating plenty of fresh fruit and vegetables. Project managers were delighted that the health interventions had been so effective. However, when asked about the vegetables they now included in their diet, many replied that potatoes were their mainstay, and since French fries at the local fast food-outlets were made of potatoes, and were convenient and inexpensive, this was their primary source of vegetables for their families.
>
> *Source*: Verbal report from field researcher to the author

the difficulties experienced when an IEC intervention was implemented with respect to healthy eating for a group of migrant women.

BCC: behaviour-change communication

A variation on the IEC theme is BCC (behaviour-change communication). This model represents a stand-alone midstream intervention that is generally not integrated with other approaches from the framework for health promotion action. The opportunity for developing countries to reach large segments of their populations with seemingly cost-effective health messages is indeed seductive. However, once again the success of such approaches is invariably limited when unsupported by infrastructure and systems change.

The proceeding photos depict the traditional Mongolian house, the ger. A recent case study (box 13.4) from Mongolia clearly illustrates some of the issues encountered when a BBC approach was employed to address a health concern.

This chapter has examined midstream interventions as depicted in the Framework for Health Promotion Action, being health education and communication strategies. It has acknowledged that health literacy and access to appropriate health education programs are important health promotion tools, and can indeed be powerful in addressing health issues and their underlying determinants. Nevertheless, health education programs, health information, and behaviour-change communication strategies, are unlikely to have sustained impact, particularly on

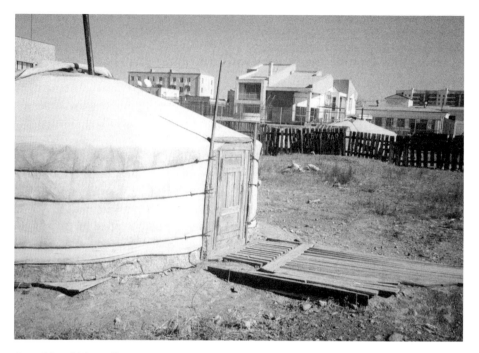

A traditional Mongolian ger

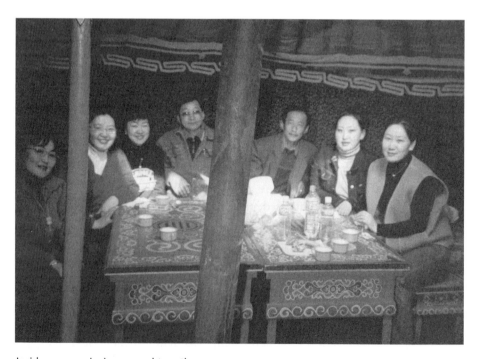

Inside a ger, enjoying a meal together

Box 13.4   Case Study 3

BBC: Behaviour, change, communication in Mongolia

Over 50 per cent of the population of Mongolia still live in traditional housing, the ger, whether in towns, cities, or nomadic. Radio coverage is widespread, and television is becoming more commonplace, particularly in the cities. People are now being exposed to BCC strategies, such as radio and television health messages. For instance, a recent campaign was conducted to encourage people to wash their hands before handling food. The intent was to raise awareness about the importance of personal hygiene, and in so doing, influence the population to adopt safer practices. However, the traditional fuel for cooking and heating is dried animal dung, which must be handled as a matter of course throughout the day. And since water is a precious commodity in this rugged country, many gers do not have access to running water or sewerage disposal. The health information being disseminated is at odds with cultural practices and infrastructure realities, and is therefore unlikely to be effective.

Source: Verbal report by a health promotion consultant
to Mongolia, to the author

---

marginalised and disadvantaged groups, without careful planning and adequate infrastructure and systems support. Further, ill-conceived interventions, which attempt to coerce individuals to adopt healthier practices, are not only unlikely to succeed, but are in fact likely to reinforce disadvantage. Well-planned and implemented midstream interventions can clearly empower individuals and improve their health, but they can also contribute to integrated approaches that influence upstream socioecological change, particularly through community and workforce development. In this sense, midstream interventions can play a vital role in challenging social and health inequities, and in so doing, are integral to the fourth dimension of health promotion described in chapter 11.

SUMMARY

- Health education programs must be carefully planned if they are to meet their objectives and have a sustained impact on participants and communities. Effective programs should *empower* individuals through knowledge and skill development to first, understand the conditions in their local contexts that contribute to their health, and second, to *enable* them to make decisions that enhance the health of themselves and their communities.

- What health education programs must *not* do is become a vehicle for expert-driven preaching, while ignoring the determinants of health and the contexts in which participants live their lives.
- Health communication strategies can influence some to adopt healthier practices, but the extent to which the changes are sustainable is largely dependent on the control that individuals can exert over their own lives. Socioeconomic status, education, and supportive networks and structures at micro and macro level, all contribute to this locus of control.
- Behaviour-change communication campaigns that target a single risk factor or health issue in silo interventions are likely to have limited impact.
- Midstream interventions, incorporating health education and communication strategies, can play an important role in integrated approaches designed to challenge social and health inequities.
- Rather than just focusing on changing unhealthy behaviours of individuals, health communication campaigns can be an effective tool in shifting an agenda with decision makers, and as such, can have the potential to influence upstream socioecological change.

DISCUSSION TOPICS

1 Use the Framework for Developing Effective Health Education Programs to plan health education programs around the following:
   a) a healthy living program for seniors in a rural setting
   b) a parenting program for first-time parents living in an urban-fringe housing development
   c) a reproductive health program for adolescents in a secondary-school setting.
2 How might a health communication campaign be used to shift an agenda among decision makers rather than target individual behaviour change?
3 Consider a health issue of relevance to your locality. Define the issue and the group you wish to target for intervention. What behaviour-change theories would influence the development of your campaign? How might your behaviour-change communication strategy be augmented by other interventions from across the Framework for Health Promotion Action spectrum?
4 Search the Internet for three difference sources of information on a health issue of your choice. How do you know whether the information presented is credible? Who is authoring the information? Who is sponsoring the web site?
5 What external factors or determinants might influence an individual who is trying to quit smoking to either sustain the new behaviour or relapse into old patterns? How might a health professional in a clinical setting use the Stages of Change model and the prerequisites for behaviour change to support a client seeking to adopt a healthier lifestyle?

6   Reflect on a health education program you have either attended or helped to conduct. What were the program objectives? What methods were utilised to deliver the program? How was it evaluated? What else would you need to know in order to assess the impact of the program?

7   Use table 13.1 to analyse the strengths and limitations of some of the more familiar health behaviour-change communication campaigns, such as those targeting road safety, exposure to the sun, and tobacco use.

14 INFORMATION ONLINE

Christine Spratt and Sarah Hopkins

Key concepts

- Information literacy
- Scholarly information
- Evaluation criteria for the World Wide Web

One of the most challenging issues you will confront as an undergraduate student is the large amount of information available in your field. This chapter is designed to help you develop strategies to search efficiently and effectively for information. Tertiary education is about coming to terms with what we call the scholarship of your discipline, and this means developing expertise in **information literacy** and the capacity to evaluate **scholarly information**. This chapter is based on our belief that the development of information literacy is integral to becoming qualified as a practitioner in any health field. You should expect to develop information literacy skills through challenging learning experiences in your course. In this chapter we begin by describing what we mean by 'information literacy'. We then focus particularly on suggesting strategies that will enable you to develop skills in finding, critically evaluating, and using online information. The information literacy skills that you develop at university will not only help define your success as an undergraduate, but also shape your approach to learning in your working life.

WHAT IS INFORMATION LITERACY?

For the purposes of this chapter, our understanding of information literacy draws on the work by the Council of Australian University Librarians (CAUL). CAUL (2001 p. 1) defines information literacy as enabling individuals to 'recognise when information is needed and have the capacity to locate, evaluate, and use effectively the needed information'. In other words, 'the information literate person is able to:

- recognise a need for information
- determine the extent of the information needed
- access the needed information effectively
- evaluate the information and its sources
- incorporate selected information into their knowledge base
- use information effectively to accomplish a purpose
- understand economic, legal, social, and cultural issues in the use of information
- access and use information ethically and legally
- classify, store, manipulate, and redraft information collected or generated
- recognise information literacy as a prerequisite for lifelong learning.'

CAUL 2001, p. 1

It is not difficult to see, given this definition, that being information literate requires the development of complex skills and knowledge. Importantly, this involves the ability to develop skills of 'critique'. Here we mean the ability to think critically, to engage actively in one's learning, and to become attuned to the idea that 'information' as 'evidence' defines what counts as valid and legitimate knowledge in health sciences and subsequently leads to developments in the field.

Table 14.1 Where you might find health information online

TYPE OF INFORMATION	EXAMPLE OF WEB SITE
Government information: Information in the public interest; contemporary research based; usually evidence based	Department of Human Services: www.dhs.vic.gov.au
Conference Papers: Some sites such as 1 (opposite) have conference proceedings listed that you can order. Others, such as 2 (opposite), have proceedings that you can download at no cost.	1 Center for Public Health Education Conference Proceedings: www.nsf.org/ cphe/cphe_confproceedings.html 2 Office of the Surgeon General Conference Reports and Proceedings: www.surgeongeneral.gov/library/ conferences.htm
Advertising: Consumer information about products; information for health professionals designed to increase sales	Novartis: www.novartis.com
Promotion of issues: Government-funded body for public health issues	VicHealth: www.vichealth.vic.gov.au
Popular culture: What is being discussed at 'grass roots' level	Oprah Winfrey web site: www.oprah.com

FINDING INFORMATION ONLINE: THE WEB AND FREE INFORMATION

A vast amount of information is available for free via the World Wide Web (the Web). This may seem like a bonus when you can type any term into an Internet search engine and find a site, but the quality of information is more varied on the Internet than in any other medium. Unlike the information that you find in books, journals, or newspapers, there is no editor or publisher checking what is available on the Web, although some sites will have strict editorial standards. This means that you have to be more rigorous about evaluating the information that you find online than from any other source.

Individuals and organisations make information available on the Web for a variety of reasons: they may be promoting a cause or issue, they may be marketing their business, it may be their job to disseminate information, or they may make information available for a select audience, for instance teaching materials for a university course.

All information that is free on the Web is free for some reason. Trying to understand *why* the information you have found has been made available is a good first step in evaluating its reliability. Some examples of different sorts of sites, which contain health information, are annotated in table 14.1.

The Web and scholarly information

The Web is also a convenient way of distributing scholarly information. Scholarly information refers to data, ideas, discussions, and conclusions drawn from 'academic research'. Such research is usually conducted under strict ethical guidelines and standards, and is always reviewed by a panel of experts before it is published. Scholarly information is usually not free. It may come from databases, books, or journals that often charge a subscription for access. These subscription sites are often available through your library. You will probably need a password—ask your health librarian what is available at your institution. The advantage of using information from these sites is that it has usually been more rigorously examined before being made available to the public. You may be accessing the online version of a journal that has a peer review process, which means that the articles have been reviewed by other experts in the field before they are published, or you may be using a database put together by an important organisation in the discipline. For example, the psychology database PsycInfo is published by the American Psychological Association and lists the contents of all major psychology publications from around the world. It is intended to be the key resource for professional psychologists as well as students. Sometimes information is available from a subscription service and for free. It may be that the information is not current, for example a number of journals allow access to the full contents of issues that are more than a year old; it may be that some parts of a publication are available for free, for example the web sites of most major daily newspapers offer a few articles to give a taste of the full publication; or the site may have been made available for a particular purpose, for instance the Medline database will be available through most university libraries from Ovid, WebSPIRS, Ebsco and similar sites, and also be searchable for free through PubMed (this latter is a health promoting strategy of the US government that is very useful to students).

EVALUATING ONLINE INFORMATION

It is always important to consider the accuracy and quality of the information you use, irrespective of its format. It is especially important to critically evaluate online resources, particularly if they are from free web sites. Using criteria to evaluate Internet sites is a key skill for all health professionals.

Table 14.2   Evaluation criteria for web sites

Who is the author?	Can you easily identify the author of the Web page or site? Does the author give their affiliations, credentials, or reason for publishing the information?
Where did the information come from?	Look at the URL or address. Where did the document originate? Is the information scholarly, governmental, from a private business or association, or an advertisement? Do other reputable Internet sites point to this one?
What is the purpose of the site?	Is the author making an argument for personal gain, offering an opinion, giving a factual report, or relaying a personal observation? What is the site's intended audience?
Does the site give references or other sources so you can cross-check the information?	Is the information from original research, experiments, observation, interviews, books, or documents? Are references provided?
Is the site contemporary?	When was the material published? Has the content been updated recently?

DEVELOPING A SEARCH STRATEGY

Good search skills will save you a lot of time and frustration whether you are looking for information in the library or on the Web. The first step of a good search is to have a *clear understanding of the topic* you are researching. In this section we will use chapter 6 on measuring population health status in Australia to illustrate some of the key skills in 'intelligent' searching that you will need to acquire as a tertiary student.

Understanding the central topic

As you can see from the title, this chapter has three main topics; population health; health services; and risk factors. If you were asked to write an essay based on the material in this chapter, you would have to start by making sure that you know what these terms mean. It's a good idea to test your understanding by try-ing to write the set question in your own words.

If an essay has been set as an assessment task, usually you will be asked to answer a question or argue for or against a statement. Make sure you know the question or statement being asked—don't write a brilliant essay on the wrong subject! When you understand the central topic, you can determine the rele-vance of all the information you find by asking yourself two key questions:

1 Does this help to answer my question?
2 Does it support or negate the argument I am making?

Combining key concepts in your search using the Web

In general, search engines, databases, and catalogues function literally. That means they search for exactly what you type in. For example, if you were look-ing for information about risk factors you would want to find articles that talk generally about risk factors and also about specific risk factors. Note that in chap-ter 6 Ackland and Catford identify four major risk factors that affect health: smoking; nutrition; alcohol consumption; and physical activity (known as SNAP). You can use these four terms in place of risk factors in your search.

Using advanced search

Some search engines allow you to type in a sentence or phrase and then try to work out what you are looking for. Searching this way usually results in a lot of

Figure 14.1   Key terms and alternative terms for searching

Key terms	Population health	Risk factors	Health services
Alternative terms	Health status	Alcohol consumption	Health care
		Smoking	Health promotion
		Nutrition	
		Physical activity	

'miss hits' or irrelevant results. A better way to search the Web is to use the advanced search option that is available on most search engines. Advanced searching allows you to choose which words and terms are most important for your search and how they should be combined. You might like to explore the advanced searching on these search engines:

Google: www.google.com.au/advanced_search?

Yahoo: http://search.yahoo.com/search/options?p=

Combining your search terms or key concepts is a very important part of intelligent searching.

Combining terms using a database

If you are searching a database through your library you can combine your terms using joining words called 'Boolean operators'. The most useful Boolean operators are AND, and OR. These words enable the database to combine the terms you have typed in and also allow you to refine your search by giving you more control over your search. In some database search software you must use Boolean operators to search for more than one word, in others it is optional.

Table 14.3 Boolean operators

AND	Both words must appear in the document.	Use for words describing two different concepts. e.g. population health AND obesity
OR	Either word can appear in the document.	Use for words describing the same concept. e.g. health service OR health care

Using Internet subject sites

In addition to looking through search engines and databases, where you choose your search terms, you can also look for information through Internet subject sites. These are sometimes called directories, portals, or gateways and may be linked from library subject web sites or from the home page of key organisations in your professional area. Directories or gateways list sites that are relevant to the subject—someone else has searched for them.

If you go to the Australian Institute of Health and Welfare web site (www.aihw.gov.au), you will see the 'Subject Portal' link on the home page. You can use this to find a diverse range of information regarding health issues facing Australians for example, in the context of the Ackland and Catford chapter we are using here, there are external links to a number of sites relevant to the risk factors the authors discuss.

Using bibliographies and references

Another way of accessing relevant research is to use the references at the end of each journal article that you use or reading lists that your lecturers give you. If the article is relevant to your topic it is likely that the articles read by the author will be relevant too. The only disadvantage of this method is that the references will always be older than the first article.

Look at the references and bibliographies at the end of journal articles or chapters in textbooks. Sometimes, authors will provide 'key references'. These are useful citations potentially valuable for you if you were required to write an essay or undertake some other form of investigation. Published authors are regarded as experts in their field and using their citations can be an invaluable starting point for your own research.

SUMMARY

- Developing skills in information literacy will be fundamental to your success as a tertiary student and will contribute to your continuing success as a lifelong learner.
- Strategies of information literacy will help you access and evaluate online health information and contribute to your development as a successful and capable student.
- You will find your library help desk, student services, and your tutors willing collaborators as you develop your skills in 'information literacy', especially in the context of health information online.

DISCUSSION TOPICS

1 Indigenous health, workplace health, and food insecurity are topics that are discussed in this text. Use the strategies introduced in this chapter to search for online information around *one* of these topics. Construct a list of the sites and articles you find, and record the steps you take to find them (e.g. record the *keywords* used in the search process so that you do not waste time repeating searches already undertaken).
2 Select one of these online sites and apply the evaluation criteria in table 14.2 to critique the site and the information presented.

USEFUL WEB SITES

The databases and scholarly sites to which we have referred (PsychInfo, PubMed Webspirs, EbscoHost) are generally accessible from most libraries, for example:
The Monash University Library: www.lib.monash.edu.au/databases

PubMed: www.ncbi.nih.gov/entrez/query.fcgi

Examples of online tutorials for information literacy skills are:

Queensland University of Technology: www.library.qut.edu.au/infolit/tutorials

University of Bristol, UK: www.vts.rdn.ac.uk The RDN Virtual Training Suite aims to help higher and further education students, lecturers, and researchers in the United Kingdom to develop their Internet information literacy and ICT skills (although it is also freely available for anyone else to use). It offers a set of free 'teach yourself' tutorials, delivered over the Web, each of which provides Internet skills training in a particular subject area. There is a tutorial for most of the subjects taught in universities and colleges.

University of Pennsylvania: www.libraries.psu.edu/crsweb/infolit/andyou/infoyou.htm

BBC Webwise: www.bbc.co.uk/webwise/learn

DETERMINANTS APPROACHES TO PUBLIC HEALTH ISSUES

PART 3

ADVOCACY, ACTIVISM, AND AWARENESS RAISING: ENCOURAGING A RELUCTANT COMMUNITY TO REDUCE ITS DEPENDENCE ON TOBACCO

Ron Borland and James Balmford

Key concepts

- Tobacco control strategies
- Public health campaigning
- Advocacy

Tobacco is the single largest cause of premature death in Australia and many other countries. In 1998, it was estimated that a little over 19,000 Australians died each year of smoking-related diseases, and between three and four million died worldwide. It is quite simply the largest killer we have (figure 15.1). Knowledge of the harms of smoking is overwhelming, with the first authoritative reviews published in the 1960s. Despite that, it has taken many years to confront the issue, with most of the activity in Australia being post the 1970s. One major reason for this is that most of the harms from tobacco occur after years of use, so there is no intrinsic fear of smoking. Coupled with the power of tobacco companies, and the high prevalence of tobacco use, this has meant that it has been all too easy to put comprehensive tobacco control in the too-hard basket. This chapter outlines what has happened in tobacco control in the last quarter of a century in Australia, and documents some of the key factors that have helped to reduce tobacco use.

Smoking has moved from being an integral part of Australian life to being increasingly socially marginalised. Starting in the late 1980s there have been marked increases in smoke-free workplaces, with most now smoke-free. Since about a decade later, smoke-free homes have become increasingly prevalent. In 2001 about half of all homes with smokers in them did not allow smoking in the home (Trotter and Mullins 2003).

Figure 15.1   Number of people who died in 1998 due to smoking compared with other causes

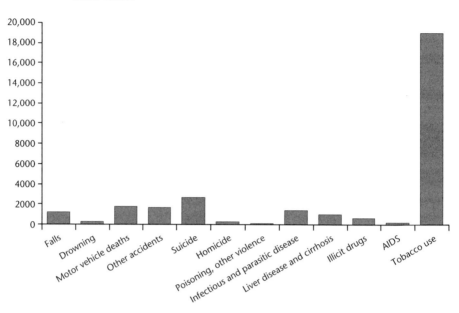

Source: ABS 1998

Since 1974, when Australian surveillance data was first systematically collected, smoking prevalence has fallen from about 36 to 22 per cent in 2000. Over the life span, smoking prevalence peaks when people are in their twenties and gradually declines thereafter as smokers quit or die prematurely. Men still smoke more than women, with a 4 per cent differential that has been fairly constant for about ten years. People from lower socioeconomic status (SES) groups smoke more and the rates among the severely disadvantaged are even higher. For example, smoking rates in 1994 in the largely disadvantaged Aboriginal and Torres Strait Islander population were 54 per cent for men and 46 per cent for women (Ivers 2001). Up until the mid 1980s there was clear evidence of increasing SES disparity in smoking prevalence, but since then smoking rates in all SES groups have declined at similar rates. Most of the SES effects are due to more people from lower SES groups ever having started smoking—percentages of ex-smokers do not differ much.

Evidence on success in reducing the uptake of smoking is less clear, but it appears that there has not been uniform progress. In the late 1960s/early 1970s there was a marked increase in the uptake of smoking while at school (Hill and Borland 1991). In 1984, the first national survey of secondary school smoking found that by age 15, 29 per cent of boys and 34 per cent of girls had smoked in the last week (Hill et al. 1987). There was an initial drop in smoking in 1987, but then a drift upwards over much of the 1990s, although the 1999 data (last available) is somewhat more positive, with 21 and 24 per cent of 15-year-old boys and girls, respectively, having smoked in the last week (Hill et al. 2002).

Unlike for adults, for much of this period girls have been more likely to be current smokers than boys, but they smoke fewer cigarettes per week.

The progress that has been made in reducing smoking prevalence can best be
attributed to a combination of public education, restrictions on promotion,
restrictions on where and when smokers can smoke, increases in the real price of
cigarettes, and increases in use of effective cessation aids. The contribution of
each of these factors is discussed below. In addition, more recently, litigation
against tobacco companies, both here and overseas, has forced them to accept
that their products cause harm and they must be seen to be concerned. However,
based on past behaviour, it will require strong public health action to ensure that
the companies act in ways that benefit public health, rather than ways that only
appear to provide benefits, such as the use of filters and light cigarettes that we
now know produce no measurable health benefit.

MASS MEDIA

Hard-hitting, realistic, anti-smoking, mass-media advertisements have played a
major role in reducing smoking prevalence. Most campaigns to reduce smoking
have been initiated at the state level. The Quit-For-Life campaigns, conducted
in New South Wales in 1983, and the Quit campaign in Victoria the following
year, were the first large-scale, coordinated, mass media-led, well-evaluated anti-
smoking campaigns in Australia. The campaigns incorporated graphic mass-media

Figure 15.2 Age-standardised smoking prevalence among males, Sydney and Melbourne,
before and after launch of Quit-For-Life campaigns

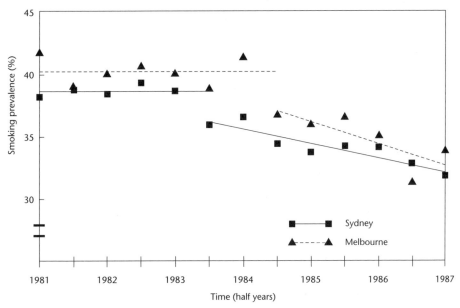

Source: Pierce at al. 1990, p. 567

advertising to raise public awareness about smoking and health, and a community agenda to promote nonsmoking by health professionals and school educators. The campaigns occurred in a context of no observable trend in smoking prevalence in either Sydney or Melbourne prior to the campaigns. Campaign onset was associated with an immediate drop in male and female smoking prevalence in both cities, with a continuing decline at least among males (Pierce et al. 1990) (See figure 15.2). The effects of the campaigns were equivalent across levels of education, halting an apparent increase in SES difference in smoking prevalence.

For the next ten years, efforts were mixed. Victoria and Western Australia, and more belatedly South Australia, ran small ongoing campaigns, NSW ran campaigns intermittently, while the other states and territories did little. In the mid 1990s, a levelling out in smoking prevalence (Hill, White, and Scollo 1998) provided the impetus for the federally funded National Tobacco Campaign (NTC), the most intense and longest-running mass-media campaign conducted in Australia to this point. The NTC was launched in mid 1997, sustained for six months at high levels, then continued on and off for the next three years. Existing state-based Quit campaigns and other partner organisations also participated. The NTC targeted young adult smokers (aged eighteen to thirty-nine), but ended up having similar effects on the whole community. It had an emphasis on relatively certain rather than less probable health effects, hence the campaign slogan, 'Every cigarette is doing you damage'. The major communication objective was to increase the perceived importance or urgency of quitting, thereby elevating it on smokers' personal agendas (Hill, Chapman, and Donovan 1998; Hassard 1999).

Evaluation of the first phase of the NTC (June to November 1997) showed that it played a significant role in reducing smoking in Australia. It achieved high levels of recall, favourable appraisal, and evoked strong affective responses, stimulating more frequent and intense thoughts about quitting. Smoking prevalence declined by 1.4 per cent following phase one of the campaign, representing approximately 190,000 fewer smokers (Hassard 1999). This reduction was sustained and built on in subsequent years (Kinsman in press).

There is no doubt, from these outcomes, that mass media works; it is highly cost-effective (although with high entry costs), and also helps keep the issue on the broader social agenda. It works at similar levels with all segments of society, and also appears to reduce smoking uptake in adolescents (one of the few interventions that achieves this).

RESTRICTING ADVERTISING AND PROMOTION

Much has been achieved since the early 1970s in reducing the capacity of the tobacco industry to advertise and promote its products. Up until the mid 1970s, tobacco was one of the most heavily advertised commodities in Australia. Between September 1973 and September 1976, direct advertising of cigarettes was phased out on Australian radio and television. In 1989 and 1992, the Federal parliament passed two waves of legislation phasing out most remaining forms of tobacco advertising by 1995 (Winstanley et al. 1995).

One contribution to the banning of tobacco advertising and promotion from billboards and print media came from the activist groups MOP UP (Movement Opposed to the Promotion of Unhealthy Products) and BUGA UP (Billboard

Figure 15.3   Examples of BUGA UP's refacing of Australian tobacco billboards

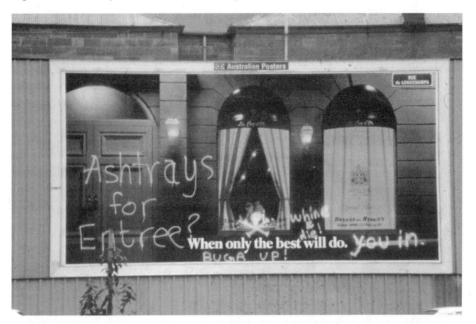

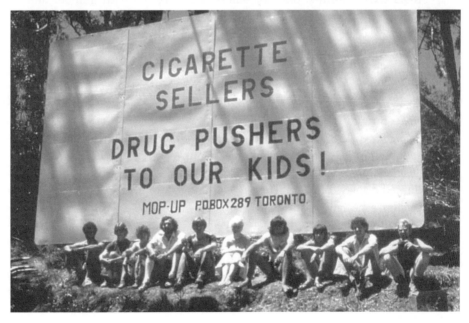

Figure 15.3 Examples of BUGA UP's refacing of Australian tobacco billboards (cont.)

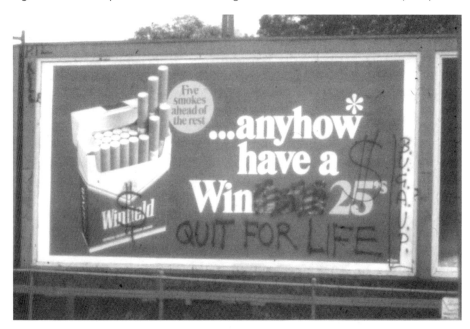

Source: Civil Disobedience and Tobacco Control: BUGA UP in Australia—
downloaded from http://tc.bmjournals.com/misc/powerpoint.shtml.

Utilising Graffiti Against Unhealthy Promotions). Both groups used community activism to highlight the inappropriateness of tobacco company behaviour. BUGA UP graffitied outdoor billboard advertising with humour and sarcasm. The group's activism was highly visible, receiving widespread news coverage, and for many years was arguably the most common anti-smoking message presented to the average Australian. Despite there being no formal evaluation of the social and political impact of BUGA UP, the movement is credited by many to have played an outstanding role in politicising the tobacco control agenda, and in changing the public perception of tobacco control and the culture of smoking in the community (Chapman 1996).

Between 1987 and 1992, outdoor advertising and advertising through sports sponsorship was progressively phased out in most states. Several states, led by Tasmania in 1999, have now banned point-of-sale advertising, but all still allow limited displays of packs. The remaining forms of promotion include some sponsorship, especially of international events; the packs themselves; a range of indirect advertising (e.g. product placement in films, product at 'image setting' events, and direct mail/email). The impact of all these restrictions has not been specifically evaluated, but international research indicates that comprehensive bans on cigarette advertising and promotion are effective in reducing smoking rates, whereas partial bans have little or no effect (Jha and Chaloupka 1999).

There have also been gradual moves to increase the strength of health warnings, especially on packaging. The first warnings in 1973 were quite weak, but improved warnings in 1987 and in 1995 were world-leading at the time. Australia is currently considering following Canada and some other countries to mandate warnings that take up around half of the surface of the pack, and which include graphic pictures of some of the harms. Prominent warnings increase the frequency of them being noticed and generating concerns, which has been linked to subsequent cessation (Borland 1997).

RESTRICTING WHERE AND WHEN SMOKERS CAN SMOKE

In 1986, the National Health and Medical Research Council published a landmark report on the health effects of passive smoking (NHMRC 1986). At this time, public knowledge of the harms of passive smoking was already high (Mullins et al. 2000), making the report an immediate stimulus for action. There has since been a substantial reduction in the proportion of people in Australia exposed to environmental tobacco smoke in workplaces and public places.

The public sector played a leading role in the adoption of smoking restrictions in the workplace. Telstra (then fully publicly owned) went smoke-free on 1 January 1988, followed by the entire Australian Public Service two months later. In Victoria in 1988, 17 per cent of indoor workers reported a total smoking ban at their workplace. By 2000, around 70 per cent of indoor workers in Victoria were protected by total smoking bans (Borland et al. 2001). The main places to resist were entertainment venues. Smoking in restaurants is now banned throughout Australia, and there are increasing restrictions in bars and gambling venues. In the USA, California has led the way with total bans on smoking in all indoor workplaces and public spaces. Australia is likely to follow over the next few years.

Litigation or fear of litigation under occupational health and safety legislation has been a major force for change, complemented by the 1991 Morling decision. In this decision, Justice Morling, of the Federal Court of Australia, found that the Tobacco Institute of Australia (TIA) had engaged in misleading or deceptive conduct in publishing a newspaper advertisement refuting evidence linking passive smoking and disease. This landmark decision established the link between passive smoking and disease among nonsmokers in a court of law, and eased the way for civil claims from people adversely affected by exposure to tobacco smoke.

Workplace smoking bans have not only protected nonsmokers, but have also led to reductions in tobacco consumption among smokers. They may also have increased quitting and reduced uptake by making workplaces less smoking-oriented (Borland and Davey in press). It seems likely that bans in other venues will augment these effects. Voluntary bans on smoking in homes are also becoming the norm, even in homes of smokers. Australia is rapidly reaching the point where smoking is socially marginalised.

INCREASES IN THE PRICE OF CIGARETTES

International research suggests that the price sensitivity of demand for cigarettes in Western countries is around –0.4; that is for every 10 per cent increase in cigarette prices, consumption can be expected to fall by about 4 per cent (Centers for Disease Control and Prevention 1998). Tax increases resulting in higher tobacco prices have been rated as the most effective single intervention available to governments to reduce demand for tobacco (Jha and Chaloupka 2000). However, the evidence base is qualitatively different to other interventions, being based on economic data rather than experimental trials. Even if we accept Jha and Chaloupka's conclusion, price rises do not occur in isolation. In many countries to get sufficient public support to enact such tax increases requires selling the policy in terms of health benefit, something that is only credible when the population is well informed about the harms of smoking and the benefit of the price increases. Health advocates have pushed for price increases and changes in pricing structures to discourage cheaper discount cigarettes.

Australian cigarette prices are now among the highest in the world (Lal and Scollo 2002). In the last twenty-five years, there have been marked increases in tobacco taxes, with the actual price of cigarettes (not discounted for inflation) now 34 per cent higher than it was in 1997 (Scollo and Borland 2002). Price has been a major contributor to both declines in smoking prevalence and in consumption among remaining smokers.

CESSATION AIDS

Most smokers who try to quit prefer to do so on their own, or with minimal assistance. However the increasing availability and sophistication of cessation aids in Australia (in particular pharmaceuticals and the national Quitline telephone support service) makes it easier for smokers wanting more intensive help to get the assistance they need, leading to an increase in use of proven aids, particularly pharmaceuticals.

Research shows that both behavioural and pharmaceutical aids increase successful cessation, and when combined, effects are typically additive. However, the contribution of cessation aids to the reduction in smoking prevalence in Australia is low, although with the marked increase in availability and use of resources, it is playing a larger role than it did before the mid 1990s. Given the difficulty of quitting due to the ambivalence caused by the addiction, getting more people to use effective programs has the potential to make an even more important contribution. This will be best done if we can find effective ways to provide only the extra help people need, rather than providing intense help regardless of need. Unless this happens, the net cost of getting smokers to quit will rise. Help for smokers is likely to make increasing use of electronic aids (telephone, Internet, electronic organisers) that have the capacity to deliver help economically. These have the potential, with or without concurrent use of pharmaceutical aids, to greatly increase the contribution of cessation aids to reducing smoking prevalence.

SUMMARY

- Public education campaigns, restrictions on advertising and promotion, and smoke-free public places, increases in tobacco taxation, and the increasing availability of cessation aids, have formed parts of a comprehensive tobacco control strategy that has reaped considerable returns.
- When one considers the burden of disease caused by tobacco use, progress in tobacco control thus far has been slow and conducted in an incremental, piecemeal fashion.
- Compared with other countries, Australia is among the leaders, with smoking rates close to the lowest in the world. However, 19,000 Australians still die each year from smoking-related illness, and more than one in five adults still smoke. We have achieved much, but still have much to do.
- There is a need to 'institutionalise' a solution to the problem. There is a need for comprehensive regulation of tobacco manufacture and sale, which eliminates the commercial incentive for selling tobacco, and ensures that less deadly products are made available to continuing smokers. Moreover, given their demonstrated effectiveness, more funds are needed for a significant ongoing, comprehensive, mass-media campaign supported by increased availability of cessation supports.
- It is likely that:
  - over the next five to ten years (from 2004) most, if not all, of those currently exposed to ETS in workplaces and public places will be protected
  - health warnings will be strengthened and models will be implemented for ensuring new information is made widely available
  - there will be further attempts to restrict the promotion of tobacco products, but tobacco companies will continue to find novel ways to subvert them
  - pressure will build to regulate tobacco products and fundamentally change the relationship between tobacco companies and consumers, and at a retail level there will be moves to remove tobacco from stores that sell products that are attractive to young people (e.g. convenience stores, cafés)
  - tobacco dependence treatment will be better institutionalised into the health care system and mass media tobacco control advertising will be a more prominent feature of the airwaves
  - by 2010, tobacco may be used at least weekly by less than 15 per cent of adults, and if all is done that could be, the figure could be closer to 10 per cent.

DISCUSSION TOPICS

1 What do we mean when we state that we 'need to institutionalise a solution to the problem'?
2 Use a health promotion framework such as the Ottawa Charter or the Framework for Health Promotion Action (see chapter 11) to help you develop an integrated plan aimed at reducing adult tobacco use to less than 15 per cent by 2010.

USEFUL WEB SITES

Action on Smoking and Health (ASH) Australia: www.ashaust.org.au
QUIT: www.quit.org.au
Tobacco Control Supersite: http://tobacco.health.usyd.edu.au
VicHealth Centre for Tobacco Control: www.vctc.org.au

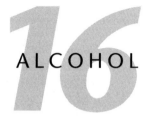

ALCOHOL

Paul Dietze and Helen Keleher

Key concepts

- Alcohol consumption and related harms
- Harm minimisation
- Mental health and alcohol use

Alcohol has a high level of social acceptance but it is a highly problematic substance for Australians. In 1998, annual costs to Australia of alcohol-caused problems were estimated to be $7.6 billion—around 22 per cent of the costs attributed to all drugs including tobacco (Collins and Lapsley 2002). While the death rate from alcohol as a single cause of death is lower than for tobacco, alcohol is one of the most fundamental contributing factors in premature and preventable death and disability in Australia, strongly implicated in cardiovascular disease, cancer, injury, violence, abuse, and mental illness (Collins and Lapsley 2002). This chapter outlines trends in alcohol use and harm, the impact of alcohol on the health and social life of Australians, determinants of alcohol use, and policy responses intended to reduce alcohol-related problems.

ACKNOWLEDGING ALCOHOL AS A PROBLEM

Australia began to consistently collect statistics on indicators for harm from alcohol misuse in the 1980s, demonstrating an emerging awareness of alcohol as a public health issue. Since then, statistics have been recorded through national surveys, data on alcohol sales, and health and law enforcement data (Heale et al. 2000). The National Alcohol Indicators Project (NAIP) has been specifically established to track trends in alcohol consumption and related harms. The indicators examined through NAIP cover a variety of health and social domains, and include: alcohol-related hospital admissions; alcohol-related mortality; per capita alcohol consumption by people 15 years of age and over; the proportion of drinking that is high risk; the proportion of people drinking harmful or hazardous quantities of alcohol; rates of violence, especially night-time assaults; and road traffic accidents (e.g. Chikritzhs et al. 2000).

About 62 per cent of the total costs attributable to alcohol are deemed to be avoidable as well as amenable to public policy initiatives and behaviour change (Collins and Lapsley 2002). Australia has developed a set of national policy approaches to control alcohol use and tackle the harm associated with its misuse. A variety of specific alcohol-related strategies, particularly the National Alcohol Strategy and National Alcohol Campaign, have been developed under the rubric of the National Drug Strategy, and a range of associated policy documents are the drivers for policy development in the states and territories. Australia has adopted a harm minimisation approach that comprises upstream policy, midstream preventative efforts at a community level through education and the provision of information, as well as downstream treatment and **harm reduction** programs. Governments also attempt to reduce harm by modifying the environment in which harmful use occurs through the widespread promotion of alcohol service guidelines and the provision of responsible serving training courses for staff involved in the serving of alcohol.

TRENDS IN ALCOHOL CONSUMPTION

Data on patterns of alcohol consumption are available through the National Drug Strategy Household Survey (NDSHS) series (AIHW 2002a). Around 82.4 per cent of respondents to the 2001 NDSHS (88.9 per cent of males and 79.1 per cent of females) were classified as current drinkers, representing a small increase on the 80.5 per cent found in the 1998 survey (AIHW 2002a). However, the 'current drinkers' found in the survey represents people who consume alcohol in a variety of ways, ranging from chronic dependent drinkers to those who report only having had a single glass in the previous year. The crucial issue concerning alcohol consumption is the number of people who consume alcohol in a fashion that places them at risk of harm. The National Health and Medical Research Council (NHMRC 2001) has developed guidelines prescribing levels of drinking that place people at low risk, risky, and high-risk for the development of alcohol-related harm.

These guidelines are based on standard drinks. A single standard drink in Australia is regarded as equivalent to 8 to 10 grams of pure alcohol (a 'pot' or 'middie' of beer, a 100ml glass of wine or drinks containing a 30ml 'shot' of spirits). Further, the guidelines segregate alcohol-related harm according to whether the harm arises in the long term (e.g. liver cirrhosis, cardiovascular disease) or short term (e.g. injury, acute pancreatitis). They also clearly stipulate the levels of alcohol consumption (low risk) that are thought to be associated with health benefits in relation to cardiovascular disease (Doll 1998). In the NHMRC guidelines, low-risk levels for the development of long-term harm include drinking up to twenty-eight and fourteen standard drinks per week for males and females, respectively. Medium-risk or 'risky' levels are defined as between twenty-nine and forty-two standard drinks per week for males, and between fourteen and twenty-nine for females. More than forty-two and twenty-nine standard drinks per week are considered high-risk for males and females respectively. The guidelines also stipulate that drinking more than six standard drinks for males, and more than four standard drinks for females, on any one drinking occasion places them at risk of developing short-term harm.

The 2001 NDSHS results suggest that the majority (72.7 per cent) of Australians consume alcohol in a manner that puts them at low risk for the development of long-term harm. Nevertheless, 7 per cent of respondents to this survey reported consuming alcohol in a manner that placed them at medium risk of long-term harm and 2.9 per cent consume alcohol in a manner that places them at high risk of long-term harm (AIHW 2002a). Further, 34.3 per cent of respondents reported consuming alcohol in a manner that placed them at risk of short-term harm in the year prior to the survey, and 6.9 per cent indicated that they did so at least weekly (AIHW 2002a).

Table 16.1 Prevalence of alcohol consumption in Australia by risk level, age, and gender, 2001

	PROPORTION OF THE POPULATION (PER CENT)						
	AGE						
LEVEL OF RISK BY GENDER	14–19	20–29	30–39	40-49	50–59	60+	ALL AGES
Males							
Low risk	64.0	77.1	81.4	79.0	75.8	71.9	75.6
Risky	6.1	9.5	5.8	6.4	7.3	5.4	6.7
High risk	2.7	5.0	3.1	3.2	4.3	2.6	3.5
Short-term risk	29.4	42.4	28.2	20.6	16.7	7.6	23.8
Females							
Low risk	62.1	75.4	78.3	76.5	73.3	66.8	72.7
Risky	8.0	10.2	6.3	7.1	6.6	4.4	7.0
High risk	3.7	4.5	2.5	2.6	2.9	1.6	2.9
Short-term risk	33.0	36.2	17.6	13.9	7.6	2.6	16.9

Source: AIHW 2002a

Table 16.1 shows the results of the 2001 NDSHS according to age, gender, and alcohol-risk categories. This table shows that males and younger people are more likely to consume alcohol at high-risk levels than females and older people respectively. However, females are slightly more likely to consume alcohol at medium-risk levels (AIHW 2002a).

One disturbing trend in alcohol consumption is the proportion of young people who report consuming alcohol in a risky manner. For example, 67 per cent of the secondary school students who reported consuming alcohol in the Australian Survey of Secondary School Students reported doing so in a way that placed them at risk of short-term harm (White, Hill, and Effendi 2003). This data suggests that risky alcohol use, in this case reflecting a propensity to drink to levels of intoxication, is fashionable among young people. Indeed, people below 25 years of age are now thought to have the riskiest drinking patterns (Heale et al. 2000). However, alcohol use is governed by other social and cultural mores for particular subpopulations. People living in nonmetropolitan areas consistently show a higher per capita consumption of alcohol than for people in metropolitan areas (Catalano et al. 2001). High levels of alcohol use are also linked to social factors such as low socioeconomic status (Jonas et al. 1999). People who use illicit drugs such as heroin often report high levels of alcohol consumption, a practice that places them at significantly increased risk of harms such as overdose (Darke and Zador 1996). Further, people suffering from mental illness and mental health problems often drink alcohol in a problematic fashion—producing a vicious cycle of **co-morbidity** between poor mental health and alcohol use (Laslett et al. 2002).

ALCOHOL-RELATED HARMS

The NAIP estimates that in 1997, 3290 Australians died from injury and disease caused by high-risk alcohol use, and 70 per cent of those deaths were males. Further, around 70 per cent of hospitalisations for alcohol due to falls, alcohol dependence, assaults, or road injuries occurred among males. Alcohol-caused death rates have decreased steadily between 1990–97 (Chikritzhs et al. 1999). It is estimated that about 30 per cent of road injuries are attributable to the risky consumption of alcohol, demonstrating that despite legislation to deter driving under the influence of alcohol, this remains a major cause of road traffic accidents and injuries (Chikritzhs et al. 2000).

Alcohol dependence is a significant alcohol-related harm that can result from excessive alcohol consumption. It has been estimated that around 3.5 per cent of the Australian population is alcohol dependent in any one year (Hall et al. 1999). This dependence results in a significant burden to the community, with around 30 per cent of all clients of Victorian government-funded specialist drug and alcohol agencies presenting for alcohol-related treatment and 22 per cent of all calls to drugs helplines in Victoria being for alcohol (DHS 2002b). While these numbers are significant, little is known about the prevalence of problems related to alcohol dependence in other settings, with most treatment for alcohol dependence probably taking place in primary care settings such as general practice (Dietze et al. 2000).

There is enormous collateral damage to society from the consumption of alcohol. Alcohol consumption is strongly associated with a number of social harms ranging from physical violence to general public order issues. While the rate of alcohol-related violent offences reported to police remained relatively stable over the 1990s, the annual rate itself is alarmingly high at around fifteen incidents per 10,000 people among people living in metropolitan Australia and twenty-three per 10,000 people living in nonmetropolitan areas. Alcohol is also linked with domestic violence and abuse, being involved in around 42 per cent of domestic incidents reported to police in Victoria in the 1999–2000 financial year (DHS 2002b).

While a picture of some of the harms associated with alcohol consumption emerges through these statistics, many of the problems associated with alcohol use such as child abuse, general and marital violence, spousal abuse, sexual aggression, neglect, and disruption go unreported. There are strong links between the effects of childhood violence on harmful alcohol use among adults. In other words, children who have either witnessed or experienced violence were greatly at risk of 'inheriting' violence. Where sexual aggression towards partners occurs, there is often violence towards children as well. However, there is a general lack of inquiry by health professionals in antenatal clinics and accident and emergency departments about domestic violence and its relation to alcohol use. Certainly, there is a case to be made that both women and children should be better protected from the consequences of problematic alcohol use.

WOMEN AND ALCOHOL

Women are more vulnerable to the effects of alcohol misuse than are males, due mainly to physiological differences (Single and Rohl 1997). Even though female alcohol-caused death rates have decreased between 1990–97, rates of alcohol-caused morbidity, as measured through hospital admissions among women, increased between the 1993–94 and 1996–97 financial years. These findings emerge in spite of the fact that the morbidity among women who suffer from alcohol dependency remains largely invisible (Nizette and Creedy 1998).

Women commonly abuse prescription medications together with alcohol. Alcohol consumption during pregnancy has a direct link with teratogenicity in the foetus, although it is not clearly established what level of alcohol consumption, if any, is safe for pregnant women (NHMRC 2001). Regardless of this there are likely to be significant public health implications surrounding alcohol consumption during pregnancy. Public awareness of the potential dangers of alcohol consumption in pregnancy is surprisingly low, while longitudinal studies in the USA examining alcohol consumption among pregnant women show that the number of women who report drinking is increasing with time (Morbidity and Mortality Weekly Report 1997).

INDIGENOUS HEALTH

The social and economic costs of the excessive use of alcohol by Indigenous Australians are significant. Although fewer Indigenous Australians drink alcohol (62 per cent)—lower than in the general population (72 per cent)—those who do drink tend to consume higher quantities, with more risky use among males in the 25 to 34 age group. Alcohol was estimated by the Royal Commissioners responsible for reviewing Aboriginal deaths in custody as being a direct cause of 10 per cent of deaths. The proportion of Aboriginal deaths considered to be alcohol related among Aboriginal people is three to four times higher than the general Australian population, with the highest mortality among middle-aged Aboriginal males where the proportion of deaths related to alcohol exceeds 30 per cent (PHAA 2000b).

Alcohol use is linked to petrol sniffing and the use of illicit drugs. Alcohol-related family violence is of particular concern to Indigenous communities. In turn, all are linked to mental health issues arising from alienation, despair, unemployment and racism (House of Representatives 1999). In remote Australia, alcohol is more easily obtainable and relatively cheaper than healthy, fresh food, impacting greatly on poor nutritional status as well as levels and severity of chronic disease (PHAA 2000a).

ALCOHOL IN THE WORKPLACE

The workplace has emerged as a major context for changing unhealthy lifestyle behaviours, and is therefore an ideal site for addressing risky drinking practices. Alcohol use compromises safety in many industries, contributing to absenteeism and reduced productivity. An approach that incorporates prevention and early intervention provides significant potential to reduce a range of alcohol-related harms. However, in order to be effective, programs must both confront and operate within the established culture of the workplace (Dietze et al. 1996).

Failure to tailor harm-reduction programs and policies to the workplace culture may result in such approaches being construed as intrusive or just plainly ignored. The Building Trades Group (2003) 'Not at Work, Mate' is an example of a successful program to deal with the maintenance of safety standards on building sites and prevention of accidents. The program has a policy framework that has informed training and education packages that come complete with videos and detailed course content, to promote safe work sites and to prevent incidents that may result from drug and alcohol use. Developed in conjunction with building workers, the program is accredited, and uses peer-based messages and training methods, delegating the identification and assessment of alcohol-impaired (and drug-impaired) workers to safety committees. Nevertheless, despite the success of properly constructed and implemented alcohol polices and programs, many workplaces do not have such policies.

Alcohol use impacts upon all workplaces, including among medical practitioners. The Nurses Board of Victoria has recently raised the issue of known or suspected drug use by registered nurses (Nurses Board of Victoria 2000). Similar problems may also occur among other medical and other health care practitioners, with costs to society of patients' morbidity and mortality as well as litigation costs (Tai et al. 1998). Nevertheless, these problems remain largely invisible.

POLICY DIRECTIONS

Policy documents cite a litany of harms associated with alcohol misuse, only a few of which have been covered in this chapter. Australia's National Alcohol Strategy 2001 to 2003–04 has a framework based on harm minimisation, the collection of information to identify the nature and extent of alcohol-related harm, and for the development of appropriate interventions. Legislative and policy responses have focused on controls on price and availability, minimum purchase ages, drink-driving laws, public education, awareness and intervention programs, and restrictions on marketing and advertising. As well, the NHMRC's guidelines on safe drinking levels have been made widely available, with the intention of increasing people's personal skills in making healthy choices about alcohol consumption.

Little is known about the extent to which Australia properly caters for the extent of alcohol-related problems in the community. Aims of alcohol policy are to reduce consumption among heavy drinkers, reduce consumption overall, and reduce harm overall. Emphasis must be placed on education, reduction of demand, and the provision of high-quality treatment services. It has long been suspected that there is a chronic shortage of alcohol treatment programs, and, as indicated, surveillance systems fail to capture the presentation of alcohol in treatment settings such as general practice—the setting where the majority of alcohol-related treatment probably takes place.

SUMMARY

- Excessive alcohol use is a problem within population groups with rural and remote populations, women, and young people particularly at risk of alcohol-related harms.
- Alcohol-related harms are a significant factor in levels of violence, especially against women and children.
- Alcohol dependence and misuse, illicit drug use, and tobacco smoking are markers of disadvantage in burden-of-disease studies, and are the biggest contributors to early and therefore preventable, death and disability in Australia.
- Stronger policy responses, and enhancement of multifaceted public health and health promotion strategies, are necessary to reduce the harms to individuals and communities from excessive alcohol use.

DISCUSSION TOPICS

1 Create a 'mind map' to conceptualise the 'collateral damage to society' from excessive consumption of alcohol.

2 Incorporate your understanding of the determinants of health in developing strategic midstream and upstream responses to binge drinking by young people in your community.

USEFUL WEB SITES

National Alcohol Strategy: www.health.gov.au/pubhlth/nds/resources/publications/alcohol_strategy.htm

National Drug Strategy: www.nationaldrugstrategy.gov.au/index2.htm

NHMRC safe drinking guidelines: www.health.gov.au/nhmrc/publications/synopses/ds9syn.htm

Curtin National Alcohol Indicators Project: http://db.ndri.curtin.edu.au/project.asp?projid=132

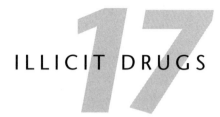

ILLICIT DRUGS

Paul Dietze and Helen Keleher

Key concepts

- Illicit drug use
- Co-morbidity
- Harm minimisation and harm reduction

Profound contradictions surround society's views on the use of psychoactive drugs. For example, while most sections of society accept the widespread distribution, sale, and use of alcohol, a number of drugs remain illicit in spite of their widespread use in the population. This fact remains, even though it is known that alcohol causes more death and disability in Australia than any drug other than tobacco (Collins and Lapsley 2002). Nevertheless, some illicit drugs create crippling, seemingly intractable problems for our social worlds and are responsible for substantial adverse health, social, and economic costs to the nation (Collins and Lapsley 2002). This chapter will address some of the issues surrounding illicit drugs, irrespective of drug type or the route of administration of the drug.

THE PREVALENCE AND EXPERIENCE OF ILLICIT DRUG USE

The prevalence of illicit drug use varies dramatically according to the particular drug under consideration. The 2001 National Drug Strategy Household Survey (NDSHS) (AIHW 2002a) shows that around 33 per cent of people surveyed report having used cannabis at some stage in their lives with 13 per cent reporting use in the twelve months prior to the survey (recent use). The prevalence of reported use of other illicit drugs is much lower, with only around 0.2 per cent, 3.4 per cent, and 2.9 per cent reporting recent use of heroin, amphetamines, and designer drugs such as ecstasy respectively. However, it should be noted that these types of household surveys most likely underestimate the true prevalence of the use of illicit drugs as: they target only households (missing other groups such as prisoners and the homeless who report high levels of illicit drug use); respondents may be reluctant to report engaging in illegal activities; and the response rates are typically low (Hser 1993). Further, changes to the 2001 survey mean that the results are not directly comparable to previous surveys in the NDSHS series (AIHW 2002a).

People who use illicit drugs can experience a variety of significant health and social harms related to their drug use that can affect not only themselves but also other parts of society more broadly. In the health domain some of the key harms include dependence, the spread of blood-borne viruses (BBVs) such as human immuno-deficiency virus (HIV) and hepatitis, and overdose, both fatal and nonfatal.

HEALTH-RELATED HARMS

Around 5 per cent of the Australian population are estimated to have met criteria for drug dependence in the twelve months prior to the conduct of the National Survey of Mental Health and Well-being in 1997 (Hall et al. 1999). Most of these respondents met the criteria for alcohol dependence (3.5 per cent) with only 0.2 per cent, 0.2 per cent, and 1.6 per cent of the population meeting the criteria for opioid (primarily heroin) stimulant, and cannabis dependence respectively. While these rates are relatively small for illicit drugs, they represent a significant pool of potential need for drug treatment services.

Beyond dependence, the measurable health-related harms associated with illicit drug use are relatively small for most drug classes. However, injecting is the preferred route of administration of heroin, in particular, in Australia among sampled drug users (Darke et al. 2002) and it is this type of drug use that is the primary focus of many media reports, policy documents, and research projects. Injecting drug use (IDU) is associated with a number of harms associated with the practice of injecting in unsterile circumstances (e.g. contaminated needles or syringes). While IDU represents the reported exposure category for only a small number of people notified as having HIV in Australia (due largely to the development and implementation of needle and syringe provision programs (see Crofts et al. 1999), IDU is a significant risk factor for the transmission of hepatitis C (HCV) with seroprevalence recorded at around 50 per cent in samples of injecting drug users tested since 1996 (National Centre in HIV Epidemiology and Clinical Research 2001).

Given that the rate of heroin use in Australia is relatively low, heroin users experience a disproportionately large amount of the harms associated with illicit drug use (Collins and Lapsley 2002). Fatal heroin overdose is the most serious consequence of heroin use. The number of heroin overdose deaths increased dramatically in Australia, peaking at around 950 in 1999. Nonfatal heroin overdose is also commonly experienced by heroin users (Darke et al. 1996), and using figures from Melbourne it can be estimated that these occur at a rate some ten times greater than heroin overdose deaths (Dietze et al. 2001). Together, these types of heroin overdose represent significant premature death and disability related to the use of illicit drugs in Australia.

ILLICIT DRUG USE AND CRIME

In contrast to legal drugs such as alcohol, the manufacture, sale, use, or possession of illicit drugs is, by definition, an offence. The sanctions that apply for these offences vary, with civil as opposed to criminal prohibition applying for some drugs in some Australian jurisdictions. The criminalisation of illicit drug offences means that significant proportions of the Australian population report engaging in illegal activities around drug use. Further, many of the harms experienced by people who use illicit drugs are limited primarily to the effects of criminal sanctions upon their social circumstances. For example, the effects of cannabis prohibition in Western Australia affects individuals who are prosecuted in the criminal system in their opportunities for work, their living circumstances, and their likelihood of further criminal involvement, when compared to the civil prohibition system operating in South Australia (Lenton et al. 1998). These effects are evident despite little evidence of any effect of criminal prohibition on the rate of cannabis use in the populations of these two states (Donnelly and Hall 1994).

The use of some illicit drugs is associated with significant levels of further criminal involvement. Heroin use in particular is associated with property crime (Makkai 2001). While the causes of this association have not been fully determined (e.g. do heroin users engage in property crime to support their drug use or is heroin use merely part of a criminal lifestyle?), the criminality associated with heroin use presents a significant burden to the Australian community (Makkai 2001).

CO-MORBIDITY

Mental health problems are more prevalent among people with drug problems than in the general population (Kessler et al. 1996). Co-morbidity rates have been increasing since the 1960s (Cuffel 1992). A large, representative US study found that the prevalence of mental health problems was as high as 65 per cent in opioid-dependent users with a risk rate that was seven times higher than in the general population (Reiger et al. 1990). The major co-morbid mental health problems found in people with problematic drug use problems are depression, anxiety disorders (e.g. panic, phobic, obsessive-compulsive, generalised anxiety, and post-traumatic stress disorders), antisocial personality disorders, and alcohol problems.

Co-morbidity has significant impact on relapse prevention and long-term treatment options. It leads to poorer clinical, personal, and social outcomes in comparison to either mental health or drug-use problems alone (Dixon et al. 1997; Lehman et al. 1993). These outcomes include: increased hospitalisation; depression and suicide; violence; incarceration; homelessness; HIV infection;

reduced ability to manage life needs; medication noncompliance; increased family problems; and higher service utilisation. There is evidence that treatment for both drug problems and mental health disorders improves prognosis, whereas continued illicit drug use intensifies mental health problems (Crome 1999). Given the range of poor outcomes, it can be argued that benefits to both individual and public health may be gained from treatment that addresses co-morbidity.

POLICY

Comprehensive public health approaches are needed if Australia is to tackle illicit drug problems. Drug use is the result of multiple social determinants and has considerable sequelae including violent experiences, poverty, unemployment, discrimination, and disadvantage. People who use drugs are often very troubled. They are people whose need for help with their health problems is very real. Australia is struggling to come to terms with these human rights issues.

There is considerable and continuing anxiety in Australia regarding illicit drugs and the most appropriate responses to the problems resulting from their use. There are three main pillars to the national policy on illicit drugs, known as harm minimisation, that was established under the National Campaign Against Drug Abuse in 1985 (AIHW 2002a). These are: supply reduction, demand reduction, and harm reduction. Nevertheless, there is tension within this policy framework as the majority of funding is oriented towards the activities of law enforcement agencies which can, at times, militate against the efforts of those working in the demand- and harm-reduction fields. This occurs in spite of available evidence of the poor outcomes associated with supply control, with estimates suggesting that only a small percentage of drugs such as heroin entering Australia are being seized by law enforcement agencies.

Prohibition is inimical to minimising the spread of HIV, HCV, and other blood-borne diseases. Supply control policy has delayed the introduction and implementation of sterile needle and syringe programs in many countries that is irreconcilable with efforts to minimise the spread of HIV infection among and from injecting drug users. Supply control policy in the opium-growing areas of the world, including South-East Asia, has led to heroin injecting replacing opium smoking, even in remote areas. This has exposed large populations to the hazards of HIV and HCV infection associated with the use of nonsterile injecting equipment. The prohibition of drugs can only effectively restrict the availability of substances if there is limited demand and little opportunity to subvert controls, and if there is no similar available drug that can be substituted. In summary, Australia's reliance on measures to control the supply of illicit drugs is expensive, ineffective, and counterproductive (PHAA 2000). Partnerships between the police, health, and welfare sectors are needed in order to reduce drug-related harm. Law enforcement can help reduce drug-related harm by adopting certain strategies, but funding to encourage projects that foster intersectoral partnerships is as likely to have an effect.

Recently in Australia there has been a shift towards considering the issues around illicit drugs within a health, rather than a law enforcement framework (Premier's Drug Advisory Committee 1996), producing law enforcement initiatives designed to divert people away from the legal system and into drug treatment. This shift reflects evidence that shows demand- and harm-reduction strategies have a greater cost-benefit to society than law enforcement practices around supply control alone. Indeed, scientific evidence from the USA has demonstrated that for every dollar invested in treatment there is a saving of seven dollars to society as a whole in terms of reduced law enforcement and imprisonment costs (Single and Rohl 1997). Within the resultant public health discourse around illicit drugs, it is harm- and demand-reduction measures that have received most attention with expanding demand-reduction initiatives such as methadone maintenance for heroin dependence and harm-reduction activities such as the provision of clean injecting equipment (through needle and syringe programs) or supervised injecting facilities. While these initiatives have been shown to be effective in relation to their stated aims (e.g. reduced heroin use, reduced blood-borne virus transmission), there is still considerable debate in the community about their value.

PRAGMATIC RESPONSES

Illicit drug markets are complex and dynamic and vary considerably as new drugs become available or people change their preferences for different drugs. For example, Australia experienced a dramatic change in the supply of heroin in early 2001 (commonly termed the heroin 'drought') that had a considerable impact upon the use of the drug and its consequences in the community (Dietze and Fitzgerald 2002). The dynamic nature of illicit drug markets, coupled with the fact that they currently operate outside of regulatory authorities and are likely to do so for the foreseeable future, requires a range of pragmatic public health responses around the effects of these markets on individuals and society more generally.

Australia has a limited number of places available within illicit drug treatment programs and a limited capacity to respond to changes in drug markets and/or drug preferences among illicit drug users (Dietze et al. 2001). Available evidence suggests that all states and territories should ensure that heroin injectors who wish to enter methadone maintenance programs and other pharmacotherapy treatments can be assessed quickly, that entry criteria are minimal, and that programs are attractive and economical. Such programs have been shown to be effective and result in high retention rates (Mattick and Hall 1993). Of the drug users surveyed in one New South Wales study, 39 per cent said they would definitely or probably start treatment tomorrow if they could and 56 per cent of these said it was the waiting list that was stopping them (Weatherburn and Lind 1999). Similar considerations apply in relation to treatment for the use of drugs other than heroin.

SOLUTION BUILDING FOR THE FUTURE

Illicit drug use is found in all social and economic groups but the harms associated with this use are found disproportionately among those most severely disadvantaged. Because the use of drugs has undesirable effects on the wellbeing of the using person, responses should be fundamentally a matter for health and welfare sectors, although, where the use of drugs has undesirable effects on the wellbeing of persons other than the user, there is a clear role for the law. As there are no optimal solutions to the problems resulting from illicit drugs, approaches should aim to identify and adopt solutions that create the least harm in the community.

SUMMARY

- Increased funding for a variety of treatment options and social support is needed, together with funding for community action to address drug problems.
- There is real need for a diversity of treatment options and for decentralised treatment availability in community health, general practice, and community hospitals. Rehabilitation programs need to be multifaceted and include skill training for longtime drug users trying to re-engage with mainstream society.
- Programs must have the capacity to deal with the social determinants of drug use.
- Persons who choose to consume or feel unable to cease consuming illicit drugs have human rights that may be threatened by policies to deal with the consequences of illicit drug use.
- Heroin overdose and blood-borne virus infection together represent the most serious potential complications of IDU for drug users and nondrug users alike; policies for illicit drugs should be at least partly considered in terms of whether they will assist or hinder efforts to control these harms.
- Further consideration is needed of the effects of the legislative framework surrounding illicit drugs in terms of the effects of prohibition on the social circumstances of individuals that may be of harm to society in the long term.
- Most evidence suggests that the current emphasis on law enforcement approaches may be misguided, and even counterproductive, especially in the face of inadequate funding for public health initiatives in the area of illicit drugs and the prevalence of illicit drug use in Australia.

DISCUSSION TOPIC

1 Evidence shows that 'demand- and harm-reduction strategies have a greater cost-effective benefit to society than law enforcement practices around supply

control alone'. With this in mind, develop *three* integrated upstream approaches to limit the harms to society that illicit drug use currently causes. What sectors have the potential to make a significant contribution to these approaches, and in what ways?

USEFUL WEB SITES

National Drug and Alcohol Research Centre: www.med.unsw.edu.au/ndarc
Population Health, Australian Department of Health and Ageing:
www.health.gov.au/pubhlth
National Drug Research Institute: www.ndri.curtin.edu.au
National Centre for Education and Training on Addiction:
www.nceta.flinders.edu.au
Turning Point Alcohol and Drug Centre: www.turningpoint.org.au
National Centre in HIV Epidemiology and Clinical Research:
www.med.unsw.edu.au/nchecr
Australian National Council on Drugs: www.ancd.org.au

18 PHYSICAL ACTIVITY AND POPULATION HEALTH

Jo Salmon, Clare Hume, and Kylie Ball

Key concepts

- Health consequences of physical activity
- Individual, social, and environmental influences on physical activity
- Physical activity guidelines

As the world becomes more urbanized, affluent and motorized, the diseases of inactivity will afflict a growing number of people. A sedentary lifestyle poses health risks for people of all ages, races, and ethnicities, for men and women alike.

(Tommy G Thompson, Secretary of US Health and Human Services)

WHAT DO WE MEAN BY PHYSICAL ACTIVITY?

As with any field of study, it is important to clearly define terminology. According to the US Surgeon General's Report of Physical Activity and Health, *physical activity* can be described as 'bodily movement produced by the contraction of skeletal muscle that increases energy expenditure above the basal level' (USD-HHS 1996, p. 20). The term 'physical activity' can be conceptualised not just as energy expenditure above the basal metabolic rate, but as a group of active behaviours that can be varied and complex. For example, active behaviours may consist of cycling, swimming, walking, sport, sweeping, or digging in the garden. The forms or types of physical activity may be grouped depending on the purpose or intent in performing the activity, such as *exercise* or *incidental physical activity*.

Physical activity can occur in a variety of contexts and settings (e.g. at home, at work, at school, during leisure time, for transport). The *type* (what sort of physical activity), *frequency* (how often), *duration* (how long), and *intensity* or

metabolic equivalents (METs) of physical activity have been shown to relate to health outcomes. METs are units used to describe the metabolic cost of physical activity as a product of the resting metabolic rate (1 MET); a brisk walking pace is usually allocated 3 METs in terms of metabolic cost.

What impact does physical activity have on population health?

The health consequences of physical activity and exercise have been extensively studied, in particular 'Epidemiologic studies of physical activity and health have compared the activity levels of people who have or develop diseases and those who do not' (USDHHS 1996, p. 85). Compared to those who are inactive, those who are moderately or vigorously active have been found to be significantly less likely to suffer premature all-cause mortality; cardiovascular diseases (CVD) such as coronary heart disease (CHD), stroke, and high blood pressure; colon and breast cancers; type 2 diabetes; overweight and obesity; osteoarthritis; and poor mental health (USDHHS 1996). Recent research has shown sedentary living is associated with 22 to 30 per cent of all cardiovascular deaths, 20 to 60 per cent of cancers, and 30 per cent of deaths from diabetes (Stone et al. 1998). Regular physical activity also confers a number of psychological benefits including increased mental performance and concentration; improved mood, sleep, energy levels; and decreased tension, stress levels, anxiety, hostility, and depression (USDHHS 1996).

What are the costs?

Physical inactivity is the second-highest ranked modifiable health-risk factor in the Australian adult population, second only to smoking as a major contributor to the overall burden of disease in this country (AIHW 1999b). Sedentary

Figure 18.1   Percent of total burden attributed to risk factors: Burden of Disease study

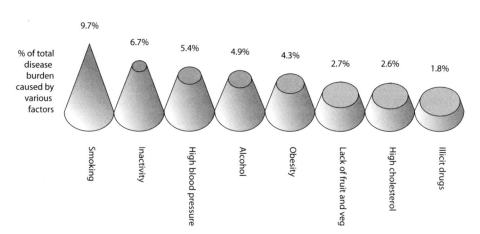

lifestyles cost the health system at least $400 million in direct health care costs and are responsible for approximately 8000 deaths per year in Australia (Stephenson et al. 2000).

How much physical activity is important for health?

As described in box 18.1, current national physical activity guidelines suggest that adults accumulate thirty minutes of moderate-intensity physical activity on five or more days per week (DHAC 1999c). Population surveys in Australia indicate declines in the proportion of adults who are meeting the physical activity guidelines (i.e. those participating in 150 minutes or more of physical activity per week), from 62 per cent in 1997 to 54 per cent in 1999 (Armstrong et al. 2000). Typically, in population surveys, those who are least active generally include women, older adults, and those who are socioeconomically disadvantaged or have lower educational attainment (USDHHS 1996). Developing strategies to reduce physical inactivity in whole populations requires an understanding of the correlates and predictors of physical inactivity.

Box 18.1   National physical activity guidelines, Australia

Think of movement as an opportunity, not as an inconvenience Be active every day in as many ways as you can Put together at least 30 minutes of moderate-intensity physical activity on most days; preferably all days. If you can, also enjoy some regular, vigorous exercise for extra health and fitness.

Source: DHAC 1999c

WHY ARE SOME PEOPLE ACTIVE AND OTHERS NOT?

As the science of explaining, predicting, and changing human behaviour is extremely complex, behavioural and social scientists often use models or theories to assist in their understanding of behaviour. A number of theories of physical activity behaviours have been developed to try and explain why some people are active and others are not. Some of these theories focus solely on psychological factors (e.g. motivation levels, enjoyment of activity). However, these models have not been very successful in explaining people's activity. This may be partly because they do not take into account broader factors that might also be important in people's choices to be active or not (Salmon et al. 2003). More recent theoretical models therefore also include social (e.g. having someone to exercise with) and environmental (e.g. having a pleasant park or bicycle track nearby) factors as possible influences on physical activity. An example of such a model is provided in figure 18.2. Note that this is just an example, not necessarily the 'best' model.

Figure 18.2 Example of an ecological model of influences on physical activity

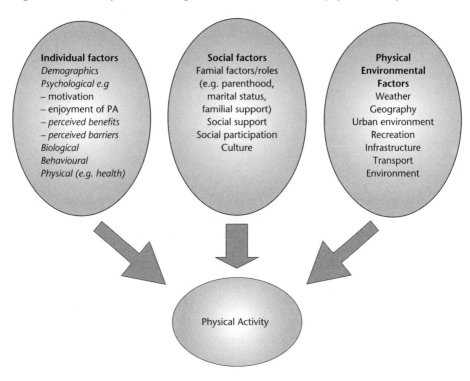

Adapted from Sallis and Owen 1999

Many hundreds of studies have examined the reasons why some people are physically active and others are not (Sallis and Owen 1999). These reasons are commonly known as 'determinants', 'correlates', or 'influences', and refer to factors that are related to participation in physical activity. It should be noted that these influences on physical activity behaviour are likely to be complex (e.g. as shown in the above model), and on the whole, we still have a relatively poor understanding of the exact reasons some people are more active than others. Nonetheless, many potential determinants of physical activity have been studied. A brief review of the literature below identifies some of the individual, social, and environmental determinants that explain differences in physical activity among adults and children.

Individual factors

Individual factors explaining physical activity include: attitudes, beliefs, and values; psychological characteristics such as enjoyment, motivation, perceived health and fitness, barriers, and physical activity **self-efficacy** (USDHHS 1996; Sallis and Owen 1999).

Perceived *enjoyment* of physical activity has been shown to predict participation in physical activities. One study of more than 1200 adults found that those reporting high enjoyment of walking were three times more likely to report walking for more than 2.5 hours a week.(Salmon et al. 2003).

An individual's *perception of their health and fitness* is also associated with participation in physical activity. Those who believe their health is poor are less likely to participate in any form of physical activity (King et al. 1992).

In relation to physical activity, *self-efficacy* is an individual's confidence in his or her ability to perform physical activity in specific conditions (Sallis and Owen 1999). Individuals may report high levels of self-efficacy regarding exercising in good weather, but not in rainy weather, and this has been shown to be an extremely strong correlate of participation in physical activity (King et al. 1992; Sallis and Owen 1999).

Barriers refer to the variety of reasons that may make it difficult or impossible for an individual to participate in physical activity. These barriers may be perceived or actual, and have been found to be associated with lower likelihood of participation. The most commonly stated barrier to physical activity participation is *lack of time;* however, those who participate in regular exercise are just as likely to report time as a barrier as are those who are sedentary (King et al. 1992). Therefore, we might question whether time is an actual barrier, or whether it reflects other factors such as a lower perceived priority for physical activity? Such ambiguity makes the investigation of barriers to physical activity an area worthy of further consideration.

Social factors

Research, both Australian and international, has shown that individuals reporting higher levels of *social support* for physical activity from family and/or friends are more likely to be physically active (USDHHS 1996; Leslie et al. 1999; Ball et al. 2001; Stahl et al. 2001).

Physical environmental factors

Physical environmental factors are among the least understood of the domains of influences on physical activity. A recent review of international literature (Humpel et al. 2002) identified three categories of physical environment factors that were found to be consistently positively associated with physical activity. These were *accessibility* of physical activity facilities in the neighbourhood environment; *opportunities* for activity in the home and neighbourhood environment; and favourable environmental *aesthetics*. Those with convenient and accessible facilities for physical activity are more likely to participate (Sallis et al. 1990; Booth et al. 2000), as are those reporting appealing aesthetics in their neighbourhood (e.g. attractive surroundings, nice gardens) (Ball et al. 2001).

The *safety of the environment* in which activity is being performed may also be an important influence on physical activity (Sallis et al. 1997). Perceived neighbourhood safety has been shown to be associated with inactivity, particularly among those aged over 65 years (Booth et al. 2000). Traffic is another aspect of safety that appears to be related to participation in physical activity, particularly among children. Parental concerns about traffic safety are thought to have led in part to decreases in children's participation in walking and bike riding activities (DiGuiseppi et al. 1997).

SUMMARY

- Studies have identified a large number of potential determinants of physical activity behaviour.
- Individual, social, and environmental factors are likely to be important, but more research into the relative influences of these factors is needed.
- A better understanding of the determinants of physical activity behaviours is required in order to effectively intervene to promote increased levels of physical activity and hence improve population health.
- In particular, research on children, older adults, culturally and linguistically diverse groups, and those with disabilities is required.

DISCUSSION TOPICS

1 Unpack the determinants of physical activity for a specific group in your own community. You might choose to study children, older adults, culturally and linguistically diverse groups, or those with a disability. Use the ecological model in figure 18.2 to guide your investigation.

2 What further information would you need before you could confidently develop a strategic plan to encourage increased physical activity for your target group?

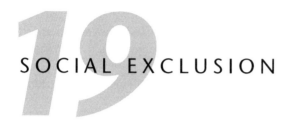

SOCIAL EXCLUSION

Helen Keleher

Key concepts

- Social exclusion
- Inequity
- Poverty

I was asked to discuss, here in Oslo, the greatest challenge that the world faces. I decided that the most serious and universal problem is the growing chasm between the richest and poorest people on earth. The results of this disparity are root causes of most of the world's unresolved problems, including starvation, illiteracy, environmental degradation, violent conflict and unnecessary illnesses that range from Guinea worm to HIV/AIDs.

President Jimmy Carter on receiving the Nobel Peace Prize, 2002

Deprivation means not being able to appear in public without shame.

Adam Smith, 1776

In the twenty-first century, people in every country of the globe are confronted by massive inequities, with increasing social exclusion recognised as a major determinant of health. The relationships between social exclusion, poverty, and poor health are not (yet) at the forefront of health policy reform in Australia. There is perhaps more easiness in analysing the material dimensions and determinants of inequality than of social exclusion, which is about nonmaterial dimensions of poverty, its effect on people's opportunities to contribute and their access to opportunities to participate in economic, social, and political life. Acceptance that social exclusion is a key determinant of health and social inequity, implies the need to make much greater investments in primary health care interventions with their progressive focus on social and economic development, rather than primary care with its focus on treatment and individualised prevention.

Certainly, there is debate, more in Australia than Europe, about whether we should use the term **social inclusion** rather than **social exclusion** and objections to the language of 'exclusion'. This chapter will provide a rationale for naming social exclusion as one of the most serious consequences of poverty and inequity, and for effective health policies and programs that are driven by principles of equity and social justice. As Carter points out above, poverty and widening gaps between rich and poor are unresolved problems of the world that have profound effects on people's health, but in order to understand the health effects of poverty and inequity, we also need to understand social exclusion. In other words, we will not achieve social inclusion unless we come to grips with the conceptualisation of social exclusion as being both constituted in poverty, deprivation, and a lack of freedoms, especially in terms of citizenship. Social exclusion is also an instrumental cause of diverse forms of the failure of capacity (to produce food for example) or capability (the possession of multiple abilities required to actively resolve problems). Definitions of inequality and inequity are explained in chapter 7, and these provide the foundation on which to discuss notions of poverty.

POVERTY

Poverty has a powerful presence in every nation of the world. Poverty can be measured instrumentally, as in the (Australian) Henderson poverty line, which is an income level that is meant to provide for basic living costs. The poverty line concept is widely criticised for its incapacity to address wealth distribution or the underlying reasons for vulnerability among some groups of people (Reiger 2000). Townsend devised a more qualitative notion of relative poverty in the late 1970s, in the United Kingdom. Relative poverty is when 'people lack the resources to obtain the types of diet, participate in the activities and have the living conditions and amenities which are customary, or are at least widely encouraged, or approved in the society to which they belong' (in Baum 2002, p. 209). Or as Adam Smith noted in the eighteenth century, deprivation results in people feeling shamed in the presence of others.

Poverty, then, is the lack of freedom to be able to do certain things that are valued (Sen 2000, p. 5). But in a wider sense, poverty creates exclusion from a whole range of opportunities including land ownership, education, and economic participation. This is known as *capability* deprivation. The capability deprivation sense of the meaning of poverty is deepened when the processes through which poverty occurs are analysed and understood, that is, the processes through which individuals or groups are wholly or partially excluded, actively or passively, from full participation in the society in which they live.

Box 19.1   Case study 1

Matt grew up in the 1960s on a mission for Indigenous people, outside a small New South Wales country town. Poverty was everywhere, as the people's main source of income was welfare. The kids from the mission used to walk 2 km to a road junction, to meet the school bus. It wasn't that the bus couldn't get to the mission, it was just that the Indigenous kids didn't want the white kids to see how they lived. Matt's white father had long gone. Matt's mother and grandmother had to go down to the river, some distance away, for fresh water. Nowadays, the mission has become a village. The houses have water supplies and gardens, there is a village green and the mission people have gone, with Indigenous people managing the village themselves. The kids of today are now proud to have the school bus come into the village to pick them up for school. Nevertheless, most of the kids grow up to experience long-term unemployment and poverty.

IMPACT OF SOCIAL EXCLUSION

The case study in box 19.1 illustrates the impact of social exclusion on the lives in Indigenous Australians.

Before reading on, write down how these experiences would make you feel. It is very difficult for most of us to have a depth of understanding of these issues, but attempt to write down what you think are the affects of these experiences on Indigenous people's lives. Now read on about the concept of social exclusion.

Notions of social inclusion and social exclusion have come primarily from the United Kingdom, Europe, and Canada. The World Health Organization (WHO) has recognised social exclusion as a key determinant of health (Marmot and Wilkinson 1998). Social exclusion has enormous economic and social consequences for people who may already be living on chronically low incomes. Populations most commonly identified as vulnerable to, or most at risk of, social exclusion include those with limited employment opportunities particularly black and ethnic minority groups, refugees, homeless people, female and male prostitutes, people living with disabilities, people living with mental illness, people living with drug addiction, and/or blood-borne viruses (HIV, hepatitis C), long-term unemployed, people living in temporary accommodation, young people (especially early school leavers), and older people (especially those living on pensions). In rural areas of Australia, there are profound class distinctions between people from the dominant culture of that area and 'outsiders' who have moved to small towns seeking cheaper housing or for lifestyle reasons.

Social exclusion is frequently related to discrimination based on difference. In the case of Indigenous Australians, discrimination has been, and often still is, based on racism. People experiencing social isolation and social exclusion demonstrate low levels of personal control (Marmot 1999; Mathers 1994), as well as loneliness and unhappiness. They demonstrate an increased need for mental health services, experience high levels of stress and higher mortality rates for all causes of death, more depression, less wellbeing and are at greater risk of pregnancy complications (Turrell et al. 1999).

Amartya Sen (2000), himself a Nobel Peace Laureate, points out that the development of conceptually adequate understandings of social exclusion has the potential to enrich causal explanations and analyses of particular aspects of poverty and deprivation. Poverty has long been understood in terms of 'capability deprivation' (since Adam Smith, if not Aristotle, understood that individual lives are inescapably part of a greater 'social' life), but Sen argues that a focus on relational processes of poverty and deprivation deepens our understanding of the meaning of social exclusion. He argues that we need to understand that social exclusion is not just the result of low social capital or poverty for example, but that there is a constitutive role of social exclusions. For example, the effects of globalisation on people insufficiently educated to have the new skills, new knowledge, or patterns of production required to compete in global markets is one of exclusion, but moreover, many such people are also excluded from maintaining their traditional forms of economic and agricultural survival. Thus by being excluded from the opportunities that globalisation might offer, the developments on which globalisation itself is constituted create others forms of exclusion.

Sen talks of both *active* and *passive* exclusions as having 'constitutive relevance and instrumental importance' (2000, p. 14). The situation of migrants and refugees can usefully illustrate the ways in which exclusion works. In any given country, there may not be deliberate attempts to exclude migrants or refugees, but they may still experience deprivation that arises from unemployment or isolation, whether social, cultural, or linguistic. Active fostering of exclusion can be instituted by governments through policies, or by others in society. Not being given a 'usable political status', delaying citizenship processes, or denial of voting rights (Sen 2000, pp. 14–15) are good examples of active exclusion.

However, in any given society, the concept of social exclusion is regarded as referring to a wide range of 'les exclus' including those with physical or intellectual disabilities, people suffering mental illness, the elderly, single mothers, vulnerable children, youth, people who abuse substances and so on. Silver adds to these examples a list of situations from which people may experience exclusion, from: 'a livelihood; secure, permanent employment; earnings; property, credit or land; housing; minimal or prevailing consumption levels; education, skills and cultural capital; the welfare state; citizenship and legal equality; democratic participation; public goods; the nation or the dominant race; family and sociability; humanity, respect, fulfilment and understanding' (in Sen 2000, p. 1).

In providing this list, Sen cautions against indiscriminate use of social exclusion as an umbrella concept to describe any situation in which a person, or group of people, find themselves left out of something, without critical examination of what insights will be provided by using social exclusion as an approach to analysis. Use of social exclusion should contribute to understanding of the nature of the problem, in identifying causal pathways, and enrich thinking for policy and social action (Sen 2000, p. 2).

The relationship between women and the labour market can also be seen as historically marked by various forms of exclusion (see for example Deacon 1989; Francis 1993). From the 1960s, the women's movement has carefully analysed the nature of sexism within families and in the workplace, its sources and causes, identified the lack of affordable, quality childcare, and the right of women to have access to the same educational opportunities afforded to males. Policy action was hard fought and while many gains have been made for Australian women, not all women have sufficient opportunities to gain the resources they need for good health and wellbeing. Sen (2000) also notes that 'the persistence of inequality between men and women is a problem that is sharper in Asia than in any other continent', and results in significant levels of social, educational, political and economic exclusion for women. Policy solutions lie in education and employment opportunities for women; these have been shown historically to have profound effects on women's health and fertility control.

Social exclusion and understanding health

There is no argument that social exclusion has significant negative effects on people's health and wellbeing. You will find additional discussion about the effects of inequity and poverty on health in several chapters in this book, which discuss various dimensions of the broader context of the determinants of health, of which social exclusion is one. Loss of health and capability are deprivations that can arise from conditions of poverty and social exclusion, but which then become a circular problem because people with poor health are limited in their capacity to access opportunities that might relieve their poverty. Understanding the meaning and many dimensions of social exclusion is critical, not just for understanding the determinants of health, but also for the development of policy action. Even for those most vulnerable, social exclusion is likely to affect psychosocial health more than physical health; yet physical health can be damaged over the long term by poor mental health. The effects of entrenched racism, deprivation, and discrimination have profoundly affected the health of Indigenous Australians:

> Morbidity and mortality statistics reflect an inheritance of loss and social upheaval that remains a central feature of Aboriginal consciousness today… Thus, health professionals who want to be effective need to 'hear' what Aborigines have to say, not just about their immediate health concerns but about the broader impediments to their wellbeing and about their own ways of tackling their concerns.
>
> Reid and Trompf 1991, pp. xxi

Health policy that actively promotes self-determination, capacity building, and community engagement will support the health of Aboriginal people.

A significant policy solution was given life in December 2002 by the National Assembly of Quebec, Canada, which unanimously passed a bill designed to cut poverty in Quebec in half over the next decade. The new law commits the provincial government to establishing an anti-poverty action plan and to giving a progress report on its fight against poverty every three years. It also sets a minimum level for social assistance payments, creates a monitoring agency, and provides funds for special anti-poverty initiatives to fight poverty and social exclusion. Every government should have such legislation.

SUMMARY

- Understanding social exclusion has relevance for health, particularly in the responsibility of health professionals to advocate for healthy public policy and social justice.
- Values about equity and social justice should be fundamental in health promotion approaches adopted by policy makers and practitioners to tackle social and health inequities.
- Health promotion approaches shape how health resources and capacity building flow through to vulnerable groups, in order to affect the determinants of health.
- In striving to overcome social exclusion and reduce health inequities, the adoption of multi-level empowerment strategies of health promotion, such as community action and community development, is necessary to enable people to have more control and decision making over their health and over the determinants of their health.

DISCUSSION TOPICS

1 Identify examples of social exclusion in your community for a particular group such as women, youth, new arrivals, older people, or Indigenous Australians.
2 Can you track the history of exclusion for this group? What measures, if any, have been implemented to address this social exclusion? In your view, what else should be done?

USEFUL WEB SITES

Inequality.org: www.inequality.org
Canadian Policy Research Networks Inc.: www.cprn.org
The University of Washington's Health and Income Equity site:
http://depts.washington.edu/eqhlth

20

FOOD INSECURITY AND THE MIGRANT EXPERIENCE

Cate Burns

Key concepts

- Food insecurity
- Nutrition promotion

Since humanity's early history, good food has been known to be important for wellbeing. Hippocrates, the ancient Greek philosopher (460–377 BC), taught that good food is good medicine. More recently, the science of nutrition has expanded our understanding of food and health. By the end of the twentieth century, scientists had identified protein, carbohydrates, vitamins, minerals, and many other micronutrients. Today, we know what you should eat, and how much, depending on your age and gender, with extra considerations being made for pregnancy and lactation (Commonwealth of Australia 1998).

However, knowing what to eat does not necessarily lead to eating the perfect healthy diet. Nutritionists would probably be the first to admit to this. Why is there a gap between knowing and eating? Basically, eating is a very complex behaviour. It is determined by many factors in addition to knowledge: food taste and texture; economic factors such as income; psychological factors such as body image; social factors such as class; and cultural factors such as the ethnic groups to which we belong, our religion, and cultural events. You can tell a lot about a person by what they put on their plate or into their supermarket trolley. As the great philosopher and gourmand, Jean Anthelme Brillat-Savarin, said, 'Tell me what thou eatest, and I will tell thee what thou art' (Brillat-Savarin 1825).

The art of **nutrition promotion** (i.e. health promotion in the area of nutrition) requires not only a broad knowledge of nutrition but also a good understanding of all the factors that determine food consumption. In this chapter, I will discuss two factors that demonstrate these other influences on food consumption that need to be taken into consideration in developing nutrition promotion or education: **food insecurity** (i.e. not having enough food or money to buy food) and migration.

FOOD INSECURITY

In most societies, the distribution of resources, including money, varies across the social strata. In many developing countries, this effect is extreme, with a great divide existing between rich and poor. In all societies, there are individuals and groups of individuals whose ability to secure food is compromised by a lack of social equity and resources.

Food security has been defined by the Expert Working Group of the American Institute of Nutrition as: 'Access by all people at all times to enough food for an active, healthy life. Food security includes at a minimum, the ready availability of nutritionally adequate and safe foods, and an assured ability to acquire acceptable foods in socially acceptable ways i.e. without resorting to emergency food supplies, scavenging, stealing or other coping strategies' (Anderson 1990). This definition indicates that people's access to food can be limited by how much money they have, whether their local shop sells nutritious and affordable food, how accessible that shop is, whether the food that is available is appropriate culturally, and whether acquisition and consumption of food conforms to social norms (e.g. it is considered socially unacceptable to have to beg or scavenge for food).

The major cause of food insecurity is not having enough income. In Australia, five adults in 100 report running out of food and not having enough money to buy more (ABS 1997). There are some people in Australia who are more vulnerable than others to food insecurity; for example, Aboriginals and Torres Strait Islanders, those on low incomes, with mental illnesses or from non-English speaking backgrounds, and those who are homeless, chronically ill, or suffering from drug or alcohol abuse. These people are said to live below the poverty line, an estimated income level that is the minimum level needed to secure the necessities of life (Pearsall 1999). For these people, food often becomes a budgetary item that can be cut back to meet accommodation, schooling, utility, or medical expenses. In these families there is less money for food and the intake of nutritious foods is poor.

The issue of poverty is essentially an ethical and economic one that largely has a political solution. In this respect, food insecurity is a societal problem. However, the experience of food insecurity at the family level in Australia is much more immediate. Studies have shown that low-income families have sound nutrition knowledge and adequate cooking skills (Crotty et al. 1992). For most, the limiting factor to eating well is lack of money. Not having enough money to buy food can result in:

- families having to rely on emergency food relief (i.e. handouts from charitable organisations)
- parents going without so that children can eat

- food purchases being dictated by the requirement that a food is cheap and filling; these filling foods are high in kilojoules but usually low in other necessary nutrients (see table 20.1 for the relative cost of 100 kilocalories (420 kilojoules) of various foods)
- a low intake of fruits and vegetables (ABS 1997)
- a lack of adequate food, which can affect concentration and learning ability among children and the ability of adults to work, as well as result in reduced school attendance for children
- increased stress in households, strained family relationships, and reduced confidence and self-esteem for the adults responsible for providing food
- increased illness and mortality.

Table 20.1 Cost of 100 kcals (420 kJ) of food

ITEM	CENTS PER 100 KCAL (420 KJ)
Mince—lean	48
Mince—low quality	30
Bananas	22
Apples	63
Oranges	77
Bread—white	18
Bread—wholemeal	19
Muesli	16
Weetbix	19
Milk—whole	40
Milk—trim	25
Milo—water	3
Sweet tea	3
Ice cream—low fat	20
Ice cream	10
Milk chocolate	29
Crème biscuits	15
Potato crisps	24

Source: New Zealand Network Against Food Poverty 2000

It is not only how much money you have that can determine how well you eat, but also where you live. The Healthy Food Access Basket Survey assessed the cost and availability of a basket of food across Queensland (Lee et al. 2002). The basket contained enough food to feed a family of six for two weeks on a diet that would meet all of their nutritional requirements. The study found that food prices were significantly higher in remote and very remote areas (20 and 31 per cent, respectively) compared with highly accessible urban areas. Basic foods were less available in the more remote stores. Another study of fast-food outlets in Melbourne showed density of population per fast food outlet was lower in the more economically disadvantaged neighbourhoods (5000 persons per outlet) as compared with higher income neighbourhoods (15,000 persons per outlet) (Reidpath et al. 2002) (figure 20.1). It is difficult to determine from this latter study whether the presence of fast-food outlets is a response to demand or if their presence drives demand, but we can say that it is easier to access fast food in poor neighbourhoods. Therefore, where you live may determine your access to healthy and unhealthy foods, and how much you pay.

Figure 20.1   The population per fast food outlet by socioeconomic status (SES), with SES 4 having the highest median individual weekly income and SES 1 the lowest

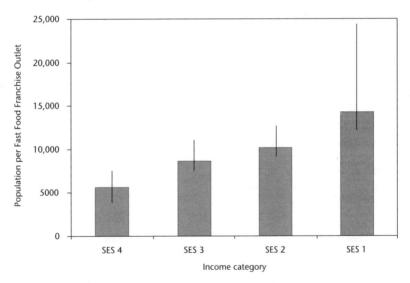

Implications of food security for health promotion

Income and environment are major determinants of food intake. Some people may not be able to afford to eat well or may live in communities where healthy foods are not available. Health promotion strategies targeting those population groups vulnerable to food insecurity would include improving income equity and ensuring a cheap supply of healthy foods.

NUTRITION IN TRANSITION/MIGRATION

Another factor that can influence eating and the adoption of healthy eating habits is migration and economic development. Migrants arrive in a new country with a food culture, beliefs about health and food, and attitudes about issues such as gender roles in food provision that are often different to those of their host country. That is not to say that migrants eat poorly. Migrants will have an understanding of health and food that may not be consistent with that of the country to which they have migrated, but that are not necessarily inconsistent with good physical and social health. In fact, most studies of people in developing countries following a traditional diet indicate that provided caloric needs are met, a traditional diet free of processed foods available in more developed countries, enhances health (Brown 1991). Many migrants from developing countries have to contend with their sudden exposure to an economically developed lifestyle. They may have experienced this in a limited sense in their countries of origin, but in the developed countries to which they migrate they are exposed to supermarkets full of cheap, processed foods and fast-food outlets, and have increased access to cars and labour-saving devices. This transition in lifestyle is known as Westernisation. It has been shown to be associated with obesity and chronic disease (Brown 1991).

Table 20.2   Typical menu for a day for a Somali man or woman living in Somalia and in Australia

SOMALIA	AUSTRALIA
Enjera (traditional bread) with sugar/oil/butter	Cereal with milk
Muufo (bread)	Bread/*enjera* with margarine
Cooked meat or egg or camel liver	Cooked meat or tuna or egg or jam
Staple (rice, pasta, polenta)	Staple (rice, pasta, polenta)
Fried, grilled, or stewed meat (camel/goat/ beef), or fish or chicken	Fried, grilled, or stewed meat (lamb/beef), or fish or chicken
Vegetable salsa	Vegetable salsa
Salad plus fruit	Salad plus fruit
Anbuulo (beans)/*muufo* with sugar/ghee/oil/sesame oil/bread	*Anbuulo*/oats/semolina with sugar/oil Bread with margarine/jam
Camel or cow milk, water, fruit juice, tea	Cow milk, water, fruit juice, tea, soft drink, cordial
Homemade cake, biscuits, chocolate, lollies, halva	Cake, biscuits, nuts, processed snacks such as potato crisps Takeaway—pizza, chicken fillet burger, halal takeaway

Let us consider migration to Australia. One in four residents of Australia was born outside Australia; a further one in four has at least one parent who was born overseas (Department of Immigration and Multicultural Affairs 1997). Every year, some 45,000 people migrate to Australia. Over 12,000 of these people come as refugees. For migrants and refugees alike, there is the adjustment to a new food system and culture. It should be noted, though, that the exchange of food cultures between host populations and migrants is a two-way process that has created a very vibrant food culture in Australia. However, migrants from developing countries, while sharing a rich food culture with their host country, can get the worst of the Australian Western food culture (Bennett 1993).

Let us take the case of Somali refugees to Australia. Somalia is a developing country in the Horn of Africa that has a particularly fragile economy. In 1991, civil war in Somalia led to a mass exodus of the population. Many were granted refugee status in Australia, Canada, and New Zealand. Table 20.2 presents some data that I collected in a study undertaken with Somali women who had migrated to Australia (Burns et al. 2000). Compare, for example, the menu for an individual for a day spent in Australia and for a day spent in Somalia. Can you spot the differences in food consumption? The differences that you may have noticed are: the substitution of lamb for camel meat and lack of camel's milk in Australia; the addition of takeaway food, breakfast cereals, and margarine; and the increase in processed snack foods. Compare also the consumption levels (i.e. the percentage of people consuming a food at least once a month) of a variety of foods eaten in Somalia and in Australia (table 20.3). What differences do you

Table 20.3 The comparative consumption of specific foods (given as the percentage of people consuming the food at least once a month) in Somalia and in Australia

	SOMALIA	AUSTRALIA
Meat		
Beef	47	49
Lamb	29	69
Camel	82	7
Goat	87	22
Fresh fish	75	56
Chicken	49	88
Processed foods		
Instant noodles	9	27
Pizza	2	27
Sweet biscuits	69	64
Chocolate biscuits	4.4	12
Pastries	7	20
Potato crisps	0	16

note? The nutritional impact of these dietary changes for Somali migrants settling in Australia would be an increase in their intake of fat, sugar, and salt.

In addition to a change in the foods selected for consumption, there are broader adjustment issues regarding food that Somalis have to contend with on migrating to Australia.

Change in food supply

Since most Somali immigrants to Australia are of the Muslim faith, meat or products containing meat derivatives can be consumed only if the animal from which they were obtained has been slaughtered according to the techniques defined in Islamic dietary law (i.e. if the food is halal). Most Somali immigrants have been accustomed to living in countries where the mainstream food supply is halal. Many indicate that they had experienced some difficulties in adjusting to a food supply that is not halal (Burns et al. 2000). For example, they may have had trouble locating suppliers of halal meats and identifying permitted foods. Also, many Somalis are unfamiliar with fruits and vegetables available on the Australian market; for example, broccoli, mushrooms, and such stone fruits as plums and peaches. The Somalis whom I interviewed were familiar with the often more expensive tropical fruits than fruits more commonly eaten in Australia but less common in Somalia, such as apples and oranges.

Change in meal times

Migrating to Australia often meant a change in the timing of the main meal of the day for the Somali immigrants in our study. In Somalia, the main meal is typically taken at lunchtime and involves the whole family. For these Somali immigrants, there were ongoing difficulties in shaping an alternative arrangement that met the dual objectives of bringing the family together and ensuring an appropriate food intake. Also, in Somalia, children come home from school to eat lunch, and many of the Somalis interviewed in my study were unfamiliar with the concept of packed school lunches.

Change in family responsibilities

In Somalia, domestic responsibilities are shared between all of the women in the extended family. For many of the Somali women interviewed, the major change on arrival in Australia was that they now had sole responsibility for food preparation. For some lone Somali men who arrived with no domestic skills, a major change was having to cook for themselves. Also, the organisation of day-to-day life in Somalia lent itself to a generally slower and more sociable pace than that experienced in Australia. Both physical activity and social interaction were integrated incidentally into everyday life in Somalia. There was a strong sense of community and interconnectedness. Further, a large amount of physical activity was expended in domestic duties and in walking (especially given that walking was the most common form of transport). In Australia, many Somalis interviewed in our study found themselves socially isolated, inactive, and prone to unaccustomed weight gain.

Implications of the migration experience for health promotion

It is important to understand the food culture of a target group in order to implement nutrition promotion programs. It is also important to understand the role that food plays in family dynamics and in the social fabric of a cultural group. The overall impact of migration can result in an increased intake of processed foods to the detriment of traditional foods, a disintegration in family eating and social networks, and a reduction in physical activity. Nutrition promotions for immigrant populations in Australia must be culturally appropriate and directed at enabling immigrants to use the food supply and understand different food customs while encouraging some retention of their own traditional eating habits.

SUMMARY

- Income and where you live have important effects on your diet and access to healthy foods.
- Migration has profound effects on the food security, food habits, and nutrition, and therefore the health and wellbeing, of migrants to Australia.
- Westernisation of the diets of migrants is related to obesity and chronic disease.
- Health promoters need to take into account issues other than the simple provision of nutrition information in order to encourage dietary habits that are consistent with health.
- Health promoters need stronger understandings of food cultures and the environments of migrant populations.

DISCUSSION TOPICS

1 Why is it that typical midstream interventions such as health education programs around healthy eating and making healthy food choices are unlikely to have a positive impact on those experiencing food insecurity in our communities?

2 How might a health professional with an understanding of the determinants of health work with new arrivals in helping them to avoid the risk of food insecurity?

21

EVIDENCE AND PUBLIC HEALTH: DATA, DISCOURSES, AND DEBATES

Jan Garrard

> ## Key concepts
>
> - Using evidence in public health practice
> - Describing the health problem
> - Identifying the causes of health problems
> - Determining the effectiveness of interventions
> - Evidence debates

A desire to understand the workings of the world and its inhabitants is an intrinsically human attribute. Questions such as 'What does it mean to *know* something?', 'How do we obtain knowledge?' and 'What should we do with it?' have been asked throughout human history. People from different walks of life answer these questions very differently. Some hold that knowledge comes from God (religious thinkers), is obtained through the rigorous application of reason and argument (the early Greek philosophers), or through systematic observation and experimentation in the 'real' world (scientists). Sir Francis Bacon, one of the powerful influences behind the scientific revolution that began in the late sixteenth century, famously stated that 'knowledge is power' and the way to knowledge involves 'the collection of data, their judicious interpretation, the carrying out of experiments, thus to learn the secrets of nature by organised observation of its regularities' ('Francis Bacon' n.d.).

Scientific ways of knowing have proven to be a powerful means of understanding, predicting, and manipulating the world of objects (physical sciences), living things (biological and behavioural sciences), and social structures and organisations (social sciences). The scientific way of knowing is now the dominant 'knowledge culture' in the world, and applied sciences such as health and medicine, are firmly grounded in scientific knowledge.

Most recently, the focus on scientific ways of knowing about health has been reflected in the growing **evidence-based medicine** (EBM) movement. 'Evidence' implies knowledge based on scientific principles and methods in contrast to information obtained from personal experience, intuition, or from anecdotal, traditional, or common-sense sources.

In the mid twentieth century, the notion that scientific method provides the one and only pathway to absolute truth came in for sustained criticism. Philosophers of science such as Thomas Kuhn (1970), Paul Feyerabend (1988), and Imre Lakatos (1978) argued that scientific facts are socially constructed rather than objectively read from nature. While some scholars adopted the extreme position that all knowledge claims are equally valid, the current widely accepted position is that scientific theories represent 'likely' rather than absolute truth. In the words of the American scientist and writer, Stephen Jay Gould (2003): 'In science, "fact" can only mean 'confirmed to such a degree that it would be perverse to withhold provisional assent.' I suppose that apples might start to rise tomorrow, but the possibility does not merit equal time in physics classrooms.' Similarly, in the health area, it is conceivable that cigarette smoking might one day turn out to be good for your health, but in the light of current evidence, medical endorsement of its use (as occurred in cigarette advertising in the 1920s) would represent an invitation to litigation.

So, despite some philosophical and methodological reservations, evidence based on scientific ways of knowing represents a powerful tool for health practice. Such evidence provides a sounder basis for action to improve health than the many health myths that can arise from sources such as the media, tradition, authority, and, most recently, the Internet.

When health researchers and practitioners apply their evidence-based thinking to health issues, they are usually attempting to answer questions such as:

- What is the nature and prevalence of the problem? (e.g. How many people in Australia experience depression?)
- What causes it? (e.g. What causes depression?)
- What can be done about it? (e.g. What strategies or interventions are effective in reducing depression?)

These three questions are associated with: *descriptive* research (describing the problem); *analytical* research (identifying causes of the problem); and *evaluation* research. When health practitioners address health problems, they try to answer these questions based on evidence. The remainder of this chapter provides an introduction to and overview of evidence-based thinking in relation to these three questions. The topic of young people and cannabis use provides a basis for this overview.

USING EVIDENCE IN PUBLIC HEALTH PRACTICE

Some statements about young people and cannabis use are listed in table 21.1. You might like to 'test' your knowledge as a stimulus to thinking about the different types of evidence required to determine whether or not these statements are true.

Table 21.1   Cannabis quiz

1	Most young adults (aged 20–29) in Australia have used cannabis	T/F
2	Cannabis use in Australia is increasing	T/F
3	More males than females use cannabis	T/F
4	The cannabis used in Australia is getting stronger	T/F
5	Cannabis use leads to psychosis	T/F
6	Cannabis use leads to poor school performance	T/F
7	Cannabis use affects driving ability	T/F
8	Cannabis use contributes to the road toll	T/F
9	Decriminalisation of cannabis leads to increased use	T/F
10	School drug education programs are an effective way of preventing young people from using cannabis	T/F

T=true; F=false.

Statements 1 to 4 are about describing the 'health problem'; statements 5 to 8 are about analytic cause and effect relationships; and statements 9 and 10 are about the effectiveness of interventions to address the problem.

DESCRIBING THE HEALTH PROBLEM

To obtain evidence-based answers to statements 1 to 4 you need to know:
- who or what organisations collect and publish or in other ways communicate this information
- how to access this information
- how to judge which information sources are reliable
- how to assess the quality of the information.

Table 21.2 summarises the processes involved in these four steps as applied to statement 1 in table 21.1, specifically: 'What proportion of young people in Australia have used cannabis?'

Table 21.2   Obtaining descriptive evidence: what proportion of young people in Australia have used cannabis?

Which people/organisations collect and publish or in other ways communicate this information	Australian Bureau of Statistics (ABS) Australian Institute of Health and Welfare (AIHW) Commonwealth and State Departments of Health Commonwealth and State Justice Departments Australian Drug Foundation

cont.

Table 21.2 Obtaining descriptive evidence: what proportion of young people in Australia have used cannabis? (continued)

How to access this information	Electronic access is the most efficient. Use a search engine such as Google and search for either the organisation (e.g. ABS) or the query (e.g. 'cannabis use among young people in Australia').
How to judge which information sources are reliable	Reliable sources include government departments, statutory authorities, accredited universities, and well-known health organisations (e.g. Australian Drug Foundation). Less reliable sources can include interest groups (e.g. the Legalise Cannabis Alliance—a registered political party in the United Kingdom), commercial interests (e.g. businesses selling drug detection kits for parents), individuals, and media reports.
How to assess the quality of the information (i.e. is it valid, reliable, trustworthy?)	The status of the organisation is a quick and usually dependable, but not infallible, way to assess quality. The only sure way to assess quality is to review a detailed report of the study methods and results. For a survey about young people's drug use, important features include sample size, method of sample selection (random), validated questionnaire items, and appropriate statistical analysis. Standard research methods texts contain details of appropriate survey research methods.

Information from the Australian Institute of Health and Welfare (AIHW), based on a national survey of approximately 27,000 people conducted under the auspices of the National Drug Strategy, states that 58.9 per cent of people aged 20 to 29 have ever used cannabis (AIHW 2002c). According to these data, there is good evidence that statement 1 is true. Data from the same source indicate that statement 3 is also true.

IDENTIFYING THE CAUSES OF HEALTH PROBLEMS

Statements 5 to 8 are categorised as analytical rather than descriptive. That is, they 'analyse' relationships between various states or conditions. For example, is it true that 'cannabis use leads to psychosis' (statement 5)? Here we are interested in a possible cause and effect relationship between cannabis use and psychosis. Two important questions need to be answered:

1 Is there an association between cannabis use and psychosis? (i.e. are young people who use cannabis more likely to experience psychosis, or are young people with psychosis more likely to use cannabis?)

2 Is the association one of cause and effect (i.e. does cannabis use *cause* psychosis?)

A recent Australian study (Degenhardt et al. 2001) reported the following prevalence of psychosis (expressed as a percentage) among four categories of cannabis users: no cannabis use (0.7 per cent); cannabis use (2.4 per cent); cannabis abuse (3.9 per cent); and cannabis dependence (6.8 per cent). These data indicate that cannabis-dependent individuals are much more likely to screen positively for psychosis.

Data like these appear very persuasive and it is tempting to conclude that cannabis use causes psychosis. But, in fact, the above evidence of association does not allow us to conclude that the relationship is causal. An appreciation of this difference frequently distinguishes 'common sense' (and often incorrect) health beliefs from the more evidence-based knowledge of health professionals.

An association such as the one described above can be interpreted in four ways:

- cannabis use causes psychosis
- psychosis causes cannabis use (e.g. psychosis sufferers may self-medicate using cannabis to relieve symptoms)
- cannabis use is associated with another factor (e.g. stress) that causes psychosis
- the association is simply an artifact (e.g. two factors may be increasing independently of each other, in much the same way as the level of credit card debt in the community has increased at the same time as the koala population in Australia has increased).

A common mistake is to accept the first interpretation without further evidence—in lay terms, jumping to conclusions. Evidence-based thinking tries to avoid this mistake by seeking further confirming or disconfirming evidence. The best evidence would come from a controlled experiment, called a randomised controlled trial (RCT). In this case, you might select a group of, say, 500 healthy young people, assign them randomly to two groups (250 participants required to smoke cannabis regularly for one year and 250 participants required to abstain), and compare rates of psychosis in the two groups. Needless to say, this experiment has never been conducted and never will be. This is an instance where the methodological requirements of good science are in serious conflict with the ethical requirement to do no harm to study participants.

Despite not being able to conduct an appropriate RCT, we can still reach an evidence-based conclusion about cannabis use and psychosis. An evidential case can be mounted, but it is more complex and less definitive than a controlled experiment. Health researchers have developed a set of criteria to help assess whether relationships between certain factors and health outcomes are in fact causal. A commonly used set was first described by Hill (1984) and includes criteria such as:

1 Is there evidence from true experiments in humans (i.e. the ethically impossible experiment described above—in this case, the answer is 'no')?
2 Is the association strong (6.8 per cent compared with 0.7 per cent is a moderately strong relationship, though the difference is smaller when adjustments are made for some demographic and other differences between the two groups)?
3 Is the association consistent from study to study?
4 Is the temporal relationship correct (i.e. does cannabis use precede psychosis?)
5 Is there a dose-response gradient (in the Degenhardt et al. 2001 study, higher levels of cannabis use were associated with increasing prevalence of psychosis)?
6 Does the association make biological sense (e.g. response of cells, tissues, organs, and organisms to stimuli—in this case, cannabis)?

Based on the findings from numerous studies conducted over the past few decades, each addressing various aspects of criteria 2 to 6, researchers are now very close to declaring that cannabis can indeed trigger psychotic episodes (Arseneault et al. 2002); thus, there is good evidence emerging that statement 5 in table 21.1 is true.

DETERMINING THE EFFECTIVENESS OF INTERVENTIONS

The third evidence-based question that health professionals often ask is whether or not interventions to address a health problem are effective. These types of questions are relevant to statements 9 and 10 in table 21.1.

A popular approach to preventing cannabis use is school drug education. But popularity is not synonymous with effectiveness, and evidence indicates that for many years some drug educators were actually contributing to the 'drug problem' rather than reducing it. Evaluation studies have demonstrated that some forms of drug education (e.g. those that emphasise the harmful effects of drug use) can lead to increased drug use, possibly by raising young people's curiosity about the effects of psychoactive substances (Stuart 1974). The now well-known fact that doing what 'feels right' (i.e. telling students about the harmful effects of drugs) may not have the desired effect is a salutary lesson in the importance of basing interventions on evidence rather than intuition, common sense, or what other people may believe or do. Similarly, it seems 'logical' that decriminalisation of cannabis would lead to increased use (statement 9), but in fact there is little evidence to support this claim (Netherlands Institute of Mental Health and Addiction 2001) and a number of Australian states are cautiously (for largely political reasons) moving towards decriminalisation (e.g. see Lenton et al. 2000).

As in the cases of evidence-based problem description and evidence-based cause and effect relationships, the research methods literature provides guidelines for distinguishing between good (i.e. valid and reliable) and poor evaluation studies. For example, a hypothetical ten-week cannabis education program ('Mull it Over') aimed at reducing cannabis use among Year 10 secondary school

Table 21.3 Recent cannabis use: the impact of Mull it Over on a Year 10 class

Pre-program cannabis use (% of students reporting recent use)	17
Post-program cannabis use (% of students reporting recent use)	25

students might measure cannabis use before and after the program (a single group, pre-post design). If the results shown in table 21.3 were obtained, would you be justified in concluding that the program was a failure? Not necessarily.

Cannabis use increases over time as students become older (called a 'maturation' effect) so the key question becomes, 'has the cannabis use of students in the program increased or decreased relative to students who did not participate in the program?'. The inclusion of a comparison (or control) group would improve the design and strengthen the evidence. Table 21.4 shows that cannabis use in such an intervention group increased less than in the comparison group, suggesting that the program was in fact successful in reducing cannabis use. In practice, researchers use statistical tests to identify whether these differences are significant.

While this design, which includes a comparison group, provides better evidence of effectiveness than the simple one-group, pre-post design, there is still room for improvement. For example, what if an event occurred in the cannabis education class that was unrelated to the drug education lessons, but impacted on cannabis use (e.g. a student being expelled for cannabis use)? This might mean that an observed change was due to a different cause (i.e. not the Mull it Over program). This problem could be addressed by conducting a large trial with multiple intervention and control classes, and by randomly assigning classes to intervention and control conditions. If the number of classes is large and classes are randomly assigned, the possibility of events other than the program causing a difference in cannabis use between the intervention and control groups is minimised. However, these requirements of 'good science' are not always feasible in practice. Meeting the demands of methodological rigour while at the same time conducting feasible and ethical research is a major challenge for public health research. The following section briefly outlines some contemporary dilemmas and debates associated with evidence in public health research, policy, and practice.

Table 21.4 Impact of Mull it Over: comparison of intervention and comparison groups

	INTERVENTION GROUP (MULL IT OVER)	COMPARISON GROUP (NO CANNABIS EDUCATION)
Pre-program cannabis use (% of students reporting recent use)	17	18
Post-program cannabis use (% of students reporting recent use)	25	33

EVIDENCE DEBATES

Unfortunately, large trials such as the one described above are expensive and disruptive to the school system. This is another example of the requirements of 'scientific validity' conflicting with the practicalities of life in the real world. It can be very difficult to impose laboratory-type controls in real-life social settings and often compromises need to be made. Problems can then arise when 'methodological purists' reject *all* forms of evidence other than that obtained from the so-called gold standard RCT. This is a crucial issue for public health and health promotion, where the most effective interventions are frequently multifaceted, community-wide strategies with a long lead time in terms of health benefits. For example, trend data indicate that Australia has successfully implemented public health strategies to reduce heart disease, lung cancer, sudden infant death syndrome (SIDS), the road toll, and HIV/AIDS (AIHW 2002b). However, public health researchers will never be able to 'prove' through RCTs that these strategies have been effective. There are, therefore, some serious limitations to transferring the rules and principles of the evidence-based medicine movement (where the 'best' evidence is considered to be that which is derived from RCTs) to evidence-based public health. Health is influenced by a range of social and environmental factors in addition to physiological factors. Accordingly, the most effective public health strategies are those that address these multiple socioenvironmental influences through interventions directed at developing healthy public policy, strengthening community action, and creating supportive environments, as has occurred, for example, in the area of tobacco control (see chapter 15).

Public health researchers are now actively involved in developing a scientifically sound and methodologically diverse evidence base for assessing the impact of public health interventions that draws on both medical science (with its emphasis on RCTs) and social science and policy analysis (which emphasise macro level trend analysis). While the Cochrane Collaboration[1] develops and disseminates systematic reviews of health interventions (including public health interventions) based on RCTs as the gold standard for evidence, the Campbell Collaboration[2] is a more recent sibling organisation established to promote systematic reviews in areas such as education, criminal justice, social policy, and social care using alternative methodologies. These sectors have much in common with public health.

SUMMARY

- As the culture of evidence evolves from its current somewhat narrow base to embrace diverse evidence-based methodologies, the public health field will benefit from more relevant, practice-oriented, and policy-friendly evidence.

> - Scientific evidence should not be the sole input into health decision making. The best available evidence should be considered within an overall context that also recognises that moral, ethical, cultural, and spiritual values impact on what we are prepared to do (and not do) to improve health. As Martin Luther King stated some forty years ago: 'Our scientific power has outrun our spiritual power. We have guided missiles and misguided men.' (King 1963)

DISCUSSION TOPICS

1 The use of hormone replacement therapy (HRT) in treating women experiencing menopause has been the subject of much debate in recent times. But what is the evidence around the use of this therapy? Conduct a search of recent articles and research findings relevant to this topic (the search skills described in chapter 14 will be useful here).

2 Now employ the strategies introduced in this chapter to analyse the information you have found around HRT. What conclusions have you made?

NOTES

1 The Cochrane Collaboration is an international nonprofit organisation involved in preparing, maintaining, and promoting the accessibility of systematic reviews of the effects of health care interventions (see www.cochrane.org).

2 The international Campbell Collaboration is a nonprofit organisation that aims to help people make well-informed decisions about the effects of interventions in the social, behavioural, and educational arenas. The objectives are to prepare, maintain, and disseminate systematic reviews of studies of interventions in these fields for policy makers, practitioners, researchers, and the public (see www.campbellcollaboration.org).

ECOLOGY, PEOPLE, PLACE, AND HEALTH

Mardie Townsend and Mary Mahoney

Key concepts

- Health and place
- Ecology and the ecological nature of health
- Nature and health
- Biophilia hypothesis

This chapter will highlight the ecological nature of human health and show the importance of place in health, using two broad areas—the family, and the human health benefits of contact with nature—as foci for discussion to illustrate important links between place and health.

THE ECOLOGICAL NATURE OF HUMAN HEALTH

Bonnie Bradford and Margaret Gwynne begin their book *Down to Earth: Community Perspectives on Health, Development, and the Environment* with this quote from Elie Wiesel, winner of the 1986 Nobel Peace Prize:

> There is a Midrashic story: A man is on a boat. He is not alone, but acts as if he were. One night, he begins to cut a hole under his seat. His neighbours shriek: 'Have you gone mad? Do you want to sink us all?' Calmly, he answers them, 'What I am doing is none of your business. I paid my own way. I'm only cutting a hole under my own seat.' What the man will not accept, what you and I cannot forget, is that all of us are in the same boat.
>
> Wiesel cited in Bradford and Gwynne 1995, p. 1

That story is about ecology. 'Ecology' is a term first coined by the German naturalist Ernst Haeckel in the 1860s. It derives from two ancient Greek words:

oikos, meaning 'house' or 'place to live', and *logos*, meaning 'study of'. Initially, the term *oikos* used to refer to the daily operation of a family household. Haeckel believed that nature, like a household, is a unified economic unit with each member working in an intimate relationship with every other member (Rifkin and Perlas 1984). The term 'ecology' has, therefore, come to mean the study of relationships between organisms and their environment (Miller 2000). However, ecology does not simply relate to the biophysical environment; rather, it provides a way of looking at *any* system by focusing on the interrelationships and interdependencies both within the system and between the system and its broader environment (including the biophysical environment).

Since the middle of the twentieth century, the notion that health is an outcome of interrelationships between humans and the individual and collective elements of their broader environments has gained in currency (McMichael 2001a). Increasingly, we are recognising that single-factor explanations of disease are not only ineffective in explanatory terms, but are also unhelpful in terms of changing health outcomes. Instead, over recent decades, a number of so-called **ecological health** models have been developed (e.g. Hancock and Perkins 1985; Hancock 1993). These models highlight the importance for health of the interrelationships and interdependencies between human beings, the 'elements' influencing or potentially influencing their health, and the broader environment in which they exist.

If we go back to the story of the man in the boat, it is obvious that the action of the man has implications for the survival of the other people in the boat, and for the boat itself. His action reflects a lack of understanding of the interrelationships and interdependencies within the system of which he is a part.

For human health to be optimised, the ecological nature of human health must be recognised.

PROMOTING HEALTHY PLACES AND HEALTHY PEOPLE

'Place' has always played a key role in human health and wellbeing, but according to Bauman (2001) and Voisey and O'Riordan (2001), in the context of rapid change and of globalisation, recognition of the importance of place and of having a sense of belonging to a particular place has increased. In the health context, the term 'place' has often been used interchangeably with the term 'setting'. Settings (e.g. schools and workplaces) have been seen as geographical areas or institutions in which health promotion may be undertaken. Settings for health are not simply spatial or physical, but may also have temporal (i.e. time-related) and cultural aspects; there has nevertheless been a tendency to ignore the ecological nature of place-related health effects. McMurray (2003, p. 21) highlighted this ecological relationship: 'People develop a sense of equilibrium within a defined context—whatever is defined as their *place*. This is an ecological relationship characterised by *mutuality*, where what happens in one aspect affects the other. People and their communal, physical environment operate in a kind of symbiotic relationship'.

Macintyre et al. (2002) suggest that the importance of place to human health can be characterised along a continuum roughly following Maslow's (1968) hierarchy of human needs. At the most basic level, humans need (unpolluted) air, (clean) water, (adequate) food, and (protective) shelter to survive. At the opposite end of Maslow's hierarchy—the end that relates to 'self-actualisation'—humans need (supportive) personal relationships, a sense of spirituality, opportunities to participate in group activities, and the chance for recreation. Macintyre et al. suggest this approach as 'a starting place for conceptualising and measuring area [place] influences on health' (2002, p. 132), and emphasise that the process of these influences is complex.

McMurray highlighted this complexity by providing the example of the relocation of older people who may be forced by ill health or other circumstances to relocate from their long-term home to a residential facility. According to McMurray (2003, p. 212), they may 'experience a loss of *place* in both the material and emotional sense', partly because of a loss of the 'material comforts' of their home but also because of the loss of what their home had come to symbolise: 'the history of establishing and sustaining the family, the sense of satisfaction that comes from providing a protective environment for loved ones, the possessions and personal touches that make the family's mark on the home, and the peculiar way the home has acted as an enclosure for their most significant moments and memories'. While the relocation may be driven by health problems, it may also create further health problems due to stress and a sense of loss.

FAMILIES AS A VITAL 'PLACE' FOR HEALTH

Until recently, surprisingly little attention has been paid by health professionals to the role of the family, a crucial 'place' influencing health status. Despite the family being included in ecological models of health, its pivotal role has not been articulated. Hogg et al. observed: 'the site of the family and the household as a focus for health education and promotion research and intervention has been relatively neglected. In many cases, the family has been seen as little more than a backdrop in efforts to change individual behaviour' (cited in Sindall 1997, p. 259).

There are three reasons for this failure to take seriously the role of the family as a crucial context for health. First, viewing the family as simply a *setting* for *promoting* health has limited the ability of professionals to notice other vital contributions it makes or roles it plays; second, the failure of professionals to look at the broader research into families that exists outside the health field has meant that valuable insights have been missed; and, third, the perceived need to determine the *exact* role or contribution of the family to health has meant that little attention has been paid to broader-based interdependencies and connections.

Increasingly, in fields other than public health and health promotion, the complex role of the family is being understood. The contribution of disciplines such as human ecology, social work, psychology, human development, and family studies in assisting this growth of understanding should be acknowledged. By studying the research in allied fields such as these, it is possible to draw out a broader understanding of the role of the family in promoting health and wellbeing.

Models for understanding the 'place' of family in human health

The most respected theoretical model for understanding the complex ecological connections between people and their environments outside the health field is the **social ecology** model for human development devised by Ure Bronfenbrenner in 1979 (and subsequently modified in 1986, cited in Bowes and Hayes 1999). His model locates the individual at the centre of a series of concentric circles that illustrate the contextual influences that impact upon an individual's development and thus the individual's health status. These contextual influences include the *microsystem* (the face-to-face settings a person engages with, such as family, school, peer group), the *mesosystem* (the interaction and interrelationship between the components of the microsystem), the *exosystem* (the broader environments that are one step removed from the individual, such as a parent's workplace), and the *macrosystem* (constituted by the broad social and cultural values that shape expectations and beliefs). These systems are all linked across time and space through the *chronosystem*.

By using an ecosystem approach such as Bronfenbrenner's to explore the influence of family on an individual, one is able to take account of the multiple factors within each level of the system that influence behaviours and outcomes, as well as the impacts of the interactions between these influencing behaviours and various aspects of the ecosystem (Sallis and Owen 1997, p. 411). The value of this ecosystem model in illustrating the role of the family in contributing to health status is that it demonstrates the *degree* of influence the family exerts—both through proximity (i.e. the close physical and personal relationships between an individual and her/his family) and magnitude (i.e. the amount of time spent within the family). Thus, based on this model, the significance of 'family' as a place-related health determinant is significantly higher than has been recognised previously, and is perhaps of greater significance than other environments.

Despite its growing popularity, Bronfenbrenner's model is limited in that it takes only the social environment into account and ignores the role of broader environmental interactions on individual and population health. Health and development are equally impacted on, and in themselves impact on, both the natural environment and the human constructed environment—that is, the physical environment we modify and the social and psychological world we inhabit (Bulbolz and Sontag 1993). A model that combines Bronfenbrenner's social ecology perspective with the environments that we interact with would be most useful.

Research on the 'place' of family in human health

Research on families is increasingly being directed towards exploring the links between healthy family or household life and individual health. The deficit approach, which involved focusing on what goes wrong in families, has gradually been replaced by an approach that involves exploring family strengths. The research shows that there are three different ways in which the family promotes or inhibits individual health:

1 through the nature of the relationships it fosters and the impacts of these
2 through the characteristics it possesses
3 through its role in mediating external forces.

There is now an understanding that resilient families help to foster resilient individuals. Resilience is the capacity of people to stay healthy and do well in the face of risk and adversity. Studies of resilience in families have explored the protective factors that families provide that ensure strong and healthy individuals. The characteristics of healthy families and households are as complex, dynamic, and diverse as family life itself, but studies of successful family relationships have consistently highlighted eight major qualities: commitment to the family; appreciation and affection; positive communication patterns; togetherness; acceptance; sharing activities; support; and resilience (Geggie at al. 2000; Patterson 2002).

Epidemiological evidence is increasingly showing that educational, economic and psychological attributes of the family have a long-term effect on the health of its members. Israel and Schurman (cited in Emmons 2000) indicated that families provide a range of support for health behaviour change, including information, appraisal, and emotional and instrumental support, but that they can also provide high levels of risk for members. Family circumstances that impact upon health status across the lifespan include (for example) educational opportunity, the risk of poverty, parental divorce, employment stability, behaviours that promote smoking, obesity, and low self-control (Wadsworth 1999).

The family's role in mediating external factors is also important to health. It involves the ability of the family to provide a buffer between external factors, such as the cumulative impacts of government policies and the health of its members. This role incorporates the role of the community in contributing to health. An important government report on the status of family life in Australia stated that the real problem facing society is not weak families, but the failure of forces outside the family to adjust to the changing realities of contemporary family life (House of Representatives Standing Committee on Legal and Constitutional Affairs 1998). In other words, there has been a breakdown in the intersection of policies and structures with the changing needs, structures, and organisation of family life. For instance, the policies and/or practices of reducing the number of aged-care facilities and discharging people from hospital to recuperate at home are based on an assumption that there is a caregiver at home to take up the gap, but that is no longer true in the majority of Australian family households. The family is now required to mediate and negotiate the expectations implied in policies and practices, and cope with the direct and indirect health consequences of such policies and practices. Considerable research is needed to understand the family's mediating role.

THE ROLE OF NATURE AS A 'PLACE' FOR HUMAN HEALTH

Over recent decades, the belief that humans are dependent on nature—not just for their material needs (food, water, shelter etc.) but also for their psychological, emotional, and spiritual needs—has gained support (Wilson 2001; Kahn and Kellert 2002). Across a wide range of disciplines (e.g. psychology, environmental health, psychiatry, biology, ecology, land-use planning, horticulture, leisure and recreation, wilderness, public health policy, and medicine), researchers and practitioners have begun to support the idea that contact with nature is beneficial for human health and wellbeing.

For example, in the early 1980s, Harvard biologist E. O. Wilson developed the **biophilia hypothesis** (Wilson 1984, 1993). This hypothesis, which has since been debated and expanded by others (e.g. Takacs 1996; Kahn 1999), suggests that because humans evolved in the company of other living organisms, they are predisposed to depend on affiliations with nature. Ecopsychologists adopt a similar view, asserting that many psychological and physical afflictions are due to withdrawal from contact with nature, and that exposure to nature can be beneficial (Scull 2001; Cohen 2000; Burns 1998).

Contact with nature appears to have a wide range of health benefits. These benefits can be accessed in a range of ways, including by interacting with nature via a garden or a pet, by being in a natural environment such as a park or a wilderness area, and even by viewing nature through a window (Maller et al. 2002). According to international research, the health effects of such contact with nature include reduced stress and tension, improved concentration, and improved psychological health. Physical health benefits can also be linked to the mental health benefits of contact with nature, as stress is a key factor in cardiovascular disease. Additionally, contact with nature has been found to have physical health benefits by contributing to heightened immunity and more rapid recovery from illness (Maller et al. 2002). Moreover, activities in natural environments may encourage increased exercise, and the air quality in the natural environments in which that exercise occurs may also result in improved respiratory health. Where contact with nature also involves contact with other humans, the health benefits may be extended beyond the individual to the community, through enhanced social capital.

A key factor identified as undermining health and wellbeing is the recent separation of people from nature (related substantially to urbanisation) (Beck and Katcher 1996). Moreover, the trends in modern society to insulate people from outdoor environmental stimuli and to expose them instead to excessive levels of artificial stimuli have been blamed for increasing exhaustion and loss of vitality and health (Stilgoe 2001). Satisfying human beings' innate affinity with the natural world may be the key to enhancing human health.

SUMMARY

- The importance of *place* for people's health and wellbeing seems so obvious in light of the preceding discussion; yet it is the very fact of its almost universal, but tacit, acceptance as important that has contributed to place (exemplified in this chapter by *family* and *nature*) often being overlooked and underrated, with less 'common or garden' explanations of differences in health taking the limelight.
- 'Family' is a significant place-related health determinant, perhaps of greater significance than other environments.
- The tacit recognition of the importance of place for health and wellbeing needs to be converted to a more explicit acknowledgment of the ways in which families and the natural environment (for example) foster positive health outcomes.

DISCUSSION TOPICS

1 Use Bronfenbrenner's ecosystem model to draw a 'map' of the role of 'family' as a determinant of health on an individual.
2 What upstream strategies specifically around 'family' and 'place' would you recommend in seeking to enhance the health of families living in your community?

MIND–BODY HEALTH CONNECTIONS

Jan Stewart

> ## Key concepts
>
> - Models of health
> - Responses to stressors
> - Coping resources
> - Mental and emotional health and wellbeing

Over the past twenty years, there has been a shift in thinking about health and wellbeing from a limited biomedical model to a more inclusive biopsychosocial model. Research within the developing field of **psychoneuroimmunology** has led to a greater understanding of the interconnections between mind and body, and demonstrated that a systemic, or holistic, approach is warranted when examining the state of our wellbeing. There is a trend in current thinking about health towards a 'wellness' perspective, which involves more acceptance of personal responsibility for improving health and wellbeing, and a greater awareness of the implications of health-related behaviours. Accordingly, wellness-focused individuals attempt to maximise their health potential, within their personal limitations (Donatelle and Davis 1997), in each of a number of key interactive dimensions, including physical, psychological, social, mental, and spiritual health (figure 23.1). Such individuals work towards creating healthy behaviour patterns, making efforts to change the controllable negative factors within their lives (Donatelle and Davis 1997). This chapter will consider the mind–body connection, focusing on the impact of stressors on health and wellbeing. Mechanisms used for coping with stressors, and the efficacy of various intervention strategies, will also be discussed.

Figure 23.1 Wellbeing model

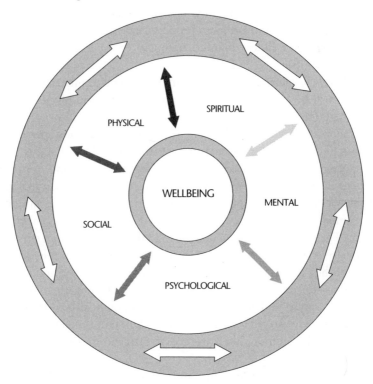

MODELS OF HEALTH

The biomedical and the biopsychosocial models of health have had a considerable influence on modern thinking about health and wellbeing.

The biomedical model

The **biomedical model** has dominated medical thinking for the past 300 years (Sarafino 1998). Proponents of this model maintain that unbalanced or abnormal physiological processes can explain all illness. The biomedical model is dualistic, in that mind and body are considered to be separate entities. Psychological and social factors are considered to be independent of the disease process. The emphasis has been disease-oriented, focusing on factors that lead to illness, rather than on health promotion.

The biopsychosocial model

During the past twenty years, there has been a gradual shift towards the **biopsychosocial model**. While biological, psychological, and social factors each have a role within the biopsychosocial model, the model also has a systemic focus:

health is considered to be a consequence of the interaction between biological, psychological, and social factors. The simultaneous study of such factors, when considering the wellness/illness process, supports interdisciplinary management of treatment for illness tailored uniquely to an individual's overall condition (Sarafino 1998).

The role of biological factors. Apart from genetic inheritance, biological functioning will be affected by physical abnormalities and physiological responses to fighting infection.

The role of psychological factors. Cognition, motivation, personality traits, and emotion are psychological factors that impact on health status (Sarafino 1998). Cognition involves perceptions, capacity to learn and remember, thought processes, and problem-solving skills. Lazarus and Folkman (1984) developed a cognitive model relating to the way events are perceived as potentially stressful. They maintained that an event will only be stressful if it is appraised as threatening. For example, some people change the meaning of an event from negative to positive (e.g. marital separation may be viewed as a release from a difficult relationship, rather than as a relationship failure). Motivation affects choices and decisions to change to positive, rather than negative, health behaviours. Personality traits and emotion have an impact on health and wellbeing; for example, people who are generally positive in their emotional responses are less likely to become ill and more likely to recover faster from disease than are people who are more negative (Kiecolt-Glaser et al. 2002a).

The role of social factors. Our interactions with others affect us, just as the way we relate to others affects them. Using a systemic approach enables us to understand that our social environment consists of several layers within the social sphere (society, community, family). The layers of the social system interact with, and affect, each other, as they do with the biological (genetics, physiology) and psychological (cognition, emotion, personality) systems. The importance of behavioural and lifestyle factors has also been recognised as impacting on health and wellbeing; for example, rate of smoking, high dietary cholesterol, and lack of exercise are related to cardiovascular disease (Sarafino 1998)./Health behaviours have been 'implicated as co-factors in the relationship between psychopathology [mental disorder] and immune function' (Kiecolt-Glaser et al. 2002b, p. 17). For example, smoking and depression combine to affect immune function (Kiecolt-Glaser et al. 2002b).

THE MIND–BODY CONNECTION

Our physiological and psychological reactions to stressful events provide clear indications of the relationship between the mind and body. Stressful events may affect the individual via several pathways (Sarafino 1998). First, there is the direct path, in which disease is promoted by the reaction of the nervous, endocrine, and immune systems to stressful situations. Because an imbalance in any of these systems can lead to physical disease, stress has the potential to cause organic damage. Second, there is an indirect path, in which the risk of developing disease may be increased through changes in behavioural responses to stress (e.g. alcohol abuse, drug use, smoking). Health-enhancing behaviours, including maintaining regular exercise and a healthy diet, protect us from developing disease. The potential impact of resource variables, such as social support and intrapsychic factors (e.g. self-esteem, sense of control), which may mediate the stress–illness relationship, also need consideration. If resources are lacking, a negative outcome (e.g. physical or mental illness) is more likely.

PSYCHOLOGICAL RESPONSES TO STRESSFUL EVENTS AND THE DEVELOPMENT OF DISEASE

The immune system guards the body against foreign invaders (antigens) (Kiecolt-Glaser and Glaser 2001). The immune system appears to be the link between the body's responses to stressful situations and a number of disorders involving the suppression of the immune system, or inappropriate functioning of the immune system. Psychoneuroimmunology is a relatively new research area that examines the interactions among specific physiological systems, and how psychological factors and health-related behaviours alter the interactive process, increasing the risk of developing immune system-related diseases like cancer, arthritis, infections, and allergies (Kiecolt-Glaser et al. 2002b). Short-term stress, such as exam stress, has an impact on the immune system, with an increase in

Box 23.1   Impact of prolonged stress on health and wellbeing

A longitudinal study examined the impact of stress in marriage. At the first stage of the study, ninety newlywed couples participated in a 'conflict resolution' session. Endocrine and immune function were measured following the session, with greater negative and hostile behaviours being associated with an increase in the level of stress hormones, greater immunological change, and decrements in immune function, during the 24 hours following the session, particularly for women. After the second year of the study, marital satisfaction was measured and found to have decreased significantly. The greatest decline in satisfaction was for women who had shown the strongest change to their immune function following the initial conflict session. There was no association between changes in men's marital satisfaction and immunological functioning. As the couples were generally quite happy, it is possible that the physiological impact of more disharmonious marriages may be considerable, especially for women. The results supported the findings of an earlier study, in which similar patterns were found in older couples married for an average of forty-two years.

Kiecolt-Glaser et al. 1997; Kiecolt-Glaser and Glaser 2001, 2002b symptoms of infectious disease being demonstrated before and after exams (Kiecolt-Glaser and Glaser 2001). Prolonged stress also impacts on health and wellbeing, with indications of suppressed immune systems for couples experiencing marital conflict (box 23.1).

A meta-analysis of stress and immunity studies showed that stress was related to immune system function, with immune suppression varying with the duration and intensity of the stressor (Kiecolt-Glaser et al. 2002b). Longer-term immune dysregulation (an interruption or interference to the normal process) may occur in situations of severe stress, for example during long-term care of a family member with Alzheimer's disease (Kiecolt-Glaser and Glaser 2001). There is also increasing evidence that emotional states, such as depression, anxiety, pessimism, and anger/hostility, impact on the disease process through altering the immune response, thus increasing the likelihood of developing certain illnesses (Kiecolt-Glaser et al. 2002a; Spielberger 2002).

COPING RESOURCES AND THE MIND–BODY RESPONSE

Not all people are affected in the same way by potentially stressful events. While stress may be a factor in disease, many people who could be at risk of becoming ill due to stressful situations do not become ill. Individuals have various internal psychological resources and external social resources for coping with stressful events. *Psychological, or intrapsychic, resources* involve thoughts and perceptions, and include personal characteristics (e.g. sense of control, optimism, self-efficacy), and coping styles (Kiecolt-Glaser et al. 2002a). People differ in the degree of control that they perceive themselves to have over aspects of their life. If people feel that life situations are beyond their control, they are at risk of developing learned helplessness, a principal component of depression (Seligman 1993). Self-efficacy is defined as having a belief that we can make a success of the things that we attempt. The likelihood of psychological and physiological strain in stressful situations increases for individuals with low self-efficacy (Bandura et al. 1992). *Social resources* are best defined as having a perception that there is available social support, which may involve tangible support (direct material assistance), emotional support (encouragement, reassurance, comfort, caring), esteem support (building self-worth, value, competence), and information support (advice, guidance, direction) (Cohen et al. 1985). The support of family and friends can be a valuable social resource, especially if the individual is satisfied with the support received (Stewart 2000). In some situations, social support will buffer the relationship between illness and stressors, providing protection against immune dysregulation (Kiecolt-Glaser et al. 2002a, 2002b). On the other hand, lower levels of social support and the disruption of close relationships have been associated with poorer immune function (Kiecolt-Glaser et al. 1997), with social isolation having been identified as a risk factor for morbidity and mortality (Kiecolt-Glaser et al. 2002a).

STRATEGIES FOR MAINTAINING EMOTIONAL AND MENTAL HEALTH

While the development and maintenance of social resources has been identified as an important factor in sustaining wellbeing, there are a number of other useful strategies. In particular, some psychological strategies (e.g. relaxation, cognitive therapy) intervene in the stress–illness relationship. A meta-analysis of research studies examined the efficacy of various psychological interventions in improving the functioning of the immune system, with mixed findings (Miller and Cohen 2001). The most reliable evidence of the beneficial effect of such interventions came from studies using hypnosis and conditioning techniques. There was also evidence of some success with stress management and disclosure techniques but, for these techniques, alteration to the immune response was related to the extent of change to relevant cognitions (appraisal and perception of events) and emotion (experience of positive or negative emotion relating to the event). In a review of intervention and coping strategies, Fredrickson (2000) supported the use of relaxation therapies, including imagery exercises, progressive muscle relaxation, and meditation, as well as cognitive and behavioural therapies, in promoting health and wellbeing. According to Fredrickson, such strategies effectively induce positive emotion, thus promoting contentment and helping individuals find meaning in, or make sense of, an event, and counteract negative emotion, thus optimising one's wellbeing. The premise for focusing on positive strategies is that emotions arise from a personal appraisal of life events. Therefore, it is important to encourage people to find positive meaning in events, perhaps by reappraising a negative event and reframing it in a positive light.

NEW DIRECTIONS

Research has confirmed the mind–body relationship in the disease process, with evidence being presented of the relationship between psychological states and dysregulation of the immune response. There is an emerging wellness orientation within current mind–body research towards finding positive meaning in potentially threatening events and developing positive emotions. Research has recently taken a new step in the direction of examining the potential for psychological interventions to affect the immune response and impact positively in the disease process. While recent findings are regarded as tentative, there is the promise of further confirmation of the efficacy of such intervention strategies. It is apparent that there will be continuing progress in this relatively new and exciting field of research.

SUMMARY

- There is increasing evidence about the mind–body relationship in understanding the determinants of health.

> - Wellbeing is determined by the interactions of physical, psychological, and social factors.
> - Research is being directed towards biopsychosocial interventions that impact positively on both states of health, and on disease processes.

DISCUSSION TOPICS

1   You can improve your ability to cope with stress in your life if you understand what makes you stressed and your own reactions to various stressors. It is a useful exercise to carry a notepad around with you for at least a week to note down the types of stressors that cause you to react, your responses to stressors, and, if possible, what you did to cope with the stressor. Your physical responses may include tenseness in your neck or shoulders, a pounding heart, or a dry mouth, while your psychological responses will be the thoughts and feelings you had as you interpreted and responded to the stressor. Some of your health behaviours may also affect your responses to a potentially stressful situation (e.g. a lack of sleep may make you feel more stressed, as might the amount of coffee or alcohol consumed, while seeking out an available friend to chat with about the situation may make you feel less stressed).

    After completing your own stress record for at least a week, you may be able to identify some patterns. Try to assess whether:
    - there was any pattern in situations or thoughts that preceded a stress response
    - your perception of the stressor affected your stress response
    - there was any noticeable pattern to your physical response, such as a specific body area that reacted more to the stressor
    - there were specific health behaviours that influenced, or were influenced by, your stress patterns
    - there were any specific coping responses you found to be effective.

2   How might these insights empower you to implement a personal action plan aimed at improving your health and wellbeing?

USEFUL WEB SITES

Wellness Inventory: www.wellnessinventory.net
The National Wellness Institute at the University of Wisconsin: http://wellness.uwsp.edu
Wellness Assessment and Standard Behaviour Change Guide: www.testwell.org/sample.htm
PsychoNeuroImmunology: An Overview: www.wellness.org.za/html1/PNI.HTM
The American Psychological Association, HelpCenter: http://helping.apa.org/sitemap.html
Wellness Associates: http://thewellspring.com

UNDERSTANDING DISABILITY

Kaye Smith and Lesley Hardcastle

> ## Key concepts
>
> - Disability
> - Medical, social, and sociopolitical discourses
> - Ecological model of understanding disability

Disability is a complex and changing phenomenon. The growth of knowledge about disability and ways of working with people with a disability has exciting implications for the development of diversity-rich and tolerant societies. There are multifaceted interrelationships between 'disability', 'health', and 'society'. In exploring these interrelationships, we will look at changes in perceptions of disability, with particular emphasis on the medical and social models of disability.

Central to the ways in which disability has been constructed at various times is the question of whether 'disability' is biologically or socially determined. Various frameworks for understanding disability have proliferated in recent years. In keeping with the 'social determinants' theme of this book, the primary focus of this chapter will be on the discourses of disability that recognise the impact of society on the experiences of people with a disability. By the term 'discourse', we mean the ways in which a society constructs meaning, the signs it uses (including language, visual images, and stories). For example, our use of the term 'person with a disability' rather than a 'disabled' or 'handicapped' person communicates to you something of our understanding of disability.

In talking about 'society' we take a broad approach. We are concerned with the social, political, cultural, economic, and physical dimensions of a society. By including 'society' as part of the relationship between disability and health, we draw attention to the serious limitations of placing disability solely within a medical framework. It was these limitations that prompted disability activists to argue for the conceptualising of disability within a multidimensional framework.

Unlike many minority groups, people who have a disability are not a clearly defined group. Disability is not confined to specific characteristics such as age, wealth, or educational level; it can affect anyone at any time. The 'differences' that categorise people with a disability are relevant to their ability to participate in certain environments. Differences in areas such as communication, mobility, and cognitive capacity mean that similar or 'equal' treatment does not necessarily mean provision of equal opportunity. For example, a person who is blind may be treated the same as anyone else when handed instructions in printed format, but obviously does not have the same opportunity as a sighted person to access that information.

HOW MANY PEOPLE HAVE A DISABILITY?

People who have a disability are a minority group, but they are the largest minority group in the world. Estimated proportions of people with a disability vary enormously. The World Health Organization, for example, has put the estimate of people who have a disability at 10 per cent of the global population (Vocational Rehabilitation Branch—ILO 1999), while Samorodov (1996) noted the reported incidence of disability in Bahrain and Austria to be 1 and 20.9 per cent, respectively. These large discrepancies are due to the lack of any collective understanding of the term 'disability' (Albrecht, Seelman, and Bury 2001; Fujiura and Rutkowski-Kmitta 2001). The Australian Bureau of Statistics (ABS) estimated that in 1998 there were more than 3.6 million people in Australia who had a disability, that is, almost one in five people, or 19.3 per cent (AIHW 1999a).

Regardless of the accuracy of these numbers, there is agreement that the proportion of the population with a disability is increasing (Vocational Rehabilitation Branch—ILO 1999; Davis 2001). Furthermore, whether we are born with a disability or acquire a disability through trauma or the ageing process, most of us will experience disability during our lives, whether it be transitory or permanent.

HISTORICAL OVERVIEW OF PERCEPTIONS OF DISABILITY

Different understandings of 'disability' have existed within different cultures and at different times. For example, prior to industrialisation, people with disabilities could be productive members of their communities. Industrialisation, however, brought demands for workers to work at set rates of production in workplaces that were often cramped and difficult to access, and those who could not meet the demands of paid employment were excluded. People with disabilities were recognised as a separate category; they were excluded from mainstream society and often segregated in institutions (Marks 1999). Marks used this relationship between industrialisation, employment, and disability to demonstrate that our understanding of 'normality' is in fact socially determined. An important aspect of any historical overview of perceptions of disability is that disability is a dynamic relational concept; one that is strongly influenced by the prevailing culture.

For the purposes of this brief chapter, we will confine our discussion to two dominant discourses, or models, of disability—the medical and the social. There are a number of models within these two dominant discourses, including the sociopolitical discourse, which we will also touch upon briefly. These models tend to overlap, and change occurs as new ways of understanding 'disability' emerge.

Medical discourse

The medical model has been powerful in shaping community attitudes towards people with a disability, by focusing on biological abnormalities and the management of symptoms and bodily functions. Identification, treatment, and prevention of illness are the major concerns, with the individual being the focus for attention and intervention. Solutions to 'problems' of disability tend to be geared towards prevention, cure, or rehabilitation for the 'patients', who are passive recipients of intervention. This model puts the 'deficit' right with the individual. The emphasis is on changing an individual rather than changing social structures or policies, and control tends to rest with the professionals, not with the individual.

The medical model understands disability as a negative deviation from what is considered to be 'normal' (Bickenbach 1993). That is, 'disability' is a relational concept that acquires meaning through an understanding of what is 'normal' or 'nondisabled'. Bickenbach, however, pointed out that '(t)he biomedical norms that underwrite impairments are idealisations that do not purport to reflect the natural course of events' (1993, p. 32). Conditions such as arthritis, although normal in an elderly person, are still considered abnormalities that require medical treatment, regardless of the person's age. Bickenbach further pointed out the lack of any direct relationship between the severity of a biomedical abnormality and the severity of any resultant limitations; that is, the severity of limitations can be counteracted by the context in which a person operates. Consider, for example, an architect who uses a wheelchair: he or she may encounter few or no restrictions in office-based employment, but could encounter several restrictions working on building sites. Participation occurs in a context. The medical model has been criticised for ignoring the impact of the environment (Barnes 1998; Williams 2001). The focus on deficit is further supported in the way political organisations categorise and survey disability populations. For example, the ABS conforms to the deficit model in its approaches to collecting data about populations with different kinds of disability. This in turn affects welfare policies and levels of support.

Whereas in the medical model power rests primarily with professionals who make decisions concerning the lives of people, in the social model of disability it is people with a disability who seek power. They advocate for equal opportunity, for the right to self-determination and inclusion in society. They see society as defining their disability and in turn restricting their personal freedom. When we consider disability as a relational concept, we are comparing an aspect of the person against a norm determined by society.

Social discourse

The social model of disability questions the relationship between personal experiences and social situations (Williams 2001). It developed from a tension between the ways in which the dominant culture and the subculture of people with a disability understood 'disability'. The social model recognises the importance of shifting the cause of disadvantage from the individual's impairment (as in the medical model) to society. In the medical model, individuals are seen to be disabled by their impairment. In the social model, people with a disability are seen to be disabled by their society.

Developing from the medical and yet connected to the social are the *charity* and *rights* discourses of disability. Social model theorists recognised in the 1960s that society catered for the needs of some but not all citizens (Marks 1999). The exclusion of people who have a disability from society is seen to result not just from the physical barriers in a society, but also from attitudinal barriers that result in lost opportunities and feelings of oppression and rejection (Barton 1998). The charity discourse defines people with disabilities as dependent, objects of pity, and needing help. It is ignorance, the charity ethic, and fear of difference that can lead to discrimination even when support is given.

With a growing awareness, particularly among disability activists in the 1980s, of the crucial role that society plays in determining the degree of disadvantage of people with a disability, there was a rejection of the medical and welfare approaches to disability and the adoption of a *'civil rights'* approach. People with disabilities became increasingly aware that many of the problems they faced were due to imposed attitudinal, architectural, and structural barriers.

The social model of disability incorporates notions of equality, inequality, and inequity. The traditional idea of equality is that everyone should be treated the same. If all people are treated equally, regardless of their differences, then inevitably some will be excluded. For example, a student with a physical disability would be excluded from an educational environment unless that environment had been designed or modified to allow their participation. Disability is a matter of inequity rather than just difference, because inequities are socially constructed and have social consequences.

The construction of disadvantage for people with a disability has been affected by exclusion from the economic, physical, social, and political domains of society, and the consequent dependence on welfare. The 'problem of disability' for governments is the cost of disability services, including: welfare support and the link with poverty; increasing expenditure on health; and the increasing costs of an ageing population.

The cost of supporting people with disability is a major focus of research and policy development. There has been much attention paid to the costs of providing services to people with a disability, but very little attention to the costs to society of not providing services, such as dependence on welfare, loss of productivity, and the consequent social costs. For example, consider the economic and social benefits that result from employment for a person with a disability.

Much of the literature of disability studies speaks not so much in terms of discrimination as of oppression. The notion of oppression is useful in highlighting the systemic disadvantage experienced by people with disabilities. For example, the systemic oppression of people with disabilities takes its most extreme form in the widespread acceptance of selective abortion where the foetus has been identified by prenatal screening as having a disability.

Sociopolitical discourse

Rather than examine disability from a single perspective, such as the social model, there is growing recognition of the important contribution many different perspectives can make to an overall understanding of disability (Fougeyrollas and Beauregard 2001; Williams 2001). These perspectives include political activism, personal narratives, and the complex relationship between people and their environments.

Although many of the disadvantages faced by people with a disability stem from society, strategies to counter these disadvantages tend to be political (e.g. disability awareness strategies, legislation). Barnes (1998) maintained that the advent of the social model of disability was the impetus for the politicisation of people with a disability; people with a disability began to see themselves as a political minority group. Personal narratives offer another perspective for understanding the range of factors that can impact on the lives of people with a disability. Many narratives are striking, not only for the similarities regarding the impact of an often hostile society on people with a disability, but also for the richness and diversity of those people's experiences.

The primary focus of health has been on issues related to the body and its functions, but there has also been increased recognition of the importance of other factors on people's sense of wellbeing. These factors will differ between individuals and include areas such as degrees of social inclusion, levels of stress, relationship issues, support networks, financial security, and job satisfaction. Both the medical and social models of disability have been criticised for ignoring the important interaction between people and their environments (Marks 1999).

Bronfenbrenner's ecological model (Bronfenbrenner 1989) provides a rationale for attending to the dynamic interrelationships between the individual and the environment. Bronfenbrenner describes an ecological hierarchy of levels ranging from the more proximal environments in which the individual operates, through to the more distal environments that are outside the normal operating contexts for the individual, but that nonetheless can impact on the person's experiences. For example, disability awareness campaigns or antidiscrimination legislation introduced at the macro level can affect day-to-day activities, such as community access.

An *ecological* understanding of disability acknowledges interrelationships between individuals and environments. That is, although environments affect the individual through the different experiences provided, characteristics of the individual also affect environments and experiences within those environments. An ecological perspective recognises that an individual's experiences and opportunities depend on characteristics of the individual (e.g. personality, past experiences, personal support networks, type and level of disability) and environmental characteristics (e.g. attitudes of others, accessibility, available resources, policies, cultural beliefs). An ecological perspective provides a more holistic approach to understanding the complex interrelationship between disability, health, and society.

SUMMARY

- Disability is considered to be part of the diversity of humankind. No one person has a complete range of abilities; rather, people are considered to have a vast range of abilities, each of which falls along a continuum from little or no mastery to full mastery.
- Disability is a worldwide human condition but, as it is experienced in our society, many unnecessary restrictions are placed on a person's freedom.
- How health professionals understand disability has ramifications for the manner in which the health sector responds to people with a disability. If disability is narrowly seen as a biomedical abnormality, then the main thrust of responses will be interventions aimed at restoring the person to the accepted norm. On the other hand, if disability is seen as socially constructed, strategies will be geared towards societal changes.
- Broader perspectives that embrace both the individual and the society in which the individual operates, and that understand disability as a phenomenon experienced by everyone, will lead to the development of integrated strategies based on holistic approaches aimed at social inclusion.

DISCUSSION TOPICS

1. Consider the relationship of language to the construction of our social understandings of disability. For instance, identify language used to *describe* and *categorise* people with a disability. In what ways can language be used to *discriminate* against people with a disability?
2. Outline the attitudinal, architectural, and structural barriers to *social inclusion* for people with disabilities in your community. You may wish to focus your attention on a particular context such as your university campus, a sporting club, your family home, or the local shopping precinct.

FROM 'DIFFERENCE' TO 'DIVERSITY': EXPLORING THE SOCIAL DETERMINANTS OF YOUTH HEALTH

Maria Pallotta-Chiarolli

Key concepts

- Identities
- Marginality
- Diversity

'The youth of today...' 'Young people at risk...' No doubt you have heard these phrases being used in the media and popular culture. But what is 'youth'? Are 'young people' a homogenous group, easily targeted for health promotion with one-size-fits-all resources and services? Which youth require what services, and why? What other factors need to be taken into account alongside 'the youth factor' if health promotion is going to effectively address the specific and multiple social determinants of diverse young people in our communities?

Think about your youth, whether you are immersed in it right now, or whether it is a reminiscence of a time long gone. What other social determinants interweaved with 'being a young adult' and with 'adolescence' made you experience the kind of youth you did? What physical, social, mental, emotional, and sexual health concerns did you experience? Were they due to your age, or were they attributable to one or more other factors/determinants that combined with your age?

This chapter will introduce you to ways of thinking about, understanding, articulating, and doing health promotion with 'youth diversity'. It will give you some theoretical frameworks, strategies, and tools with which to plan, develop and implement health promotion and health services for 'diverse young people'. Think about it as a tool-kit of checklists and questions, as well as some fancy words that you can pull out and apply to any group of young people you will be working with.

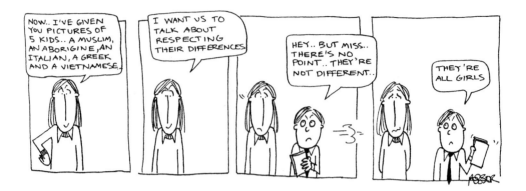

A DIVERSITY OF DIFFERENCES

- What are the differences *between* young people?
- What are the differences *within* groups of young people?
- What are the differences among young people that go *beyond* dominant social constructions and hierarchical dualities?
- What are the differences among young people *against*, or challenging, dominant assumptions and prejudices?

Most discussion of difference refers to a comparative model: the difference between two or more groups or individuals. However, as Burbules (1997) writes, this comparative model can still be based on the limiting assumption that the groups on each side of that either/or fence are homogenous, and that one side is superior or 'normal' in comparison to the other 'inferior' or 'abnormal' side. Think about how this hierarchical dualism, in relation to masculinity, sexuality, and disability, is apparent in the harassment that Andrew, 15, writes about in the following:

> I get called gay because I've got cerebral palsy and my right hand and wrist hangs limp...They think I'm different because I've got cerebral palsy and they think I'm different because I don't play sport and they think I'm different because I'm not drinking and I'm not doing drugs.
>
> Martino and Pallotta-Chiarolli 2001a, p. 14

Similarly, health workers may talk about young people being from an 'ethnic' or 'Anglo' background. But what about the differences within those two categories. Which ethnic group? Which 'Anglo': Scottish, English, Irish, Celtic? Who are third generation 'ethnic-Australians' and who are newly arrived? Are they migrants, refugees, or international students? How would all these specificities impact upon health and the way health workers develop resources for young people?

What about the differences beyond what society has come to accept as 'normal' and 'natural' differences? What if our frameworks of 'difference' do not allow for certain intermixtures and boundary-blurring? What if the differences we come across in youth groups are in excess of dominant ways of thinking and speaking about a health issue or group? For example, we may be doing youth work in relation to gender and sexuality that still positions certain determinants as oppositional. Youth are either boys or girls, either heterosexual or homosexual. What about young people that are beyond those categories, such as bisexual young people? What about young people who are intersexed, transgendered, or transsexual, or just like to play with and perform a wide repertoire of genders?

> People pick on me sometimes because I'm different to other boys. I call myself 'a tomgirl' because I sometimes dress up like a girl...When I'm wearing girls' clothes I always walk around wiggling my butt and walking sort of curvy. When I walk as a boy I just walk up and down, straight. I prefer bobbing up and down in the middle of both...I'm neither a boy or a girl... I'm in the middle, right in the middle. I'm both...I'm better off, I suppose. I can do a bit of both.
>
> Stephen, 13, in Martino and Pallotta-Chiarolli 2001a, p. 17

Finally, how do some young people's experiences critique and challenge the gaps and assumptions of dominant youth and health discourses? For example, some dominant discourses about young people with physical and/or intellectual disabilities include that they are asexual, or heterosexual, or that sex is a 'dangerous' issue to raise with them. Yet, the actual sexual lives, desires, and identities of young people with physical and intellectual disabilities work against these assumptions and prejudices. Thus, health workers face a very important decision: do we work with the realities of these young people's lives, or do we ignore and silence these realities in order to comply to the dominant discourses of disability and sexuality?

Working from within a framework of 'diversity' means that instead of imposing simplistic, hierarchical, and either/or classifications, health workers:

- allow for variation and degree
- become self-reflexive, questioning their own systems and assumptions of difference, what they mean for them as health workers and what they mean for their clients
- study and learn about different social groups, and the multiplacement of individuals within these groups
- set up respectful dialogues and engagements with their clients, listening to them *on their own terms*, to understand how they live their realities, and how they understand what they are living
- become informed about who the community gatekeepers are, and which key informants and groups provide alternative views.

THE INTERWEAVING OF DIFFERENCES

Based on the work of Gilbert and Gilbert (1994), here are five theoretical frameworks for exploring social diversity, community expectations, and individual agency in young people in order to more effectively develop and implement health programs:

Intracategory heterogeneity. This means avoiding homogenising practices such as stereotyping and essentialism that may be used to disguise or deny the diversity of individual experiences within a group. Health workers need to be aware of how they may be working with particular stereotypes of a community. **Essentialism** is a particular form of stereotyping that attributes group characteristics or group cultures to biological or innate reasons. Thus, 'that's the way boys are' is a phrase often used to justify young men's aggression and risk-taking behaviours as hormonally driven rather than exploring the sociocultural and discursive factors that construct male aggression and risk taking as 'normal' and 'natural'. Is it 'natural' for boys to take drugs and binge-drink? Many boys like Paul, 17, in the following quote, indicate that social constructions and stereotypes of 'normal' masculinity are a key factor in boys' behaviours, and therefore can be resisted:

> Some guys see that they've got to prove themselves by drinking silly. ...They think, 'Hey it's masculine to drink. I mean I don't like the taste of it but it's something I've got to do because I'm a guy and everyone else is drinking'...I don't drink because I just don't feel like it whereas other people will say, 'Hey, everyone else is drinking...I've got to catch up'.
>
> Martino and Pallotta-Chiarolli 2001a, p. 45

Interweaving of categories. This means drawing attention to how focusing on one category of identity may distract from or deny attention to the relationships between various conditions and constructs such as ethnicity, class, gender, sexuality, religion, geographical location, and education. As we have seen, the individual identities of the young people we work with are sites of the intermixture of categories such as ethnicity, indigeneity, sexuality, disability, rurality/urban location, and gender (Pallotta-Chiarolli 1999a). Many gay, lesbian, bisexual, and transgender (GLBT) people from diverse backgrounds experience feelings of inhabiting cultural borderlands, where they must negotiate the codes and regulations of:

- an ethnic family, community, and culture
- a predominantly Anglo-Australian GLBT community and culture
- a predominantly Anglo-Australian society and popular culture that privileges 'whiteness' and heterosexuality. (Pallotta-Chiarolli 1998b, 1999b).

For example, tertiary GLBT students from culturally diverse backgrounds may feel alienated from the ethnic clubs on campus but also from GLBT organisations, as Eric, 22, explains in the following:

> I remember the very first year at uni... I just stopped thinking about fitting in the so-called mainstream society or the Anglo culture and ...I joined the Hong Kong student association. Nothing happened. I didn't go to their functions because

they're all a whole bunch of, like, straights ...and I don't know how to tell them...
I feel a little bit devastated, 'Oh what happened to me, I don't fit in here, I don't
fit in there, I'm not in the gay community, I'm not in the Chinese community'...I
[eventually] joined a queer social group on campus... But because I was the only
Asian guy there ...sometimes I didn't know what they were talking about, you
know, the slang, and they laughed ... and I felt left out

(Pallotta-Chiarolli et al. 1999, pp. 24–5).

Connecting marginalities. This means identifying the links and overlaps
between various forms of discrimination and **marginality** (i.e. being socially positioned as inferior) such as racism, sexism, ageism, classism, ableism, lack of education, and homophobia. Consider the following words of Matteo, a young gay
man of Italian background. The connected marginalities within his parents that
make Matteo feel he can't come out are war, poverty, and migration, and a lack
of education and familiarity with sexual diversity. How would you undertake a
consultative process with gatekeepers and alternative key informants within
Italian health and welfare services, Italian community groups, and the Italian
media? What work could you do within the gay community to support Matteo?

It's harder for gay men and lesbians from Italian backgrounds to come out. I love my
parents and don't want to hurt them. I say things like 'Of course I'll get married one
day, I'm just waiting for the right girl'. How can two old people who'd need to have
the word 'homosexual' explained to them ever come to terms with their gay child?
They'd think it was something we'd picked up from Australian friends. They've lived
through poverty, war, hunger. They come to a country where they have to start again
in everything. They make a thousand sacrifices for the kids they cherish. After all
that, I haven't got it in me to break their hearts. Some might handle it.

Pallotta-Chiarolli 1991, p. 23

Contextualisation. This means rendering definitions and identities as in constant processes of shifting and fluxing rather than static by referring to shifting
and multiple contexts of time, place, and space. As health workers, we need to
be aware of shifting historical, cultural, and political contexts in relation to young
people's health concerns. For example, what and who gets problematised and
pathologised tends to be socially constructed. Thus, until 1973, homosexuality
was listed as a psychiatric disorder. This meant that medical interventions and
shock therapy were considered appropriate to treat this so-called pathology in
young people. Today, thankfully, this is no longer the case as mental health
research and social thinking have progressed to the point where the heteronor-
mative society (in which heterosexuality is privileged as the 'normal' and superior sexuality) around a GLBT young person is increasingly problematised.

However, we are still struggling with medical terms such as GID (Gender
Identity Disorder) that are premised on a system of gender that constructs people as being *always* and *only* either male or female. Thus, young people such as

Stephen might be pathologised as having GID rather than being a creative and insightful young person who understands and enacts the performativity of gender without doing years of academic reading on the subject (Martino and Pallotta-Chiarolli 2003). Historical and cross-cultural studies of gender also contextualise our gender duality system as being socially and culturally specific as various cultures over time, place and space have defined various 'gender systems'.

Self-ascription and personal agency. This means acknowledging the subjective perceptions, definitions, and agency of the persons who have been assigned labels and slotted into categories, and their efforts to negotiate them. Rather than assigning labels and making assumptions about a group of young people, health workers need to ask them how they wish to be labelled, what meanings do they give to certain cultural, gendered, sexual, and other behaviours and beliefs. Thus, rather than saying, 'You are...because I have read about you/seen a film about you and therefore I know you do/believe/expect/...', we need to turn our external ascriptions into questions and empower our clients to have agency in self-ascription: 'What do you call yourself? What does this word mean to you? How do you see yourself? Am I correct or incorrect in thinking that...? I've read or seen a film where young people like you are depicted as... what do you think/how real is that for you?'

Consider the similarities and differences in the way the following Muslim young women self-ascribe. Karima is from a Lebanese Muslim background and chooses not to wear a hijaab:

> It is Islam that enables me to achieve all my goals as it teaches me that a Muslim woman should not be aggressive or submissive...you should never judge Islam by a few people. I realised how misunderstood 'True Islam' was and still is. It is shielded by this male-dominated cultural interpretation of Islam that is so damaging
>
> ...
>
> I am an Australian Muslim Woman
> I am me...
>
> Pallotta-Chiarolli 1998a, pp. 208–9

Ayse is from a Turkish Sunni Muslim background and found her own family were shocked and disapproving when she chose to wear a hijaab:

> I could never have imagined that a one metre square piece of chiffon could have made such a dramatic difference...I believe in rights for women...I *am* a feminist... I am not a victim, and certainly not a second class citizen as you may think Islam classifies me...I was born in Australia, have lived in Australia, in fact have never left the east coast of Australia but I'm too dark to be an 'Aussie' I guess...And, well, I do wear the hijaab, so I am considered a 'radical Muslim' by my family and Turkish community. Therefore, they do not consider me 'one of them'...[And] glossy magazines [only] recount tales of 'honour killings and female circumcision'.
>
> Pallotta-Chiarolli 1998a, pp. 205–6

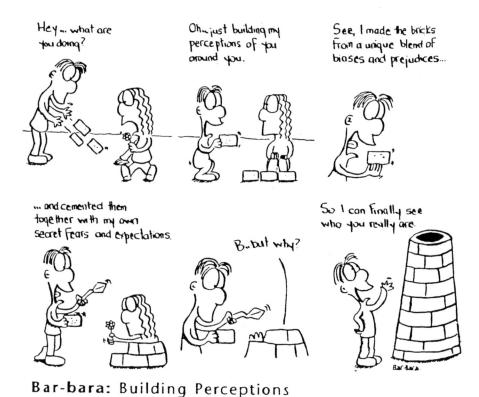

Bar-bara: Building Perceptions

SUMMARY

- Each young person deserves the right to live the various facets of their identities and their lives, and inhabit diverse social spaces, in emotionally, sexually, mentally, socially, and physically healthy ways.
- In a socially diverse society, we need to be aware of and understand how social determinants of health such as cultures, religions, traditions, sexualities, genders, socioeconomics, and lifestyle options, impact on specific individuals and communities, and thereby impact on the wider society.
- As health workers, we need to develop skills of perception and interrogation, critical thinking, and the negotiation of differences. We need to engage with social diversity rather than reconstruct it as homogeneity or simplify it as comparative difference.

DISCUSSION TOPICS

1 Identify barriers in your own community or workplace for young people seeking to live in 'diverse social spaces in emotionally, sexually, mentally, socially, and physically healthy ways'.

2 What knowledge, understanding, and skills do you believe health workers need to develop in order to genuinely engage with social diversity and promote health?

ACKNOWLEDGMENTS

I wish to thank the many young people who have worked with me and taught me so much over the years. I admire and respect their strengths, insights, and determination.

SOCIAL DETERMINANTS OF MENTAL HEALTH FOR YOUNG SAME-SEX ATTRACTED MEN

Damien Ridge

Key concepts

- Mental health
- Homophobia
- Conformity and resistance
- Structure and agency

While there are many different ways to understand 'culture', in a nutshell, culture is about the various networks of 'beliefs, attitudes, behaviours, and histories that are prevalent among communities of people' (MindMatters 2001, p. 15). We know that cultural ways are learnt, although our ways of doing things often seem natural to us. For instance, while it seems natural to some cultures to prioritise the individual and their rights (e.g. to universal human needs, to consume, to compete in a market), in other societies it makes little sense to talk about rights without linking such discussions to responsibilities (e.g. to contribute to society, to work collectively, to support aged relatives). Cultural ways of doing things are often unconscious, since we learn them at very early ages. We also know that cultures are not static—they tend to change. It is clear that some cultural ways are more acceptable (dominant), while others are less acceptable (subordinate) in our society. In this chapter, we will focus on one specific social group that, historically, has been labelled and subordinated in Australian culture. We will examine how cultural and structural forces impact on members of this group, and what implications this might have for their mental health. Not only this, but we will also look at the issue of human agency—the capacity to make choices, resist, and overcome constraints.

The group we will discuss to illustrate social determinants that shape mental health is young same-sex attracted men, and the mental health impacts we will focus on include depression and suicidality. The kinds of social forces we will investigate are homophobia in the school yard as well as the pressures to conform in commercialised gay spaces such as bars and nightclubs. In terms of personal agency, we will consider resistance to bullying and pressures to conform in schools and contemporary gay life.

HOMOPHOBIA

As was pointed out in chapter 25, diversity refers to the many ways in which we differ from one another, including in our ethnicity, gender, character, identity, and education. In the twenty-first-century Western world, it is becoming much more possible to talk about and acknowledge the differences between people, and there are a range of indicators for this. When I was a young boy growing up in the 1970s, men were encouraged to behave something like Paul Hogan did on TV—ocker, rugged, sexually available. Now, there are more ways to express maleness emerging in Australia, for example artistic, sensitive, bisexual, gay (Connell 1995). The MindMatters (2001) strategy currently used in secondary schools in Australia to promote mental health, specifically supports the notion of valuing our diversity—including our sexual and gender diversity—as a way to reinforce student wellbeing. Additionally, in recent times, there have been high-profile cases of bullying at school based on perceived sexuality, and schools are under pressure to tackle homophobia and to support sexual diversity (Williams 2002).

There are a range of indicators for this rapid change. It may be easy to forget that it wasn't until 1973 that homosexuality was removed as a diagnostic category from the *Diagnostic and Statistical Manual of Mental Disorders*, used by psychiatrists to classify psychiatric disease. It was only recently that some Australian states decriminalised homosexuality. Now, rather than problematising homosexuality, the problems with homosexuality are being viewed more and more as resting not in the individual, but in society at large (Plummer 2001). And the diagnosis is a severe case of collective 'homophobia'—the irrational fear and hatred of homosexuality. Until only a few years ago, it was quite possible for conservative elements in Australian society to get away with statements that young people could not be same-sex attracted. As the rhetoric went, if they were attracted to the same sex, then it was just a 'phase', or they were 'innocent children' who had been somehow 'brainwashed' and recruited into a homosexual lifestyle by adults. However, Korfiadis (2001) has shown that conservative opponents to the recent controversial VicHealth Sexual Diversity Projects (that aimed to support young people's sexual diversity) have shifted their rhetoric and acknowledged the reality of young same-sex attracted youth. Additionally, the popular US television series *Queer as Folk* (SBS 2002–03) portrayed in explicit detail the story of a 17-year-old boy having a sexual relationship with a 29-year-old man. The series was a cultural marker of a much bigger social phenomenon—never before has information about being non-heterosexual been so widely available in the public domain, particularly in the media and on the Internet.

Never before has it been so possible for young men and women to come out as non-heterosexual. Indeed, as early as the late 1980s, research was showing that students in industrialised countries were 'coming out' as non-heterosexual at earlier and earlier ages, and that they were increasingly finding it possible to 'come out' at school (Plummer 1989; Murray 1992; Prestage et al. 1995).

Nevertheless, despite massive social changes in public acknowledgment of sexual diversity (particularly since the advent of the AIDS epidemic forced uncomfortable issues about sex into the public domain), homophobia is still one of the key kinds of social discrimination that students experience in Australian schools. David Plummer (2002) working from the University of New England in New South Wales, has recently shown that homophobia is in fact not present in certain traditional and modern settings—that is, it is not an essential part of human nature. Nevertheless, homophobic terms of abuse such as 'poofter' and 'faggot' come into play in Australian primary school playgrounds in the very early years, and in a most powerful way (Plummer 1999). These terms are used as the worst possible insults available to boys, and are deployed against boys who are somehow 'different', for example not masculine enough, not sporty enough, don't wear their hair right, or who are interested in art. The implication is that all boys who do not fit a narrow range of masculine styles are at risk of this form of abuse. Plummer found that this homophobic abuse causes enormous anxiety and fear for boys, beyond that of other forms of abuse.

In general, schools are still not friendly places for same-sex attracted young people. In a recent national study of over 700 same-sex attracted young people in Australia, half reported being verbally and/or physically abused because of their sexuality, and most of this abuse took place at school (Hillier et al. 1999). Nevertheless, in recognition of the enormous challenges in coming out and the duty of care of schools, some Australian school environments now offer more support to gay and lesbian students (see table 26.1 for recommended ways of supporting sexual diversity in schools). For instance, there are cases documented of school staff intervening in the 'downward spiral' that many young people are caught in by naming incidents as homophobic, and framing such incidents as a problem of the school culture (and not the individual), thus helping lesbian and gay students to feel respected and safe (Hillier et al. 1999). One problem in tackling homophobia in schools is that it is quite easy to unwittingly position heterosexuality as the norm (Letts and Sears 1999). For instance, removing the student for counselling may be appropriate, but it may also imply that the problem lies in the individual student, rather than in the school culture itself (Pallotta-Chiarolli 2000; Seal 1999).

Even though homophobia becomes less overt as young people move from the playground into adult settings, surveys show that homophobic discrimination is widespread in adult spaces, including in workplaces and when same-sex attracted people approach health care professionals (Victorian Gay and Lesbian Rights Lobby 2000). It seems that the relative 'political correctness' of adults compared to children drives the enduring system of homophobia underground, rather than

Table 26.1   Recommendations for primary schools to support sexual diversity

---

Guarantee a safe environment
  Actively identify safety zones
  Actively protect targets

Neutralise danger zones
  Actively identify danger zones
  Pay special attention to isolated areas e.g. play areas, change-rooms,
  boarding houses, camp

Actively advocate for and support different children
  Affirm difference
  Provide positive role models
  Provide opportunities to network and seek support

Name and explicitly reject homophobia
  Monitor and intervene in homophobia
  Accept that the process is continual and requires strategy and effort
  Continual in-group/out-cast dynamics will need regulating

Be careful to differentiate between peer groups, alienated and rival groups, and loners
  Peer groups emulate and enforce orthodox masculinity
  Alienated groups represent competing masculinities
  Loners represent the 'other' and are targeted by all of the above groups

Consider replacing sex education with misogyny and homophobia education
  Provide a safe environment in which boys can discover their identity. Consider abandon-
  ing sex education unless it can: (i) deconstruct masculinity, homophobia, and misogyny;
  (ii) be sex positive; (iii) provide relationship skills; and (iv) emphasise physical, emotional,
  and sexual safety.

Be aware of the growing likelihood of legal action if the school fails to respond adequately

---

Source: Plummer 2001

dismantling it (Plummer 1999). Now that we have established some key features about the nature of homophobia, let us turn to the potential mental health impacts of homophobia.

MENTAL HEALTH IMPACTS OF HOMOPHOBIA

Homophobia is often expressed through bullying, particularly in schools. Bullying (e.g. ignoring, name calling, teasing, emotional abuse, physical violence) is an aggressive behaviour that involves a power imbalance that favours the aggressor; it is unjust, repeated, and experienced by the victim as oppressive (Rigby 2002). Bullying impacts negatively on mental health. In the short term, bullying is associated with anger, stress, depression, difficulty concentrating, tiredness, withdrawal, and loss in confidence (Eslea and Smith 1998). In the long term, a proportion of (but not all) victims of bullying will become fearful of others and suffer low self-worth and depression continuing into adulthood.

As with other forms of abuse and bullying, the mental health implications of young people being subjected to homophobia are becoming increasingly clear. Homophobia has been linked to outcomes such as personal harm, psychological disorders, and substandard health care for same-sex attracted young people (Hillier et al. 1998; Robertson 1998; Fergusson et al. 1999; Plummer 1999). Psychosocial outcomes of homophobia include shame, anxiety, isolation, lack of self-worth, devalued sense of masculinity, emotional confusion and turmoil, possible rejection by family and friends, homelessness, and elevated risks of HIV/AIDS (Ridge 1997; Hillier et al. 1998; Robertson 1998; Meyer 2001). Not surprisingly, research indicates that harm resulting from homophobia can translate into actual psychological disorders (Robertson 1998; Diaz et al. 2001; Sandfort et al. 2001). Compared to their heterosexual counterparts, same-sex attracted people are at an increased risk for a range of conditions, including depression, anxiety, suicide attempts, and multiple disorders (McDonald and Cooper 1998; Fergusson et al. 1999). For instance, a study of 408 gay men in Adelaide found that 27 per cent had major depression (eight times the wider population) (McNair et al. 2001). Additionally, there is a consistent picture emerging in overseas research that an unusually high proportion of non-heterosexual young people (roughly 20 to 50 per cent, with most studies reporting approximately 30 per cent) have reported an attempted suicide (Roesler and Deisher 1972; Plummer 1989; Kruks 1991; Remafedi et al. 1991). The narratives of young same-sex attracted people who attempt suicide suggest they do so for a range of reasons linked to homophobia, such as to avoid being seen as homosexual, to cope with bullying and rejection, and to avoid emotional pain (Emslie 1996; Ridge 1997).

While not all of the kinds of mental health problems experienced by same-sex attracted young people can and should be linked to homophobia, it does make sense that many problems of same-sex attracted people at least have some origin in homophobia. Plummer (1999) has likened the experience of homophobia to surviving torture (after all, there are currently few places to hide from homophobic abuse in the school yard). Interestingly, the outcomes of anxiety, depression, and suicidality among same-sex attracted people are similar to what we see among survivors of torture and abuse.

SOCIAL CONSTRAINTS AND RESISTANCE

There is a common mythology that young same-sex attracted men—particularly when they escape the homophobia of the school ground—go through stages of coming to terms with their sexuality, and then 'come out' into a 'gay community' that provides some refuge from homophobia and support for emotional wellbeing (Troiden 1989). There is an assumption that emotional issues resulting from homophobia are somehow resolved through coming out, and that the transition alleviates, rather than presents, new challenges for wellbeing (Ridge 1997). However, research that focuses on the narratives of men regarding their actual experiences challenge this 'coming out' narrative (Ridge et al. 1997; Ridge et al. 1999). What the research shows is that social problems such as isolation are not necessarily resolved by integrating into new gay-friendly networks. When men move into gay networks, they are actually 'coming in' to particular cultural contexts and new challenges to wellbeing can arise (Connell 1992). For instance, as outlined in table 26.2, gay networks based in commercialised spaces such as bars and nightclubs (this is frequently what same-sex attracted men are talking about when they mention 'the scene') may be experienced by men as alienating, hierarchical, and exclusionary (Ridge et al. 1997). Young men who do not understand or fit in with certain codes and styles may feel excluded or pressured to

Table 26.2 Features of the gay scene and associated mental health implications

KINDS OF ISSUES ENCOUNTERED IN COMMERCIAL GAY ENVIRONMENTS BY YOUNG MEN	REPORTED HEALTH/MENTAL HEALTH IMPLICATION OF SCENE CULTURE
Varying social status of participants and hierarchical social relations based around certain styles of appearance, class, group memberships, perceived masculinity, ethnicity.	Compulsive behaviours, e.g. sexual, substances, body control strategies. Emphasis on individualism. Discrimination, e.g. against ethnic minorities.
Pleasure is foremost, e.g. dancing, celebrating, sex, substance use.	Isolation and feelings of alienation. Feeling pressured to 'fit in' to restrictive styles and codes.
Uniform styles and codes, e.g. youthful, muscular, low body fat.	Body image concerns, use of steroids, unhealthy body control strategies.
Friendships as limited, e.g. 'good time friends'.	Going 'full on' into the scene and associated issues, e.g. increased drug use, loss of employment.
Predominant styles of communication, e.g. gossip.	Negative self-talk.
Sexualisation of relations, e.g. prominence of cruising, sex on premises venues, issues of negotiating sexual safety.	Sexual risk taking. The need to negotiate boundaries.
Particularly initially, men look for 'community' and meaning on the scene, but frequently become more realistic about what it can offer.	

change (Ridge et al. 1999). For instance, young men report intense pressures to conform to particular youthful styles, such as having a muscular and non-fat body appearance. With such pressures within the scene to attain certain standards, some men can have difficulties in being caring towards themselves, and instead become self-critical.

SOCIAL STRUCTURE AND HUMAN AGENCY

Importantly, despite the pervasive social structures of homophobia in schools and perceived lack of diversity on the commercial 'gay scene', young men are not powerless. Men can and do find ways to negotiate and even budge the seemingly solidified social structures in these environments. Giddens (1984) called this situation the 'dialectic of control', where human agency is important in all forms of social life: even the less powerful can resist social control. Within the school yard, young same-sex attracted boys and men are successfully fighting back against homophobic bullies (Williams 2002). And we must not forget that all boys eventually get out of the school yard anyway.

Many men move into the much more sexually affirming gay scene, and this involves agency but also bravery. Within the gay scene, many men become realistic about what the scene itself can offer, and in the words of one young man, come to understand and use the scene as a space that provides 'a good night out with pitfalls for the unwary', rather than attempt to look for any real social support within that scene. Other men might play with the available structures and codes, perhaps even subverting them, such as by wearing male 'drag'—putting on muscular bodies and demeanours that gay men are supposed to be excluded from (Butler 1990). Still other men might move away from the perceived constraints of the gay scene, and perhaps develop significant relationships with their lovers (Butler and Clarke 1991). However, as Wright (2002) has found, if these relationships break down, then the separation itself can be highly traumatic, with high levels of suicide attempts and a lack of social support. Nevertheless, men do bounce back from separations and find ways to regain their strength—frequently using autonomous coping strategies (e.g. cutting ties, immersion in work activities, keeping a journal, reading).

More widely than the questioning and reworking going on in the gay scene, since the gay liberation movement of the 1960s and 1970s, queer politics in the West has involved challenges to the 'gay identity' and everything that has come to be associated with it, including 'body fascism', ethnocentricity, and uniformity. Today, many younger same-sex attracted men are detached from the notion of gay identities and communities, avoiding the gay ghetto to go 'where the music is good' (Reynolds 2002). They are finding meaning in 'a jumble of identities, relationships and circumstance' (e.g. ethnicity, work, relationships, consumption), rather than what may appear as tired and even 'zombie'-like gay identities.

SUMMARY

- Homophobia and discrimination are strong determinants of health for same-sex attracted people.
- It is clear that people actively grapple with the social factors that impact on their health in order to find better outcomes and determine their own understandings of health.
- Supportive and safe environments are a key determinant of mental health for young same-sex attracted men.

DISCUSSION TOPICS

1 Consider the recommendations of the Plummer (2001) report in table 26.1. Use these recommendations to help you construct an integrated health promotion action plan designed to support sexual diversity in schools. Which elements of your plan are specifically targeted upstream?

2 Identify the key stakeholders in implementing this action plan. What roles would each stakeholder play?

WORKPLACE HEALTH

Andrew Noblet

Key concepts

- Traditional approaches to combating stress
- Organisational sources of job stress
- A settings approach to addressing workplace stress

The aim of this chapter is to highlight the shortcomings of the traditional approach to promoting health in the workplace and to provide a conceptual framework for developing a settings-based approach for addressing the determinants of health at work. As a means of illustrating the differences between the traditional and settings-based approaches, this chapter will focus on one of the most critical issues affecting the health of workers: occupational stress. **Occupational stress** occurs when external demands and conditions don't match a person's needs, expectations or ideals or exceed their physical capacity, skills, or knowledge for comfortably handling a situation (adapted from French et al. 1982). Chronic occupational stress is regarded as both a serious public health concern and a major barrier to organisational success. In human terms, prolonged exposure to stressful situations at work is associated with a range of physical (e.g. cardiovascular disease), psychological (e.g. depression), social (e.g. interpersonal conflict), and behavioural (e.g. alcohol and other drug abuse) health problems (Levi 1996). For organisations, occupational stress can contribute to a number of outcomes that are critical to their success, including absenteeism, labour turnover, and job performance (Spector et al. 1988; Yagil 1998). The human and economic costs of job stress strongly suggest that it is in everybody's interests—employees, employers, and the community at large—that steps be taken to build healthier and less stressful working environments.

THE TRADITIONAL APPROACH TO COMBATING STRESS AT WORK

The traditional approach to addressing stress in the workplace is to focus on individual employees and provide them with information and guidance on how to adapt to, or cope with, the pressures and demands faced in everyday work life. Typically these interventions include one-to-one counselling, relaxation training, lifestyle education, and other behaviour change strategies. Reviews of job stress interventions indicate that individual-orientated strategies are by far the most common approach to job stress (Giga et al. 2003; Murphy 1988).

This traditional approach has been strongly criticised by organisational health practitioners, employee representatives, and occupational stress researchers. Before examining the specific criticisms that have been directed at this approach, read the following case study (box 27.1). The Opticom case study is based on a program in which the author was briefly involved in the late 1990s. Consider why the program failed to achieve the aim of reducing absenteeism and identify the major weaknesses of the traditional approach to combating stress at work.

The Opticom case study is a typical example of where an organisation has undertaken health promotion in a setting (Baric 1993). The majority of initiatives were aimed at identifying individuals who are at risk of developing lifestyle-related diseases (e.g. cardiovascular disease), and encouraging them to adopt healthier lifestyles. The health impact of the setting itself—including social, organisational, and physical conditions—was largely overlooked.

Box 27.1   Stress at Opticom (part 1)

The operator-assisted services (OAS) section of Opticom is a 24-hour call centre located in the Perth Central Business District. Approximately 200 employees are employed across three shifts to attend to local and international enquiries. Opticom recently appointed a new manager to the OAS unit who, in her first review of the unit's operations, found that it was experiencing high absenteeism (most of which was sick leave), increasing customer complaints, and low morale. Anecdotal evidence from a number of employees also suggested that stress levels were high.

The manager was determined to reduce the high rates of sick leave and immediately sought the services of a corporate health promotion company. This company introduced a series of health checks and follow-up counselling covering such issues as diet, blood pressure, fitness, and stress. In the case of stress, all staff were also given the opportunity to attend relaxation classes twice a week.

After six months, an evaluation of the program revealed that it had very little impact on absenteeism. While the screening sessions held during work hours were well attended, the relaxation classes were not.

The individual approach to occupational stress has been heavily criticised for blaming the victim. Fisher and Cotton (1994) report that individual symptoms of stress are often manifestations of organisational-level problems rather than personal coping deficiencies. Thus, by trying to teach employees to cope with stressful working conditions, proponents of this approach can be seen to be blaming the victim of poor communication channels, inadequate training, autocratic management styles, and other common sources of workplace stress. Deflecting blame onto the individual implies that nothing can or will be done to change these organisational sources of stress (Quinlan and Bohle 1991). Individual-level strategies have also been criticised for failing to achieve long-term outcomes. Research examining the benefits of employee-centred strategies have found that such strategies tend to result in shorter-term psychological benefits that are not sustainable over a longer period (Michie 1992; Whatmore et al. 1999).

ORGANISATIONAL SOURCES OF JOB STRESS

There is considerable variation in the way individuals perceive and respond to the environments in which they work. Personal (e.g. personality type and coping skills) and situational (e.g. previous experiences and support from work colleagues) variables will influence the onset and duration of job stress and what one person finds demanding and stressful others will perceive as challenging and stimulating (Cooper and Marshall 1976). Despite this variation, a range of physical, social, organisational, and economic conditions have been identified as common sources of job stress (table 27.1). These conditions, referred to as **job stressors**, are the physical, social, organisational, or economic conditions at work that contribute to stress.

Table 27.1 Common job stressors

WORK CHARACTERISTIC	JOB STRESSOR
Organisational function and culture	Poor communications
	Poor problem-solving environment
	Poor development environment
Participation	Low participation in decision making
Career development and job status	Career uncertainty or career stagnation
	Poor-status work or work of low social value
	Poor pay, job insecurity, or redundancy
Role in organisation	Role ambiguity or role conflict
	Responsibility for others or continual contact with other people

cont.

Table 27.1 Common job stressors (continued)

WORK CHARACTERISTIC	JOB STRESSOR
Job content	Lack of variety
	Fragmented or meaningless work
	Underutilisation of skills
Workload and work pace	Quantitative work overload or underload
	Qualitative work overload or underload
	Lack of control over pacing
Work organisation	Inflexible work schedule
	Unpredictable hours
	Long or unsocial hours
Interpersonal relationships at work	Social or physical isolation
	Lack of social support
	Interpersonal conflict and violence
Home–work interface	Conflicting demands of work and home
	Low social or practical support from home
	Dual career problems

Adapted from Cox and Cox 1993

After the corporate health program was found to have little impact on the health and performance of OAS employees at Opticom, informal discussions with employees found there were a number of organisational factors that were particularly stressful for workers. Read part 2 of the Opticom case study (box 27.2) and, in conjunction with organisational and psychosocial stressors listed in

---

Box 27.2   Stress at Opticom (part 2)

There are many problems inherent within the OAS unit. The task of attending to public enquiries is extremely repetitive. In the domestic section, for instance, operators would receive an average of 175 calls per eight-hour day, with each lasting between 30 seconds and five minutes. They often have to attend to irate and sometimes abusive callers and receive next to no training in dealing with this sort of conflict. There is a top-down style of management and operators have virtually no say in decisions directly affecting what they do, despite the fact that they are generally in the best position to identify problems and generate ideas for overcoming them. Exacerbating the situation is an unpredictable style of supervision that swings erratically from overbearing to nonexistent.

table 27.1, identify the specific conditions that were likely to be making significant contributions to the stress experienced by members of the OAS unit.

THE SETTINGS APPROACH TO ADDRESSING STRESS AT WORK

The settings approach to health promotion provides valuable opportunities for dealing with both the sources and effects of occupational stress. The settings approach focuses on the physical, social, and organisational environments in which people spend their time and aims to create settings (i.e. schools, hospitals, workplaces, and communities) that support and enhance health (Baric 1993). This approach represents a significant shift from traditional health promotion methods that seek to use settings as a venue for promoting healthier lifestyles (e.g. exercise more, reduce caffeine intake, and avoid high-fat foods). The settings approach recognises the importance of traditional, individual-focused methods, but emphasises that these strategies should complement (not replace) efforts to identify and address settings-based sources of ill health (Noblet and Murphy 1995).

Job stress prevention strategies aim to achieve one or a combination of the following goals: prevent the development of potentially stressful situations (i.e. stressors); reduce the intensity of, or exposure to, these stressors; and help equip people with the knowledge, skills, and resources to cope with stressful conditions.

A conceptual framework that reflects the settings approach to health promotion and which can be used to develop specific stress prevention strategies is DeFrank and Cooper's (1987) typology of job-stress interventions. DeFrank and Cooper classified interventions according to the level in the organisation that the strategy targeted: the individual employee, the organisation, and the organisation–individual interface. The aim of individual-level interventions is to address the individuals exhibiting stress symptoms, create greater awareness of the adverse effects of chronic strain, and teach arousal reduction skills and coping techniques. The next level of stress intervention refers to the interface between the individual and the organisation and encompasses role ambiguity, relationships at work, person–environment fit, and employee involvement in decision making. Examples of specific individual–organisation level strategies include co-worker support groups, role clarification mechanisms, and participatory decision-making programs. The third level of interventions addresses areas in the physical, organisational, and social environments that may produce stress. Interventions that target the organisation include organisational restructuring, selection and placement, training, and job redesign. It should be noted that the intervention levels are not independent of each other and there is overlap between the three levels.

Strategies involving both individual and organisational interventions are more likely to lead to longer-term improvements in employee health and business performance than those that focus solely on the individual (Cartwright et al. 2000; Bond and Bunce 2001). However, recent research involving participatory action

Box 27.3   Stress at Opticom (part 3)

After Opticom realised that its strategies had not worked, it decided to undertake a more inclusive and systematic investigation into why OAS was not performing as well as it should. A small committee, consisting of management and employee representatives, was formed to guide and oversee this assessment. The committee quickly found that the unit's performance fluctuated significantly and a period when error rates were particularly high was mid afternoon on a weekday. Informal discussions with a cross-section of employees later found that a major source of poor performance was mothers worrying about whether their children had got home from school safely. OAS employed a large number of mothers with dependent children and action needed to be taken to address their needs. Through the ideas generated by employees, Opticom gave their operators a 10-minute break around 4 p.m. so they could call home to make sure that the kids had arrived safely. This strategy alone resulted in a significant improvement in the service quality and morale. The timing of the relaxation classes was also changed to better accommodate the work and personal commitments of employees.

research (PAR) indicates that the single most important factor in determining the success of job-stress programs is the extent that the initiatives match the needs of employees (Bond and Bunce 2001). Participatory action research reflects the empowerment approach to health promotion (Naidoo and Wills 1994) and provides all levels of the organisation, particularly shop-floor employees, with the opportunity to identify their own needs and then develop strategies for addressing these needs.

Part 3 of the Opticom case study (box 27.3) is a good example of where all three levels of job-stress interventions have been implemented simultaneously. The work schedule was modified to better accommodate the nonwork commitments of employees (organisational-level intervention); employees were involved in the decision-making processes that led to the development of the new strategies (individual–organisational level intervention), and employees were given the opportunity to develop and apply relaxation skills that could help them cope with stressful conditions and events (individual-level intervention). The empowerment approach has also enhanced the capacity of the organisation to address other workplace stressors (i.e. erratic supervision, poor conflict resolution skills, and monotonous workloads). OAS now has a structure (i.e. coordinating committee) and a system (i.e. employee and organisational needs assessment) in place to identify health-related issues. Furthermore, the enthusiasm and trust that has been established with the success of the first strategy will give the committee the confidence required to drive this system and help it achieve effective, long-term outcomes.

SUMMARY

- The pressures associated with increasingly competitive and cost-conscious marketplaces will continue to place enormous demands on organisations and their members.
- Excessive job stress is therefore an issue that is likely, at some stage, to impact on the lives of all employees, irrespective of their position in the organisational hierarchy or the industry in which they work.
- While individual level strategies can offer short-term solutions, the settings approach to health promotion provides a more effective and sustainable framework for addressing the sources and symptoms of job stress.

DISCUSSION TOPICS

1 Consider the workplace where you work (or have worked in the past). What organisational and psychosocial conditions are (or were) common sources of stress for you?

2 How did these conditions affect your wellbeing? Make sure you take into account physical, psychological, behavioural, and social dimensions of health when considering these affects.

3 Focus on one of the stressors you have experienced and use DeFrank and Cooper's (1987) typology of job-stress interventions to develop a comprehensive series of strategies that can eliminate or significantly reduce the impact of this stressor.

28 PROMOTING HEALTHY AGEING

Helen Keleher

Key concepts

- Determinants of healthy ageing
- Socioeconomic status, social connectedness, and social isolation
- Health promotion strategies with older people
- Challenges arising from an ageing population

AGEING: NOT FOR THE FAINT-HEARTED!

> Will you still need me,
> Will you still feed me,
> When I'm sixty-four?

The Beatles sang these words in the late 1960s, perhaps long before you were born. While they sang of experiences that we all face as we pass through life, not many of us contemplate in our youth, what ageing is really like. Old age seems so far away—our parents and grandparents have always seemed like 'oldies' compared to our own youthfulness! So it can be surprising to realise that they were once young, with photographs or stories revealing the energy and beauty of our parents and our grandparents in their younger years. But we can also be shocked to realise that their youthfulness and sense of adventure was often tied to terrible experiences such as war, or the deprivations of massive economic depression or famine. These experiences will be quite foreign to many people born in Australia since the 1950s, while others will have dealt with the health effects of war, migration, or refugee experiences. Many of the older people alive today were small children during the Great Depression of the 1930s with its associated economic hardship and deprivation (Byles 2001). Byles reminds us that the adolescence and adulthood of today's older people were dominated by the Second World War, followed by the boom economic period of the 1950s with full employment and the push towards home ownership. Nevertheless, sex-role stereotypes determined social values and constrained opportunities. The sexual division of labour meant that few adult women had choices outside home and family, and men were expected to be full-time breadwinners. Male values dominated workplaces and domestic situations (Germov 2002).

Considerable social change has occurred in Australia since the 1960s, bringing more relaxed attitudes to social boundaries, increased social diversity and multiculturalism, improved levels of education, greater mobility, and increased workforce participation. Past generations did not expect to live much more than 64 years of age, and if they did, their health was generally much less robust than the older people of the early twenty-first century. Life expectancy has risen considerably. A demographic shift is under way in Australia and in most developed countries, towards a higher proportion of people aged over 60 years. Today's older people are taller, fitter, and healthier than previous generations—in other words, they are more robust. Moreover, people of today are preparing to live longer than any other generation in history. This requires new understandings of what it means to have large numbers of people living to be 80, 90, or even 100 years of age, in what has become known as 'the third age'.

To promote healthy ageing and to overcome ageist discriminatory attitudes, the United Nations declared 1999 to be the International Year of Older People, during which Australia actively promoted the theme of 'Celebrating Ageing'. The celebrations and activities through that year were based on nineteen United Nations' principles about older people's rights to a good quality of life. Those principles include dignity, participation, self-esteem, independence, and valuing older people's productivity and contributions to society (VicHealth 1996). Nevertheless, our social systems, particularly health, must continue to develop the capacity of staff and programs to be responsive to older people's needs, and to gain the knowledge and skills required for effective service delivery to our older generations.

HEALTH SYSTEM CHALLENGES FROM AN AGEING POPULATION

Our longer life expectancy and the health needs of increasing numbers of older people in Australia pose considerable challenges for health and community services (Duckett 2001), because as we get older, we become prone to illness and diseases. The number of people aged over 65 years doubled between 1971 and 1991, and by 2010 will increase by one-third again (Swerissen and Duckett 2002), with higher proportions of older women than men. Currently, about 12 per cent of the population is aged 65 years or older, but by 2051, that proportion is predicted to rise to 25 per cent (ABS 1999). This changing age structure will be accompanied by growing levels of chronic illness, poor mental health, and widening health and social inequalities (Mathers 1994; Turrell et al. 1999). The incidence and prevalence of chronic, complex diseases among older populations places a significant burden on individuals, communities, and health services (NPHP 2001).

Differences in mortality rates for cardiovascular diseases (CVD) have been found among men with higher rates of ischaemic heart disease related to low incomes, single parent families, and those in public rental accommodation. Rates of colon cancer mortality are higher in middle-class areas and lower in low SES areas. People of low SES report higher levels of chronic illness and dental health, especially missing teeth (Turrell et al. 1999).

Challenges arise not just from the increasing prevalence of chronic disease but also from the complexities of co-morbidities, that is, having more than one illness at a time. The prevalence of chronic illness is compounded by the increasing numbers of older people living on low incomes, increasing workforce participation by women who have otherwise traditionally provided care for older family members, as well as the gradual loss of social connectedness that arises from social isolation (Palmer and Short 2000; NPHP 2001). As discussed in previous chapters, type 2 diabetes, CVD, stroke, cancers, neurological disorders, renal disease, chronic respiratory disease, and arthritis cause the major burden of disease and disability for older people. Many older people experience more than one of these diseases, but it is also common for older people's chronic diseases to be complicated by social conditions, including mental health problems, particularly depression and anxiety; grief and loss; poor nutrition; smoking; and inadequate income to maintain a satisfying quality of life.

The combination of social and health issues raises questions about how we should provide caring services for populations of elderly people who will gradually need various forms of support. Although only 7 per cent of older people live in residential aged care, governments are becoming increasingly concerned about the rising costs of formal care and are seeking mechanisms to contain the costs of hostel and nursing home beds. On the other hand, older people themselves value their independence, often expressing a desire to stay in their own communities. Thus, there are challenges in providing the maintenance and support services required by older people to enable them to live at home.

Other pressure points in the care and support of older people arise from the increasing sophistication of biomedical technology combined with the increasing pressure on hospitals to shorten lengths of stay and reduce inpatient costs. Further, there is increasing emphasis by governments on reducing hospital admissions that are deemed to have been preventable, and this is providing an impetus for chronic disease management in the community. **Carers** themselves have become politicised through groups such as the Carers Association of Australia, members of which are active in the pursuit of policies to support carers (Creelman 2002). While governments have increased investment in community care and in support for carers, there is no doubt that there are trends towards facilitating the unpaid work of carers and increasing government reliance on the informal caring sector (Hancock and Moore 1999; Creelman 2002). Families are increasingly called upon to provide continuity of care for older people, not just for those who are recovering from illness or disease, but on an ongoing basis. Yet, families are not always available to provide ongoing care of older family members, so the provision of social support services for older people is critical. However, in Australia, support services are widely regarded as inadequate (Palmer and Short 2000).

DETERMINANTS OF HEALTHY AGEING

A key principle of the Ottawa Charter is to create supportive environments that will promote health. The World Health Organization's Healthy Cities program describes the basis of this principle in terms of the provision of clean, safe, high-quality, sustainable physical environments; the building of strong, mutually supportive, and nonexploitative communities with a high degree of public participation in which the provision of affordable, accessible public transport is integral to mobility. The quality of the environment impacts on older people's capacity to remain active and independent, with a supportive environment enabling participation in the everyday social interactions of communities without reliance on a driver's licence and a private car. Without such access, older people are particularly prone to social isolation. Ageing populations, especially in rural areas, are often isolated by a lack of transport options. The provision of public transport, one vital element in supportive environments, is a prominent determinant of health for older populations. Another aspect of a supportive environment is the quality of urban structures, as these determine people's access to opportunities for physical activity (as discussed in chapter 18). Footpaths and cycling paths become a means to physical activity and the development of recreational and fitness opportunities. Participation in physical activity helps to minimise the symptoms of type 2 diabetes, cardiovascular diseases, cancers, and arthritis.

Older people whose health status is more vulnerable to illness and disease are those who have lived on, and retire on, lower incomes; older women; and those living alone. In later life, the distribution of resources and increasing vulnerability of older people reflect wider social structures and inequalities, including those related to gender. There are strong associations between life experiences and our likely health status as an older person. Chronic disease is increasingly understood as being associated with exposure to risk or suboptimal experiences across the life-course (NPHP 2001). Older people from low socioeconomic backgrounds demonstrate significantly lower levels of social interaction, higher levels of overweight, and lower levels of physical activity than do their counterparts from higher socioeconomic groups. Low-income older people also tend to make greater use of general practitioner services and are more likely to have a prescribed medication.

Proponents of the public health determinants approach understand that much of the burden of chronic, complex disease is preventable and that we should be actively promoting healthy ageing. This requires an understanding of relationships between determinants of health and health promotion programs. For example, falls prevention is the focus of major public health investment because falls are a leading cause of injury in people over the age of 65 years. Risk factors include disability, medication, chronic disease, and environmental hazards. Deaths from falls are usually the result of the after-effects of the injury sustained (AIHW 1998). Nevertheless, a focus on falls prevention in isolation of other determinants of health is likely to produce only limited outcomes. Integrated health promotion programs built on engagement with communities of older people are much more likely to produce sustainable, effective outcomes than programs that focus on a single disease or condition.

Given that older people have become a priority population for government prevention and health promotion programs, increased emphasis on capacity building within communities is required, as a more holistic, socioenvironmental approach to health is much more likely to improve the health of older population groups. Community capacity building entails acknowledging the important role that older people can play in the planning, implementation, and evaluation processes of programs that address their health status. Despite the knowledge base of the principles for good public health and health promotion, community health programs targeted at older people still tend towards silo approaches that address specific health issues or contributing risk factors in isolation. Top-down approaches that 'do health promotion' on individuals are more common than those with a socioenvironmental approach.

While some governments have forecast doom and gloom for health budgets because of the predicted growth in the proportion of older people in Australia, some health economists hold substantial doubts that the proportion of aged people will cause significant increased demand for health services (Palmer and Short 2000). Rather, healthy ageing is being promoted as a cause for celebration.

SUMMARY

- Ageing is a normal life experience, not a medical or social problem.
- Socioeconomic status, lack of transport options, access to health services, and the availability and quality of social supports, are key determinants of the ageing experience.
- The quality of people's ageing experience depends very much on healthy public policies that acknowledge the needs of older people in planning and community action to ensure that healthy ageing is possible for all Australians.

DISCUSSION TOPIC

An increased 'emphasis on capacity building within communities is required' if we are to improve the health of older populations. Imagine the year is 2015, and you are looking back over the past ten years or so to track and celebrate significant achievements with respect to capacity building within communities. What changes would you hope to observe over that period, and what impact would you expect these changes to have on the health of older people?

GLOSSARY

absolute poverty
The notion of absolute poverty is based on the idea that there is a fixed income point and if one earns more than that fixed amount then one is not poor and if one earns less than that fixed amount one is poor (see relative poverty).

advocacy
A process which openly aims to change laws, regulations, policy, and organisational practices that impact on the ability of individuals and communities to make healthy choices.

anaemia
A condition characterised by a deficiency in haemoglobin (the oxygen-carrying component of the blood).

atherosclerosis
Disease process characterised by a gradual build up of cholesterol and other material underneath the lining of the artery.

behaviour change communication (BCC)
Aims to inform and influence individuals about the adoption of healthier behaviours.

biomedical model
The scientific medical model that is focused on disease, diagnosis and treatment of individuals.

biophilia hypothesis
The assertion that because humans evolved in the company of other organisms, they are predisposed to depend on affiliations with nature.

carer
A person such as a family member, friend, or neighbour who provides regular and sustained care and assistance to another person with or without payment of a government pension or benefit.

co-factor
A nonprotein substance that must be combined with the protein portion of an enzyme before the enzyme can act.

community action
The empowerment of communities, their ownership and control of their own endeavours and destinies. This is often the outcome of community engagement and capacity building.

community development
Active involvement of people sharing in the issues which affect their lives, by drawing on existing human and material resources to enhance self-help and social support.

co-morbidity

Two or more coexisting disease or illness conditions that may be related or unrelated.

consumer engagement

Seeks to increase the uptake of health services by a diverse range of consumers, particularly vulnerable population groups, and those experiencing disadvantage and/or social exclusion.

culture

A group's construction of shared values, traditions, histories, knowledge, rituals, customs, language, foods and other facets that distinguish them from other cultural groupings.

death rate

The number of deaths per million people in each year; the lower the mortality rate, the healthier is the population—this is the opposite logic from life expectancy!

deoxyribonucleic acid (DNA)

DNA molecules are the building blocks of genes. Specific genes are composed of a particular sequence of DNA molecules that provide the code for protein synthesis.

depression

A group of illnesses characterised by excessive and long-term lowered mood that causes significant ongoing distress and/or impairment.

determinant of health

A factor or characteristic that brings about a change in health, either for the better or for the worse (also see distal determinant of health and proximal determinant of health).

Disability Adjusted Life Year (DALY)

A measure of population health based on the calculation of the number of years of life lost due to premature mortality, and the number of less than healthy years of life lived due to premature morbidity.

distal determinant

A distal determinant of health is one that is distant either in time or place from the change in health status. Distal determinants of health are also referred to as 'upstream factors' (see also proximal determinant).

distal factors

Remote from the point of reference. For example, increasingly distal determinants of lung cancer are: DNA damage from tobacco smoke; smoking behaviours; availability and price of cigarettes; and tobacco control policies.

DNA base pairs

The nitrogen base components of nucleic acids. Bonds between complementary bases hold together the two strands of a double-stranded DNA molecule.

downstream public health interventions

Those at micro level including treatment systems, disease management, and investment in clinical research.

ecological fallacy

The ecological fallacy occurs when one infers that a relationship that holds at a population level between two ecological factors, such as DALYs per capita and

GNP per capita, is also true for two individual factors, such as personal health and personal wealth.

ecological health

Health is the outcome of complex interrelationships and interdependencies between human beings, the determinants of health, and the broader environment in which they exist.

ecologically sustainable development (ESD)

An intergovernmental policy with a set of guiding principles recognising the need to integrate environmental protection with economic and social development (Brown 1997; Nicholson et al. 2002). As a practice, an approach to using, conserving, and enhancing natural resources so that ecological processes, on which all life depends, are maintained, and the total quality of life, now and in the future, is improved. Health is central to the concept (Brown 1997; Nicholson et al. 2002).

environmental health

Those aspects of human health determined by physical, chemical, biological and social factors in the environment. Environmental health is about creating and maintaining environments which promote good public health.

environmental health justice

The right to a safe, healthy, productive, and sustainable environment. Environmental health justice requires the pursuit of equal justice and protection in legislation, regulations, government policy, and actions.

enzyme

A protein that is produced by a cell and acts as a catalyst in a specific cellular reaction.

epidemic

The occurrence in a community or region of cases of an illness, specific health-related behaviour, or other health-related events clearly in excess of normal expectancy. The community or region and the period in which the cases occur are specified precisely (Last 2001).

epidemiology

The study of the patterns and causes of disease in populations.

equity

The fair distribution of resources in relation to needs. See the entries under health equity, inequity, and inequalities.

essentialism

A particular form of stereotyping that attributes group characteristics or group cultures to biological or innate reasons.

evidence-based medicine

Involves the judicious use of current best evidence from health care research in the treatment and management of individual patients.

exegesis

Critical explanation and interpretation that is one of the fundamental tasks and skills of historians, and it is usually missing from heroic, individualised and decontextualised historical stories.

food security

The ready availability of nutritionally adequate and safe foods, and an assured ability to acquire acceptable foods in socially acceptable ways without the need for coping strategies such as begging, stealing, or scavenging for food.

globalisation

A set of processes leading to the creation of a world as a single entity, relatively undivided by national borders or other types of boundaries, such as cultural, economic, and temporal boundaries.

harm reduction

A strategy, with demand reduction and supply reduction, to reduce harms associated with hazardous substance use.

HDL cholesterol

High-density lipoproteins (HDL) collect cholesterol from low-density lipoprotein and take it back to the liver for excretion as bile acids. A high concentration of HDL cholesterol reduces the risk of cardiovascular disease.

health and place

The impact of locality and connectedness on the health and wellbeing of individuals and communities.

health equity

The rights of people to have equitable access to services on the basis of need, and the resources, capacities and power they need to act upon the circumstances of their lives that determine their health.

health literacy

The knowledge gained from experiences, values, beliefs, and attitudes that promote recognition and appropriate help-seeking, knowledge of health-related issues including factors that create health and how to seek health information, the ability to recognise specific disorders, of self-treatments, and how to find professional help.

health promotion

The process of enabling people to take control over factors that determine their health.

healthy public policy

An explicit concern for health and equity in all areas of policy and by an accountability for health impact, with aims to create supportive environments to enable people to lead healthy lives and the building of policies particularly in non-health sectors, to support health.

heterozygous

Having a different allele (version) of a particular gene on each chromosome of a chromosome pair. For two versions of a gene, S and s, the heterozygous state would be Ss.

homozygous

Having the same allele (version) of a particular gene on each chromosome of a chromosome pair. For two versions of a gene, S and s, the homozygous states would be SS or ss.

inequalities

Measurable differences or variations in some condition such as health or income levels.

inequities
> Those inequalities that are deemed to be unfair or stemming from some form of injustice. Inequities involve relations of equal and unequal power (political, social and economic) as well as justice and injustice.

information, education, and communication (IEC)
> Midstream intervention that delivers health education and behaviour change campaigns based on evidence about the health of a group.

information literacy
> Enables individuals to recognise when information is needed and have the capacity to locate, evaluate, and use information effectively.

job stressors
> The physical, social, organisational, or economic conditions at work that contribute to stress.

Knowledge, attitude, behaviour change (KAB)
> A theory of behaviour change suggesting that increasing a person's knowledge will lead to attitudinal change leading to change of behaviour.

LDL cholesterol
> Low-density lipoproteins (LDL) are the main carrier of cholesterol from the liver to the cells. A high concentration of LDL cholesterol increases the risk of cholesterol deposition under the arterial lining and therefore increases the risk of cardiovascular disease.

life expectancy
> The average length of life for people in a community.

lipoproteins
> Transport particles made up of lipids and proteins that carry cholesterol and other fats through the blood.

macrophages
> Scavenger cells that engulf extracellular material via a process called phagocytosis.

marginality
> Social positioning outside, on the borders, or 'in the margins', of groups and communities that is politically, culturally and economically upheld and sanctioned as mainstream, central, dominant and 'normal'.

mental health literacy
> The ability to recognise specific disorders; know how to seek mental health information; knowledge of risk factors and causes; knowledge of self-treatment and of professional help available; and having an attitude that promotes recognition and appropriate help-seeking skills and behaviours.

messenger ribonucleic acid (mRNA)
> mRNA is a transcript of one of the two strands of a DNA molecule. It carries the code for protein synthesis.

metabolic equivalents (METs)
> Units used to describe the metabolic cost of physical activity as a product of the resting metabolic rate.

methyl donor

Donates a methyl (-CH3) group in a chemical reaction.

midstream public health interventions

Intermediate level interventions focused on lifestyle, behavioural and individual pre-vention programs.

mutation

A change in the sequence of a gene that results in the protein produced being severely altered or nonfunctional.

node

A connecting point at which several lines come together.

occupational stress

Occurs when external demands and conditions don't match a person's needs, expec-tations, or ideals or exceed their physical capacity, skills, or knowledge for comfortably handling a situation.

pandemic

An epidemic occurring worldwide, or over a very wide area, crossing international boundaries, and usually affecting a large number of people (Last 2001).

place

In situational and relational terms, place is defined as locality (the family, the natural environment) and also as the connections formed with and within those localities.

polymorphism

A difference in a gene that is common within a population (i.e. occurring in >1% of people).

population health

An approach to health that aims to improve the health of the entire population and to reduce health inequities among and between specific population groups. Action is directed at the health of an entire population or sub-population, rather than individ-uals through policies, programs, research and interventions designed to protect and enhance health.

prevalence

The percentage of the population suffering from a disorder at a given point or period of time.

primary care

An episode of care for diagnosis, treatment of illness, or disease management, as well as an entry point into the health system for people who are seeking help.

primary health care/development

Community-based health care practice based on the social model of health, guided by principles of equity, acceptability, cultural competence, affordability, and universalism, and a commitment to community and health development.

proximal determinant

A determinant of health that is proximate or near to the change in health status. By 'near' one can mean near in either time or distance, but generally it refers to any determinant of health that is readily and directly associated with the change in health status. Proximal determinants are also referred to as 'downstream factors' (see distal determinant).

psychoneuroimmunology
Examines the interactions among specific physiological systems, and how psychological factors and health-related behaviours alter the interactive process, increasing the risk of developing immune system-related diseases such as cancer, arthritis, infections, and allergies.

psychosocial
The inter-relatedness of social perspectives with behavioural and psychological factors and an emphasis on midstream interventions.

public health
A field of both policy and practice that is necessary for the health of populations. Public health involves a vision and planning for the future that addresses inequities and the needs of vulnerable groups, and those with the most disadvantaged health status.

relative poverty
How wealth is distributed between the members of a society, and not about the absolute amounts held by each person. Thus a person could earn a lot, but relative to everyone else in the society earn very little.

risk factor
A variable that potentially increases the susceptibility of developing a condition or disease. For example, physical inactivity and social isolation are risk factors for cardiovascular disease.

scholarly information
The information about your discipline area that is generally reviewed by experts in the field in a process known as peer review.

self-efficacy
Having a belief that we can make a success of the things that we attempt.

settings
Spatial or physical locations or institutions such as schools or workplaces in which health promotion may be undertaken and which addresses institutionally determined norms and factors that impact on health such as bullying, discrimination and environments. Settings may be also classified as contextual (e.g. cities, islands, villages) or as elemental (e.g. workplaces, schools, homes).

silo intervention
A stand-alone intervention that tends to isolate a health issue, group, or risk factor, and in so doing, fails to recognise the wider context.

social capital
Commonly defined in terms of the norms of trust and reciprocity and the level of social cohesion that operate in a society. Societies that exhibit high levels of trust among the community, a preparedness to help each other, and a general sense of belonging are thought to possess high levels of social capital.

social ecology

An ecological model developed by Ure Bronfenbrenner that takes account of multiple factors that influence behaviours and outcomes for individuals.

social exclusion

A social determinant of health related to systematic discrimination and forms of exclusion.

social justice

An ethical concept concerned with unfairness and inequity in society.

social model of health/socioecological approach

An approach to health promotion and community development that addresses the broader determinants of health and acts to reduce social inequalities and injustices, with an emphasis on community engagement and participation, and empowerment of individuals and communities.

sustainability

Refers to continuation of aspects of health promotion such as issues, programs, changes, or partnerships; sustainable development is development that meets the needs of the present without compromising the ability of future generations to meet their own needs.

universal health services

Those services funded centrally that are provided for, and available to everyone, on the basis of need.

upstream public health interventions

Those at the macro level including government policies, global trade agreements and investment in population health research.

web of causation

A model of causality showing the interconnections between multiple causal factors.

REFERENCES

ABS 1996, *The 1995 National Nutrition Survey: User's Guide*, Australian Bureau of Statistics, Canberra.

ABS 2001a, *Births Australia, 2000*, Australian Bureau of Statistics, Canberra.

ABS 2001b, *Causes of Death, 2000*, Australian Bureau of Statistics, Canberra.

ABS 1999, 'Australia now—A Statistical Profile', <www.abs.gov.au>, 30 November 2002.

ABS & Department of Health and Family Services 1995, *National Nutrition Survey: Selected Highlights*, Australian Bureau of Statistics, Canberra.

ABS & Department of Health and Family Services 1997, *National Nutrition Survey, Selected Highlights, Australia 1995*, Commonwealth of Australia, Australian Government Publishing Service, Canberra.

The *Age* 2002, 'Tougher penalties for drink-drivers', Melbourne, 2 February, p. 6.

Agyeman, J. and Evans, R. 2002, 'Environmental quality and human equality', *Local Environment*, 7:1, pp. 5–6.

AIHW 1998, 'Social Atlas', <www.aihw.gov.au>, 30 November 2002.

AIHW 1999a, *Open Employment Services for People with Disabilities 1997–1998*, Australian Institute of Health and Welfare Publications Unit, Canberra.

AIHW 1999b, *The Burden of Disease and Injury in Australia*, Australian Institute of Health and Welfare, Canberra.

AIHW 2000, *Australia's Health 2000*, Australian Institute of Health and Welfare, Canberra.

AIHW 2001a, *Chronic Diseases and Associated Risk Factors in Australia 2001*, Australian Institute of Health and Welfare, Canberra.

AIHW 2001b, *Heart, Stroke and Vascular Diseases: Australian facts 2001*, Australian Institute of Health and Welfare, Canberra.

AIHW 2002a, *2001 National Drug Strategy Household Survey: first results*, Drug Statistics Series no. 9, AIHW Cat. No. PHE 35, Australian Institute of Health and Welfare, Canberra.

AIHW 2002b, *Australia's Health 2002*, Australian Institute of Health and Welfare, Canberra, <www.aihw.gov.au>, 5 January 2003.

AIHW 2002c, *2001 National Drug Strategy Household Survey: Detailed Findings*, Australian Institute of Health and Welfare, Canberra.

Albrecht, G., Seelman, K., and Bury, M. 2001, 'Introduction: The Formation of Disability Studies', in G. Albrecht, K. Seelman and M. Bury (eds), *Handbook of Disability Studies*, Sage, Thousand Oakes.

Allotey, P. and Ravindran, T. K. S. 2003, 'Gender Analysis in the Control of Malaria: The Insecticide', in C. Garcia-Mareno and R. Snow, *Gender Analysis and Health*, World Health Organization, Geneva.

Ancion, C. 2002, 'Europe supports health promotion as a method to tackle social inequalities in health', *Eurohealth*, vol. 8, no. 3, pp. 5–7.

Anderson, S. A. (ed.) 1990, 'Core indicators of nutritional state for difficult to sample populations', *Journal of Nutrition*, vol. 120, no. 11S, pp. 1557–600.

Armstrong, T., Bauman, A., and Davies, J. 2000, 'Physical activity patterns of Australian adults. Results of the 1999 National Physical Activity Survey', Australian Institute of Health and Welfare, Canberra.

Arseneault, L., Cannon, M., Poulton, R., Murray, R., Caspi, A. and Moffitt, T. E. 2002, 'Cannabis use in adolescence and risk for adult psychosis: longitudinal prospective study', *British Medical Journal*, vol. 325, pp. 1212–13.

Atkisson, A. 2000, *Believing Cassandra. An Optimist Looks at a Pessimist's World*, Scribe Publications, Carlton North, Victoria.

Ball, K., Bauman, A., Leslie, E., and Owen, N. 2001, 'Perceived environmental aesthetics and convenience and company are associated with walking for exercise among Australian adults', *Preventive Medicine*, vol. 33, no. 5, pp. 434–40.

Bailie, R., Siciliano, F., Dane, G., Bevan, L., Paradies, Y., and Carson, B. 2002, *Atlas of Health-Related Infrastructure in Discrete Indigenous Communities*, Aboriginal and Torres Strait Islander Commission, Melbourne.

Bandura, A., Reese, L., and Adams, N. E. 1992, 'Microanalysis of action and fear arousal as a function of differential levels of perceived self-efficacy', *Journal of Personality and Social Psychology*, vol. 43, no. 1, pp. 5–21.

Baric, L. 1993, 'The settings approach: implications for policy and strategy', *The Journal of the Institute of Health Education*, vol. 31, no. 1, pp. 17–24.

Barnes, C. 1998, 'The Social Model of Disability: A Sociological Phenomenon Ignored by Sociologists?', in T. Shakespeare (ed.), *The Disability Reader: Social Science Perspectives*, Continuum, London.

Bartley, M., Blane, D., and Davey Smith, D. (eds) 1998, *The Sociology of Health Inequalities*, Blackwell Publishers, Oxford.

Barton, L. 1998, 'Sociology, Disability Studies and Education: Some Observations', in T. Shakespeare (ed.), *The Disability Reader: Social Science Perspectives*, Continuum, London.

Baum, F. 2001, 'Health, equity, justice and globalisation: some lessons from the People's Health Assembly', *Journal of Epidemiology and Community Health*, vol. 55, pp. 613–16.

Baum, F. 2002, *The New Public Health*, 2nd edn, Oxford University Press, Melbourne.

Baum, F. and Keleher, H. 2002, 'Public health update', *Medical Journal of Australia*, Special Issue, 7 January, 176: 36.

Bauman, Z. 2001, *Community: Seeking Safety in an Insecure World*, Polity Press, Cambridge, UK.

Beaglehole, R. and Bonita, R. 1993, *Basic Epidemiology*, World Health Organization, Geneva.

Beck, A. and Katcher, A. 1996, *Between Pets and People: The Importance of Animal Companionship*, Purdue University Press, West Lafayette, Indiana.

Bennett, S. A. 1993, 'Inequities in risk factors and cardiovascular mortality among Australia's immigrants', *Australian Journal of Public Health* , vol. 17, no. 3, pp. 251–61.

Berkman, L. F. and Kawachi, I. (eds) 2000, *Social Epidemiology*, Oxford University Press, New York.

Bettcher, D. and Lee, K. 2002, 'Globalisation and public health glossary', *Journal of Epidemiology and Community Health*, vol. 56, pp. 8–17.

Bickenbach, J. 1993, *Physical Disability and Social Policy*, University of Toronto Press Inc., Toronto.

Bjorntorp, P. and Rosmond, R. 2000, 'Neuroendocrine abnormalities in visceral obesity', *International Journal of Obesity Related Metabolism Disorders*, vol. 24 (Supp 2), pp. S80–S85.

Bolander-Gouaille, C. 2000, *Focus on Homocysteine*, Springer, Paris.

Bond, F. and Bunce, D. 2001, 'Job control mediates change in a work reorganization intervention for stress reduction', *Journal of Occupational Health Psychology*, vol. 6, no. 4, pp. 290–302.

Booth, M. and Samdal, O. 1997, 'Health promoting schools in Australia: models and measurement', *Australian and New Zealand Journal of Public Health*, vol. 21, no. 4, pp. 365–70.

Booth, M. L., Owen, N., Bauman, A., Clavisi, O., and Leslie, E. 2000, 'Social-cognitive and perceived environment influences associated with physical activity in older Australians', *Preventive Medicine*, vol. 31, no. 1, pp. 15–22.

Borland, R. 1997, 'Tobacco health warnings and smoking-related cognitions and behaviors', *Addiction*, vol. 92, pp. 1427–35.

Borland, R. and Davey, C. In press, 'Impact of Smoke-free Bans and Restrictions', in P. Boyle, N. Gray, S. Henningfield, J. Seffrin, and W. Zatonski (eds), *Tobacco: The Public Health Disaster of the Twentieth Century*.

Borland, R., Balmford, J., Farquharson, K., Lal, A., Liberman, J., and Scollo, M. 2001, 'Environmental Tobacco Smoke in Australia: What is Being Done and What More Could Be Done to Reduce Exposures'. Report prepared for the Commonwealth Department of Health and Aged Care, VicHealth Centre for Tobacco Control, <http://www.health.gov.au/pubhlth/strateg/drugs/tobacco/resources.htm>, 10 December 2002.

Bowes, J. and Hayes, A. 1999, *Children, Families and Communities: Contexts and Consequences*, Oxford University Press, Melbourne.

Bradford, B. and Gwynne, M. (eds) 1995, *Down to Earth: Community Perspectives on Health, Development, and the Environment*, Kumarian Press, West Hartford, Connecticut.

Brewster, D. 1999, 'Environmental management for vector control', *British Medical Journal*, vol. 319, pp. 651–2.

Brillat-Savarin, J. A. 1986, *1825—The Physiology of Taste, or Meditations on Transcendental Gastronomy*, trans. M. F. K. Fisher, North Point Press, San Francisco.

British Medical Journal 2001, 'Social exclusion: old problem, new name', *British Medical Journal*, vol. 323, (Editor's choice).

Bronfenbrenner, U. 1979, *The Ecology of Human Development*, Harvard University Press, Cambridge, Massachusetts.

Bronfenbrenner, U. 1989, 'Ecological systems theory', *Annals of Child Development*, vol. 6, pp. 187–249.

Brown, P. J. 1991, 'Culture and the evolution of obesity', *Human Nature*, vol. 2, pp. 31–57.

Brown, V. A. 1999, 'Top Down, Group Up or Inside Out? Community Practice and the Precautionary Principle', in R. Harding and E. Fisher (eds), *Perspectives on the Precautionary Principle*, The Federation Press, Sydney.

Brown, V. A., Ritchie, J. A., and Rotem, A. 1992, 'Health promotion and environmental management: the partnership for the future', *International Journal of Health Promotion*, vol. 7, no. 3, pp. 219–30.

Brown, V. A., Nicholson, R., and Stephenson, P. 2002, 'Environmental Health Policy in a Time of Change', in H. Garner and S. Barraclough (eds), *Health Policy in Australia*, 2nd edn, Oxford University Press, Melbourne.

Brown, V. A., Nicholson, R., Stephenson, P., Bennett, K. J., and Smith, J. 2001, *Grass Roots and Common Ground: Guidelines for Community-based Environmental Health Action— a discussion paper*, Occasional Paper No. 2, Regional Integrated Monitoring Centre, University of Western Sydney, Richmond.

Building Trades Group, 'Training on Alcohol and Other Drug Safety in the Workplace', <www.btgda.org.au/trainingeducation.html>, 10 February 2003.

Bulbolz, M. and Sontag, M. S. 1993, 'Human Ecology Theory', in P. Boss (ed.), *Source Book of Family Theories and Methods*, Plenum Press, New York.

Burbules, N. C. 1997, 'A grammar of difference: some ways of rethinking difference and diversity as educational topics', *Australian Educational Researcher*, vol. 24, no. 1, pp. 97–116.

Burn, A. R. 1956, *Pericles and Athens*, English Universities Press, London.

Burns, C., Webster, K., Crotty, P., Ballinger, M., Vincenzo, R., and Rozman, M. 2000, 'Easing the transition: food and nutrition issues of new arrivals', *Health Promotion Journal of Australia*, vol. 10, no. 3, pp. 230–6.

Burns, G. W. 1998, *Nature-Guided Therapy—Brief Integrative Strategies for Health & Well-being*, Brunner/Mazel, Philadelphia.

Bush, R. 2002, 'Community engagement', VicHealth Letter, 2001, Inequalities in health, 11 March, pp. 18–19.

Butler, J. 1990, *Gender Trouble*, Routledge, New York.

Butler, M. and Clarke, J. 1991, 'Couple Therapy with Homosexual Men', in D. Hopper and W. Dryden (eds), *Couple Therapy: A handbook*, Open University Press, Buckingham.

Byles, J. 2001, 'Older Women: Over the Hill, or Picking up Speed?', in C. Lee (ed.), *Women's Health Australia: What do we know? What do we need to know? Progress on the Australian Longitudinal Study on Women's Health 1995–2000*, Women's Health Australia, Research Centre for Gender and Health, University of Newcastle, Newcastle.

Cameron, M. 1993, 'Evaluation of Transport Accident Commission Road Safety Television Advertising', Monash University Accident Research Centre, Melbourne.

Cartwright, S., Cooper, C., and Whatmore, L. 2000, 'Improving communications and health in a government department', in Murphy, L. and Cooper, C. (eds), *Healthy and Productive Work: An International Perspective*, Taylor and Francis, London.

Catalano, P., Chikritzhs, T., Stockwell, T., Webb, M., Carl-Johan, R., and Dietze, P. 2001, *Trends in per capita alcohol consumption in Australia 1990/91–1998/99*, National Alcohol Indicators Project, Bulletin no. 4, National Drug Research Institute, Curtin University, Perth.

Catford, J. 1991, 'Primary environmental care: an ecological strategy for health', *Health Promotion International*, vol. 6, no. 4, pp. 239–40.

Catford, J. 1993, 'Auditing health promotion: what are the vital signs of quality?', *Health Promotion International*, vol. 8, no. 2, pp. 67–8.

Catford, J. 1996, 'Moving into the next decade—and a new dimension?', *Health Promotion International*, vol. 11, no. 1, pp. 1–3.

Catford, J. 1997, 'Developing leadership for health: our biggest blind spot', *Health Promotion International*, vol. 12, no. 1, pp. 1–4.

Catford, J. 2002, 'Health inequalities—a new optimism for health promotion research, policy and services', *Health Promotion International*, vol. 17, no. 2, pp. 101–4.

Centers for Disease Control and Prevention (CDC) 1998, 'Response to increases in cigarette prices by race/ethnicity, income and age groups—US, 1976–1993', *Morbidity and Mortality Weekly Report*, vol. 47.

Chapman, S. 1996, 'Civil disobedience and tobacco control: the case of BUGA UP', *Tobacco Control*, vol. 5, pp. 179–85.

Chikritzhs, T., Heale, P., Dietze, P., and Webb, M. 2000, *Trends in alcohol-related road injury in Australia, 1990–1997*, National Alcohol Indicators Project, Bulletin no. 2, National Drug Research Institute, Curtin University, Perth.

Chikritzhs, T., Jonas, H., Heale, P., Dietze, P., Hanlin, K., and Stockwell, T. 1999, 'Alcohol-caused deaths and hospitalisations in Australia, 1990–1997', *Bulletin no. 1*, National Drug Research Institute, Curtin University, Perth.

Chu, C. and Simpson, R. (eds) 1994, *Ecological Public Health: From Vision to Practice*, Griffith University, Nathan, Queensland.

Cohen, M. J. 2000, 'Nature connected psychology: creating moments that let earth teach', *Greenwich Journal of Science and Technology*, vol. 1, pp. 1–22.

Cohen, S., Mermelstein, R., Karmack, T., and Hoberman, H. N. 1985, 'Measuring the Functional Components of Social Support', in I. Sarason and B. Sarason (eds), *Social Support: Theory, Research, and Applications*, Martinus Nijhoff, Dordrecht, Netherlands.

Collins D. J. and Lapsley H. M. 1991, 'Estimating the economic costs of drug abuse in Australia', National Campaign Against Drug Abuse, Monograph Series no. 15, Australian Government Publishing Service, Canberra.

Collins, D. J. and Lapsley, H. M. 2002, 'Counting the cost: estimates of the social costs of drug abuse in Australia in 1988–9', National Drug Strategy, Monograph Series no. 49, Australian Government Publishing Service, Canberra.

Commonwealth of Australia 1998, *The Australian Guide to Healthy Eating*, Australian Government Publishing Service, Canberra.

Connell, R. W. 1992, 'A very straight gay: masculinity, homosexual experience, and the dynamics of gender', *American Sociological Review*, vol. 57, no. 6, pp. 735–51.

Connell, R. W. 1995, *Masculinities*, Allen & Unwin, Sydney.

Cooper, C. and Marshall, J. 1976, 'Occupational sources of stress: a review of the literature relating to coronary heart disease and mental ill health', *Journal of Occupational Psychology*, vol. 49, no. 1, pp. 11–28.

Council of Australian University Libraries 2001, *Information Literacy Standards*, Library Publications, Underdale, SA, <www.caul.edu.au/caul-doc/InfoLitStandards2001.doc>.

Cox, T. and Cox, S. 1993, 'Occupational health: control and monitoring of psychosocial and organisational hazards at work', *Journal of the Royal Society of Health*, vol. 113, no. 4, pp. 201–5.

Coyne, T. 2000, 'Lifestyle diseases in Pacific communities', Secretariat of the Pacific Community, Noumea, New Caledonia.

Creelman, A. 2002, 'Carer policy in Aged Care: A Structural Interests Perspective', in H. Gardner and S. Barraclough (eds), *Health Policy in Australia*, Oxford University Press, Melbourne.

Crofts, N., Aitken, C. K., and Kaldor, J. M. 1999, 'The force of numbers: why hepatitis C is spreading among Australian injecting drug users while HIV is not: the hepatitis C virus requires expanded strategies to control its spread', *Medical Journal of Australia*, vol. 170, pp. 220–1.

Crome, I. B. 1999, 'Substance misuse and psychiatric comorbidity: towards improved service provision', *Drugs: Education, Prevention and Policy*, vol. 6, no. 2, pp. 149–74.

Crotty, P. A., Rutishauser, I., and Cahill, M. 1992, 'Food in low income families', *Australian Journal of Public Health*, vol. 16, no. 2, pp. 168–74.

Cuffel, B. J. 1992, 'Prevalence estimates of substance abuse in schizophrenia and their correlates', *Journal of Nervous and Mental Disease*, vol. 180, pp. 589–92.

Darke, S. and Zador, D. 1996, 'Fatal heroin "overdose": a review', *Addiction*, vol. 91, no. 12, pp. 1765–72.

Darke, S., Ross, J. and Hall, W. 1996, 'Overdose among heroin users in Sydney, Australia: Prevalence and correlates of non-fatal overdose', *Addiction*, vol. 91, pp. 405–11.

Darke, S., Topp, L., Kaye, S., and Hall, W. 2002, 'Heroin use in New South Wales, Australia, 1996–2000: 5 year monitoring of trends in price, purity, availability and use from the Illicit Drug Reporting System (IDRS)', *Addiction*, vol. 97, no. 2, pp. 179–86.

Davis, L. 2001, 'Identity Politics, Disability, and Culture', in G. Albrecht, K. Seelman, and M. Bury (eds), *Handbook of Disability Studies*, Sage, Thousand Oakes.

Deacon, D. 1989, *Managing gender: The State, the New Middle Class and Women Workers 1830–1930*, Oxford University Press, Melbourne.

Deakin University and Department of Education, Employment and Training 2000, *Health Promoting Schools in Action: A Guide for Schools,*. Deakin University, Department of Education Employment and Training and VicHealth, Melbourne.

DeFrank, R. and Cooper, C. 1987. 'Worksite stress management interventions: their effectiveness and conceptualisation', *Journal of Managerial Psychology*, vol. 2, no. 1, pp. 4–10.

Degenhardt, L., Hall, W., and Lynskey, M. 2001, 'Alcohol, cannabis and tobacco use among Australians: a comparison of their associations with other drug use and use disorders, affective and anxiety disorders, and psychosis', *Addiction*, vol. 96, pp. 1603–14.

Department of Health and Aged Care 1999a, *Implementation Guide for Outcomes Based Funding*, Divisions of General Practice Program, Department of Health and Aged Care, Canberra.

Department of Health and Aged Care 1999b, *Mental Health Promotion and Prevention National Action Plan*, under the Second National Mental Health Plan: 1998–2003, Department of Health and Aged Care, Canberra.

Department of Health and Aged Care 1999c, *National Physical Activity Guidelines for Australians*, Commonwealth Department of Health and Aged Care, Ausinfo, Canberra. Department of Human Services 1998, *Improving Health Promotion—Actions for the Southern Metropolitan Region—Leadership and Infrastructure for Quality Health Promotion*, Department of Human Services, Victoria, Australia.

Department of Human Services 1999, The Victorian Burden of Disease Study, <www.dhs.vic.gov.au/phd/bod>, 5 January 2003.

Department of Human Services 2001, The Victorian Ambulatory Care Sensitive Conditions Study: Opportunities for Targeted Interventions, <www.dhs.vic.gov.au/phd/acsc>, 5 January 2003.

Department of Human Services 2001a, Improvement in the Life Expectancy of Victorians, The Chief Health Officer's Bulletin, 1:16–19, <www.health.vic.gov.au/chiefhealthofficer/chobulletin/downloads/vol1no1july2001/lifeexpectancy.pdf>.

Department of Human Services 2002a, Victorian Population Health Survey 2001: Selected Findings, <www.dhs.vic.gov.au/phd/healthsurveillance>, 5 January 2003.

Department of Human Services 2002b, *The Victorian Drug Statistics Handbook 2001: Patterns of Drug Use and Related Harm in Victoria*, Rural and Regional Health and Aged Care Services Division, Melbourne.

Department of Immigration and Multicultural Affairs (DIMA) 1997, *Immigration Update, June Quarter 1997*, Department of Immigration and Multicultural Affairs, Canberra.

Diaz, R. M., Ayala, G., Bein, E., Jenne, J., and Mann, B. V. 2001, 'The impact of homophobia, poverty, and racism on the mental health of gay and bisexual Latino men: findings from 3 US cities', *American Journal of Public Health*, vol. 91, no. 6, pp. 927–32.

Dietze, P., Rumbold, G., Cvetkovski, S., Hanlin, K., Laslett, A. M., and Jonas, H. 2000, 'Using population-based data on alcohol consumption and related harms to estimate the relative need for alcohol services in Victoria, Australia', *Evaluation and Program Planning*, vol. 2, no. 4, pp. 429–36.

Dietze, P. M., King, T., Rumbold, G., and Crowley, S. 1996, 'Recommendations for dealing with alcohol and other drugs in the workplace: conducting, researching and funding programs'. Published in the Research Report series of the National Campaign Against Drug Abuse, Commonwealth Department of Health and Aged Care, Canberra.

Dietze, P. and Fitzgerald, J. 2002, 'Interpreting changes in heroin supply in Melbourne: droughts, gluts or cycles?', *Drug and Alcohol Review*, vol. 21, pp. 295–303.

Dietze, P., Fry, C., Rumbold, G., and Gerostamoulos, J. 2001, 'The context, management and prevention of heroin overdose in Victoria, Australia: the promise of a diverse approach', *Addiction Research & Theory*, vol. 9, no. 5, pp. 437–58.

Dietze, P., Richards, J., Rumbold, G., and Aitken, C. (in press), *Treatment utilisation by heroin dependent persons in Australia: Implications for treatment service systems: Draft Report*, Turning Point Alcohol & Drug Centre, Melbourne.

DiGuiseppi, C., Roberts, I., and Li, L. 1997, 'Influence of changing travel patterns on child death rates from injury: trend analysis', *British Medical Journal*, vol. 314, no. 7082, pp. 710–13.

Dixon L., McNary, S., and Lehman, A. 1997, 'One-year follow-up of secondary versus primary mental disorder in persons with comorbid substance use disorders', *American Journal of Psychiatry*, vol. 154, no. 11, pp. 1610–12.

Doll, R. 1998, 'The benefit of alcohol in moderation', *Drug and Alcohol Review*, vol. 17, pp. 353–63.

Doll, R. and Hill, A. B. 1964, 'Mortality in relation to smoking: ten years' observations of British doctors', *British Medical Journal*, vol. 1, pp. 1399–1467.

Donatelle, R. and Davis, L. 1993, *Access to Health*, Prentice-Hall, Englewood Cliffs, NJ.

Donatelle, R. J. and Davis, L. G. 1997, *Health: The Basics*, Allyn & Bacon, Sydney.

Donnelly, N. and Hall, W. 1994, *Patterns of Cannabis Use in Australia, National Drug Strategy Management Series no. 27*, Australian Government Publishing Service, Canberra.

Dowsett, G. and Aggleton, P. 1999, *Contextual Factors Affecting Young People's Risk Related Sexual Behaviour in Developing Countries—A Comparative Analysis of Findings*, UNAIDS, Geneva.

Dreman, S. (ed.) 1997, *The Family on the Threshold of the 21st Century—Trends and Implications*, Lawrence Erlbaum Associates, Mahwah, New Jersey.

Duckett, S. 2001, *The Australian Health System*, Allen & Unwin, Sydney.

Dunstan, D., Zimmet, P., Welbourne, T., Sicree, R., Armstrong, T., Atkins, R., Cameron, A., Shaw, J., and Chadban, S. 2000, 'Diabesity and associated disorders in Australia: the accelerating epidemic', *The Australian Diabetes, Obesity & Lifestyle Report*, International Diabetes Institute, Melbourne.

Dunstan, D. W., Zimmet, P. Z., Welbourne, T. A., Cameron, A. J., Shaw, J., de Courten, M., Jolley, D., and McCarty, D. J. 2001, *The 1999–2000 Australian Diabetes, Obesity and Lifestyle Study (AusDiab)*, International Diabetes Institute, Melbourne.

Durning, A. T. 1995, 'Are We Happy Yet?', in T. Roszak, M. E. Gomes, and A. D. Kanner (eds), *Ecopsychology: Restoring the Earth, Healing the Mind*, Sierra Club Books, San Francisco.

Emmons, K. 2000, 'Health Behaviors in a Social Context', in L. Berkman and I. Kawachi (eds), *Social Epidemiology*, Oxford University Press, New York.

enHealth Council 1999, National Environmental Health Strategy, Commonwealth Department of Health and Aged Care, Canberra.

Emslie, M. 1996, 'Ignored to death: representations of young gay men, lesbians and bisexuals in Australian youth suicide policy and programs', *Youth Studies Australia*, vol. 15, no. 4, pp. 38–42.

Eslea, M. and Smith, P. 1998, 'The long-term effectiveness of anti-bullying work in primary schools', *Educational Research*, vol. 40, no. 2, Summer, pp. 203–18.

Ewan, C., Bryant, E., and Calvert, D. 1990, 'Health implications of long term climate change. Volume 1: effects and responses'. Discussion document commissioned by the National Health and Medical Research Council, University of Wollongong, NSW.

Falk, R. 2000, 'Stress in Working Life', in L. Skiold (ed.), *A Look into Modern Working Life*, National Institute for Working Life, Stockholm, pp. 272–6.

Farmer, P. 1996, 'Social inequalities and emerging infectious diseases', *Emerging Infectious Diseases*, vol. 2, no. 4, pp. 259–69.

Farmer, P. 1999, 'Pathologies of power: rethinking health and human rights', *American Journal of Public Health*, vol. 89, no. 10, pp. 1486–96.

Feachem, R. 2001, 'Globalisation is good for your health, mostly', *British Medical Journal*, vol. 323, pp. 504–6.

Fergusson, D. M., Horwood, L. J., and Beatrais, A. L. 1999, 'Is sexual orientation related to mental health problems and suicidality in young people?', *Archives of General Psychiatry*, vol. 56, no. 10, pp. 876–80.

Feyerabend, P. K. 1988, *Against Method*, Verso, London.

Fisher, B. and Cotton, P. 1994, 'Stress and wellbeing at work', *The Australian Psychological Society*, National Occupational Stress Conference 1994, Gold Coast, p. 22.

Ford, E. S., Smith, S. J., Stroup, D. F., Steinberg, K. K., Mueller, P. W., and Thacker, S. B. 2002, 'Homocyst(e)ine and cardiovascular disease: a systematic review of the evidence with special emphasis on case-control studies and nested case-control studies', *International Journal of Epidemiology*, vol. 31, no. 1, pp. 59–70.

Fougeyrollas, P. and Beauregard, L. 2001, 'An Interactive Person-environment Social creation', in G. Albrecht, K. Seelman, and M. Bury (eds), *Handbook of Disability Studies*, Sage, Thousand Oakes.

Francis, R. 1993, *The Politics of Work: Gender and Labour in Victoria 1880–1939*, Cambridge University Press, New York.

Francis Bacon (1561–1626), <www.oregonstate.edu/instruct/phl302/philosophers/bacon.html>, 29 January 2003.

Frankish, C. J. et al. 1996, *Health impact assessment as a tool for population health promotion and public policy*, Institute of Health Promotion Research, University of British Columbia, Vancouver.

Fredrickson, B. L. 2000, 'Cultivating positive emotions to optimize health and well-being', *Prevention and Treatment*, vol. 3, Article 1, <http://journals.apa.org/prevention/volume3/pre0030001a.html>, 8 November 2002.

French, J., Caplan, R., and Harrison, R. 1982, *The Mechanisms of Job Stress and Strain*, Wiley, Chichester, UK.

Frenk, J. and Gomez-Dantes, O. 2002, 'Globalisation and the challenges to health systems', *British Medical Journal*, vol. 325, pp. 95–7.

Frost, W. H. (ed.) 1936, *Snow on Cholera*, The Commonwealth Fund, New York, p. xxxvi.

Fujiura, G. and Rutkowski-Kmitta, V. 2001, 'Counting disability', in G. Albrecht, K. Seelman, and M. Bury (eds), *Handbook of Disability Studies*, Sage, Thousand Oakes.

Funk, M., Ostfeld, A. M., Chang, V. M., and Lee, F. A. 2002, 'Racial differences in the use of cardiac procedures in patients with acute myocardial infarction', *Nursing Research*, vol. 51, pp. 148–57.

Gardner, L. I. Jr., Stern, M. P., Haffner, S. M., Gaskill, S. P., Hazuda, H. P., Relethford, J. H., and Eifler, C. W. 1984, 'Prevalence of diabetes in Mexican Americans. Relationship to percent of gene pool derived from Native American sources', *Diabetes*, vol. 33, no. 1, pp. 86–92.

Geggie, J. DeFrain, J., Hitchcock, S., and Silberberg, S. 2000, *Family Strengths Research Project*, Family Action Centre, Newcastle, Australia.

Germov, J. 2002, 'Theorising Health: Major Theoretical Perspectives in Health Sociology', in J. Germov (ed.), *Second Opinion: an Introduction to Health Sociology*, Oxford University Press, Melbourne.

Giddens, A. 1984, *The Constitution of Society: Outline of the Theory of Structuration*, Polity Press, Cambridge.

Giga, S., Noblet, A., Faragher, B., and Cooper, C. 2003, 'Organisational stress management interventions: a review of UK-based research', *The Australian Psychologist*, vol. 38, no. 2, pp. 158–64.

Gilbert, R. and Gilbert, P. 1994, 'Discourse and disadvantage: studying the gender dimensions of educational disadvantage', Annual Conference of the Australian Association for Research in Education, November 1994, Newcastle.

Gilles, P. 1998, 'Effectiveness of alliances and partnerships for health promotion', *Health Promotion International*, vol. 13, no. 2, pp. 99–120.

Gracey, M. 1987, 'The state of health of Aborigines in the Kimberley region', *Medical Journal of Australia*, vol. 146, no. 4, pp. 200–4.

Graham, H. (ed.) 2000, *Understanding Health Inequalities*, Open University Press, Buckingham.

Guest, C., Douglas, R., Woodruff, R., and McMichael, A. J. 1999, 'Health and the environment', *TELA: Environment, Economy and Society*, no. 1, Australian Conservation Foundation & Australian Medical Association, Victoria.

Hall, J. and Taylor, R. 2003, 'Health for all beyond 2000: the demise of the Alma-Ata Declaration and primary health care in developing countries', *Medical Journal of Australia*, vol. 178, pp. 17–20.

Hall, W., Teeson, M., Lynskey, M., and Degenhardt, L. 1999, 'The 12-month prevalence of substance use and ICD10 substance use disorders in Australian adults: findings from the National Survey of Mental Health and Well-Being', *Addiction*, vol. 94, pp. 1541–50.

Hancock, L. and Moore, S. 1999, 'Caring and the State', in L. Hancock (ed.), *Health Policy in the Market State*, Allen & Unwin, Sydney.

Hancock, T. 1993, 'Health, human development and the community ecosystem: three ecological models', *Health Promotion International*, vol. 8, no. 1, pp. 41–7.

Hancock, T. 1994, 'Sustainability, Equity, Peace and the (Green) Politics of Health', in C. Chu and R. Simpson (eds), *Ecological Public Health: From Vision to Practice*, Griffith University, Queensland.

Hancock, T. and Perkins, F. 1985, 'The mandala of health: a conceptual model and teaching tool', *Health Education*, Summer 1985, pp. 8–10.

Hanna, K. and Coussens, C. (eds) 2001, *Rebuilding the Unity of Health and the Environment. A New Vision of Environmental Health for the 21st Century*, National Academy Press, Washington, D.C.

Hardoy, J. E., Mitlin, D., and Satterthwaite, D. 2001, *Environmental Problems in an Urbanizing World: Finding Solutions for Cities in Africa, Asia and Latin America*, Earthscan Publications Ltd, London.

Hassard, K. (ed.), 1999, *Australia's National Tobacco Campaign, Evaluation Report Volume One*, Commonwealth Department of Health and Aged Care, Canberra.

Heale, P., Stockwell, T., Dietze, P., Chikritzhs, T., and Catalano, P. 2000, *Patterns of alcohol consumption in Australia, 1998, National Alcohol Indicators, Bulletin no. 3*, National Drug Research Institute, Perth.

Hearn, B., Henderson, G., and Houston, S. 1993, 'Water supply and Aboriginal and Torres Strait Islander health: an overview', *AGSO Journal of Australian Geology and Geophysics*, vol. 14, no. 2/3, p. 135.

Hickie, I. 2002, 'Responding to the Australian experience of depression', *Medical Journal of Australia*, <www.mja.com.au/public/issues/176_10_200502/hic10078_fm.html>.

Hill, A. B. 1965, 'The environment and disease: association or causation?', *Proceedings of the Royal Society of Medicine*, vol. 58, pp. 295–300.

Hill, A. B. 1984, *Short Textbook of Medical Statistics*, 11th edn, Hodder and Stoughton, London.

Hill, D. J. and Borland, R. 1991, 'Adults' accounts of onset of regular smoking: influences of school, work and other settings', *Public Health Reports*, vol. 106, no. 2, pp. 181–5.

Hill, D. J., Chapman S., and Donovan, R. 1998, 'The return of scare tactics', *Tobacco Control*, vol. 7, pp. 5–8.

Hill, D. J., White, V. M., and Effendi, Y. 2002, 'Changes in the use of tobacco among Australian secondary students: results of the 1999 prevalence study and comparisons with earlier years', *Australian and New Zealand Journal of Public Health*, vol. 26, no. 2, pp. 156–63.

Hill, D. J., White, V. M., and Scollo, M. 1998, 'Smoking behaviours of Australian adults in 1995: trends and concerns', *Medical Journal of Australia*, vol. 168, pp. 209–213.

Hill, D. J., Willcox, S., Gardner, G., and Houston, J. 1987, 'Tobacco and alcohol use among Australian secondary schoolchildren', *Medical Journal of Australia*, vol. 146, pp. 125–30.

Hillier, L., Dempsey, D., Harrison, L., Beale, L., Matthews, L,. and Rosenthal, D. 1998, *Writing Themselves In: A National Report on the Sexuality, Health and Well-Being of Same-Sex Attracted Young People, Monograph Series No. 7*, National Centre in HIV Social Research, La Trobe University, Melbourne.

Hillier, L., Harrison, L., and Dempsey, D. 1999, 'Whatever happened to duty of care? Same-sex attracted young people's stories of schooling and violence', *Melbourne Studies in Education*, vol. 40, no. 2, pp. 59–74.

HM Government 2003, Victorian Britain Exhibition, Public Record Office, <www. learningcurve.pro.gov.uk/victorianbritain>.

Hosman, C. and Lopis, E. M. 2000, 'Mental health promotion', in *The Evidence of Health Promotion Effectiveness: Shaping Public Health in a New Europe*, 2nd edn, IUPHE, Paris.

House of Representatives Standing Committee on Aboriginal Affairs 1979, *'Aboriginal Health', Report from the House of Representatives Standing Committee on Aboriginal Affairs*, Australian Government Publishing Service, Canberra.

House of Representatives Standing Committee on Family and Community Affairs 1999, 'Inquiry into Indigenous Health', Discussion Paper, Commonwealth of Australia, Canberra.

House of Representatives Standing Committee on Legal and Constitutional Affairs 1998, *To Have and to Hold, Strategies to Strengthen Marriage and Relationships*, Parliament of the Commonwealth of Australia, Canberra.

Hser, Y. I. 1993, 'Prevalence estimation: summary of common problems and practical solutions', *Journal of Drug Issues*, vol. 23, no. 2, pp. 335–43.

Human Genome Program 1992, *Primer on Molecular Genetics*, United States Department of Energy, Washington D. C.

Humpel, N., Owen, N., and Leslie, E. 2002, 'Environmental factors associated with adults' participation in physical activity. A review', *American Journal of Preventative Medicine*, vol. 22, no. 3, pp. 188–99.

International Committee of the Red Cross 1998, *Banning anti-personnel mines: The Ottawa treaty explained*, International Committee of the Red Cross, Geneva.

Intergovernmental Panel on Climate Change 2001, 'Climate change 2001: the scientific basis', WG I contribution to the IPCC Third Assessment Report, Summary for Policymakers, <www.ipcc.ch/pub/spm22-01.pdf>, 18 January 2003.

Ivers, R. 2001, 'Indigenous Australians and tobacco: a literature review', Cooperative Research Centre for Aboriginal and Tropical Health, Darwin.

Jha, P. and Chaloupka, F. 1999, 'Curbing the epidemic: governments and the economics of tobacco control', The World Bank, Washington.

Jha, P. and Chaloupka, F. 2000, 'The economics of global tobacco control', *British Medical Journal*, vol. 7257, pp. 358–61.

Joint Health Survey Unit 2001, *Health Surveys for England, 2000*, National Centre for Social Research and the Department of Epidemiology and Public Health, University College London, London.

Jonas, H., Dietze, P., Rumbold, G., Hanlin, K., Cvetkovski, S., and Laslett, A. 1999, 'Associations between alcohol-related hospital admissions and alcohol consumption in Victoria, Australia: influence of sociodemographic factors', *Australian and New Zealand Journal of Public Health*, vol. 23, no. 3, pp. 272–80.

Jones, A., Montgomery, H. E., and Woods, D. R. 2002, 'Human performance: a role for the ACE genotype?', *Exercise and Sport Reviews*, vol. 30, no. 4, pp. 184–90.

Jones, J., Kickbusch, I., and O'Byrne, D. 1995, 'Improving health through schools', *World Health*, vol. 48, no. 2, p. 10.

Kahn, P. H. 1999, *The Human Relationship with Nature: Development and Culture*, MIT Press, Cambridge, Massachusetts.

Kahn, P. H. and Kellert, S. R. (eds) 2002, *Children and Nature: Psychological, Sociocultural, and Evolutionary Investigations*, MIT Press, Cambridge, Massachusetts.

Katzmarzyk, P. K. 2002, 'The Canadian obesity epidemic, an historical perspective', *Obesity Research*, vol. 10, no. 7, pp. 666–74.

Kawachi, I., Kennedy, B. P., Lochner, K., and Prothrow-Stith, D. 1997, 'Social capital, income inequality, and mortality', *American Journal of Public Health*, vol. 87, pp. 1491–8.

Kawachi, I. and Kennedy, B. 2002, *The Health of Nations: Why Inequity Is Harmful to Your Health*, The New Press, New York.

Kawachi, I., Subrimanian, S., and Almeida-Filho, N. 2002, 'A glossary for health inequalities', *Journal of Epidemiology & Community Health*, (Glossary), vol. 56, no. 9, p. 647.

Keleher, H. 2000, *Australian Nursing: For the Health of Medicine or the Health of the Public?*, School of Sociology, Politics and Anthropology, La Trobe University, Bundoora.

Keleher, H. 2001, 'Why primary health care offers a more comprehensive approach for tackling health inequities than primary care', *Australian Journal of Primary Health*, vol. 3, no. 3, pp. 59–67.

Keleher, H. and Murphy, B. 2002, *Report of Outer East Alliance Social Determinants of Health Project*, Outer East Alliance, Ringwood.

Kellert, S. R. 1997, *Kinship to Mastery: Biophilia in Human Evolution and Development*, Island Press, Washington, D. C.

Kellert, S. R. and Wilson, E. O. 1993, *The Biophilia Hypothesis*, Shearwater Books/Island Press, Washington, D. C.

Kendler, K. S. and Eaves, L. J. 1986, 'Models for the joint effect of genotype and environment on liability to psychiatric Illness', *American Journal of Psychiatry*, vol. 143, no. 3, pp. 279–89.

Kennedy, B. P., Kawachi, I., and Prothrow-Stith, D. 1996, 'Income distribution and mortality: cross sectional ecological study of the Robin Hood Index in the United States', *British Medical Journal*, vol. 312, pp. 1004–7.

Kessler, R. C., Nelson, C. B., McGonagle, K. A., Edlund, M. J., Frank, R. G., and Leaf, P. J. 1996, 'The epidemiology of co-occurring addictive and mental disorders: implications for prevention and service utilization', *American Journal of Orthopsychiatry*, vol. 50, pp. 36–43.

Kickbusch, I. 1989a, 'Approaches to an ecological base for public health', *Health Promotion*, vol. 4, no. 4, pp. 265–8.

Kickbusch, I. 1989b, *Good Planets are Hard to Find: Approaches to an Ecological Base for Public Health. In A Sustainable Health Future Towards an Ecology of Health*, Commission for the Future and La Trobe University, Melbourne.

Kickbusch, I. 1997, 'Think health: what makes the difference?', *Health Promotion International*, vol. 12, no. 4, pp. 265–72.

Kickbusch, I. and Buse, K. 2001, 'Global Influences and Global Responses: International Health at the Turn of the Twenty-first Century', in M. Merson, R. Black, and A. Mills (eds), *International Public Health*, Aspen Publishers Inc., Gaithersburg.

Kiecolt-Glaser, J. K. and Glaser, R. 2001, 'Stress and immunity: age enhances the risks', *Current Directions in Psychological Science*, vol. 10, no. 1, pp. 18–21.

Kiecolt-Glaser, J. K., Glaser, R., Cacioppo, J. T., MacCallum, R. C., Snydersmith, M., Kim, C., and Malarkey, W. B. 1997, 'Marital conflict in older adults: endocrinal and immunological correlates', *Psychosomatic Medicine*, vol. 59, no. 4, pp. 339–49.

Kiecolt-Glaser, J. K., McGuire, L., Robles, T. F., and Glaser, R. 2002a 'Emotions, morbidity, and mortality: new perspectives from psychoneuroimmunology', *Annual Review of Psychology*, vol. 53, no. 1, pp. 83–107.

Kiecolt-Glaser, J. K., McGuire, L., Robles, T. F., and Glaser, R. 2002b, 'Psychoneuroimmunology and psychosomatic medicine: back to the future', *Psychosomatic Medicine*, vol. 64, no. 1, pp. 15–28.

King, A. C., Blair, S. N., Dishman, R. K., Dubbert, P. M., Marcus, B. H., Oldridge, N. B., Paffenbarger, R. S. Jr., Powell, K. E., and Yeager, K. K. 1992, 'Determinants of physical activity and interventions in adults', *Medicine and Science in Sports and Exercise*, vol. 24, supp. 6, pp. S221–36.

King, M. L. Jr. 1963, *Strength to Love*, Fontana Books, London.

Kinsman, T. (ed.) In press, *Australia's National Tobacco Campaign, Evaluation Report Volume Three*, Commonwealth Department of Health and Aged Care, Canberra.

Kirkpatrick, S. 1994, *Evaluating training programs: The four levels*, Berrett-Kolehler, San Francisco.

Knowler, W. C., Bennett, P. H., Hamman, R. F., and Miller, M. 1978, 'Diabetes incidence and prevalence in Pima Indians: a 19-fold greater incidence than in Rochester, Minnesota', *American Journal of Epidemiology*, vol. 108, no. 6, pp. 497–505.

Koos, E. L. 1954, *The Health of Regionville*, New York, Columbia University Press.

Korfiadis, V. 2001, 'Exploring the discourses deployed around controversial VicHealth Sexual Diversity Projects: implications for health promotion', Unpublished Honours Thesis, School of Health Sciences, Faculty of Health & Behavioural Sciences, Deakin University, Melbourne.

Krieger, N. 1994, 'Epidemiology and the web of causation: has anyone seen the spider?', *Social Science and Medicine*, vol. 39, no. 7, pp. 887–903.

Kruks, G. 1991, 'Gay and lesbian homeless/street youth: special issues and concerns', *Journal of Adolescent Health*, vol. 12, no. 7, pp. 511–18.

Kuhn, T. S. 1970, *The Structure of Scientific Revolutions*, 2nd edn, University of Chicago Press, Chicago.

Labonte, R. 1997, *Power, Participation and Partnerships for Health Promotion*, VicHealth, Melbourne.

Lakatos, I., Worrall, J., and Curry, G. (eds) 1978, *Mathematics, Science and Epistemology*, Cambridge University Press, New York.

Lal, A. and Scollo, M. 2002, 'Big Mac index of cigarette affordability', *Tobacco Control*, vol. 11, pp. 280–2.

Laslett, A. M., Donath, S., and Dietze, P. 2002, 'Long-term Consequences of Alcohol Consumption', in Commonwealth Department of Health and Ageing (ed.), *National Alcohol Research Agenda*, Commonwealth Department of Health and Ageing, Canberra.

Last, J. 2001, *A Dictionary of Epidemiology*, 4th edn, Oxford University Press, New York.

Last, J. M. 1987, *Public Health and Human Ecology*, Appleton and Lange, Connecticut.

Lazarus, R. S. and Folkman, S. 1984, *Stress, Appraisal, and Coping*, Springer, New York.

Lee, A., Darcy, A., Leonard, D., Groos, A. D., Stubbs, C., Lowson, S., Dunn, S. M., Coyne, T., and Riley, M. 2002, 'Food availability, cost disparity and improvement in relation to accessibility and remoteness in Queensland', *Australian and New Zealand Journal of Public Health*, vol. 26, no. 3, pp. 266–72.

Lehman, A. F., Myers, C. P., Thompson, J. W., Cortey, E. J. 1993, 'Implications of mental health and substance use disorders: a comparison of single and dual diagnosis patients', *Journal of Nervous and Mental Disease*, vol. 181, pp. 365–70.

Lenton, S., Christie, P., Humenuiuk, R., Brooks, A., Bennett, M. and Heale, P. 1998, *Infringement versus Conviction: The Social Impact of a Minor Cannabis Offence Under a Civil Penalties System and Strict Prohibition in Two Australian States* (National Drug Strategy Monograph No. 36), Australian Government Publishing Service, Canberra.

Lenton, S., Heale P., Erickson, P., Single, E., Lang, E., and Hawks, D. 2000, *The Regulation of Cannabis Possession, Use and Supply: A Discussion Document Prepared for the Drugs and Crime Prevention Committee of the Parliament of Victoria, RI Monograph No 3*, National Drug Research Institute, Curtin University of Technology, Perth.

Leslie, E., Owen, N., Salmon, J., Bauman, A., Sallis, J. F., and Lo, S. K. 1999, 'Insufficiently active Australian college students: perceived personal, social, and environmental influences', *Preventive Medicine*, vol. 28, no. 1, pp. 20–7.

Letts, W. J. and Sears, J. T. (eds) 1999, *Queering Elementary Education: Advancing the Dialogue about Sexualities and Schooling*, Oxford Rowman and Littlefield Publishers Inc., Lanham, Boulder and New York.

Levi, L. 1996, 'Spice of Life or Kiss of Death', in C. L. Cooper (ed.), *Handbook of Stress, Medicine, and Health*, CRC Press, New York.

Leviticus 1954, The Holy Bible: Leviticus, authorized version, J. Stirling, London, The British & Foreign Bible Society.

Lilley, S. 2000, 'What determines health? An annotated bibliography on indicators for the determinants of health', Health Canada, <www.hc-sc.gc.ca/hppb/phdd/determinants/e_deter_biblio.html>.

Lister-Sharp, D., Chapman, S., Stewart-Brown, S., and Sowden, A. 1999, 'Health promoting schools and health promotion in schools: two systematic reviews', *Health Technology Assessment*, vol. 3, p. 22.

Listorti, J. A. and Doumani, F. M. 2001, *Environmental Health: Bridging the Gaps*, World Bank Discussion Paper No. 422.

Lillioja, S., Mott, D. M., Howard, B. V., Bennett, P. H., Yki-Jarvinen, H., Freymond, D., Nyomba, B. L., Zurlo, F., Swinburn, B., and Bogardus, C. 1988, 'Impaired glucose tolerance as a disorder of insulin action. Longitudinal and cross-sectional studies in Pima Indians', *New England Journal of Medicine*, vol. 31, no. 19, pp. 1217–25.

Lowe, I. 2002, 'Ecological health promotion: some principles', *Health Promotion Journal of Australia*, vol. 13, no. 1, pp. 5–9.

London School of Hygiene & Tropical Medicine 1990, *Epidemiology Lecture Notes*, London School of Hygiene & Tropical Medicine, London.

Lvovsky, L., Cropper, M., Listorti, J. A., Elmendorf, E., Chandra, C., Lampietti, J., Subida, R., Klees, R., Hughes, G., and Dunleavy, M. 2000, *Health and Environment*, Draft for discussion, World Bank Group.

Lynch, J. W., Davey Smith, G., Kaplan, G. A., and House, J. S. 2000, 'Income inequality and mortality: importance to health of individual income, psychosocial environment, or material conditions', *British Medical Journal*, vol. 320, pp. 1200–4.

MacArthur, I. 1999, 'Introduction to Environmental Health', in W. H. Bassett (ed.), *Clay's Handbook of Environmental Health*, 18th edn, E & FN Spon, London.

MacArthur, I. and Bonnefoy, X. 1998, *Environmental Health Services in Europe 2: Policy options*, WHO Regional Office for Europe, Copenhagen.

Macintyre, S., Ellaway, A., and Cummins, S. 2002, 'Place effects on health: how can we conceptualise, operationalise and measure them?', *Social Science & Medicine*, vol. 55, pp. 125–39.

Makkai, T. 2001, 'Patterns of recent drug use among a sample of Australian detainees', *Addiction*, vol. 96, pp. 1799–808.

Maller, C., Townsend, M, Brown, P. and St Leger, L. 2002. *Healthy Parks Healthy People: The Health Benefits of Contact with Nature in a Park Context*, Report to Parks Victoria and the International Park Strategic Partners Group, Deakin University Social and Mental Health Priority Area Occasional Paper Series, vol. 1, Deakin University Faculty of Health and Behavioural Sciences, Melbourne.

Marks, D. 1999, *Disability: Controversial Debates and Psychosocial Perspective*, Routledge, London.

Marmot, M. 1999, 'Multilevel Approaches to Understanding Social Determinants', in M. Marmot and R. Wilkinson (eds), *Social Determinants of Health*, Oxford University Press, Oxford.

Marmot, M. 2001, 'Multilevel Approaches to Understanding Social Determinants', in L. Berkman and I. Kawachi (eds), *Social Epidemiology*, Oxford University Press, New York, pp. 349–67.

Marmot, M. and Wilkinson, R. G. (eds.) 1998, *Social Determinants of Health*, Oxford University Press, Oxford.

Marshall, B. and Maher, S. 2001, *Understanding Health Modules 1, 2 and 3: Study Guide and Reader*, Deakin University, Geelong.

Marshall, B., Sheehan, M., Northfield, J., Maher, S., Carlisle, R., and St Leger, L. 2000, 'School-based health promotion across Australia', *Journal of School Health*, vol. 70, no. 6, pp. 251–2.

Martens, P. and McMichael, A. J. (eds) 2002, 'Environmental Change, Climate and Health', in P. Martens and A. J. McMichael (eds), *Environmental Change, Climate and Health. Issues and Research Methods*, Cambridge University Press, Cambridge.

Martino, W. and Pallotta-Chiarolli, M. 2001a, *Boys' Stuff: Boys Talking About What Matters*, Allen & Unwin, Sydney.

Martino, W. and Pallotta-Chiarolli, M. 2003, *So What's A Boy?: Issues of Masculinity in Education*, Open University Press, London.

Maslow, A. 1968, *Toward a Psychology of Being*, 2nd edn, Van Nostrand, New York.

Mathers, C. 1994, *Health Differentials Among Adult Australians Aged 25-64 years*, Health Monitoring Series No 1, Australian Institute of Health and Welfare, Australian Government Printing Service, Canberra.

Mathers, C., Vos, T., and Stevenson, C. 1999, *The Burden of Disease and Injury in Australia*, Australian Institute of Health and Welfare, Canberra.

Mattick R. P. and Hall, W. (eds) 1993, *A Treatment Outline for Approaches to Opioid Dependence: Quality Assurance in the Treatment of Drug Dependence Project*, National Campaign Against Drug Abuse No. 21, Canberra.

McDonald, R. and Cooper, T. 1998, 'Young gay men and suicide: a report of a study exploring the reasons which young gay men give for suicide ideation', *Youth Studies Australia*, vol. 17, no. 4, pp. 23–7.

McKeown, T. 1976, *The Modern Rise of Population*, Edward Arnold Publishers Ltd, London.

McKinlay, J. B. 1979, 'A Case for Refocusing Upstream: The Political Economy of Health', in E. G. Jaco (ed.), *Patients, Physicians and Illness*, Macmillan, Basingstoke, UK.

McMichael, A. J. 1993, *Planetery Overload: Global Environmental Change and the Health of the Human Species*, Cambridge University Press, Cambridge.

McMichael, A. J. 2001a, 'Global climate change and health: research challenges, ecological concepts and sustainability', *The Journal of the Australian Institute of Environmental Health*, vol. 1, no. 4, pp. 13–15.

McMichael, A. J. 2001b, *Human Frontiers, Environments and Disease: Past Patterns, Uncertain Futures*, Cambridge University Press, Cambridge.

McMichael, A. J. and Beaglehole, R. 2000, 'The changing global context of health', *The Lancet*, vol. 356, pp. 495–9.

McMichael, A. J. and Kovats, R. S. 2000, 'Global environmental change and health: approaches to assessing risk', *Ecosystem Health*, vol. 6, no. 1, pp. 59–66.

McMichael, T. 2001, *Human Frontiers, Environments and Disease: Past Patterns, Uncertain Futures*, Cambridge University Press, Cambridge, UK.

McMichael, T. 2002, 'The biosphere, health and "sustainability" ', *Science*, vol. 297, p. 1093.

McMurray, A. 2003, *Community Health and Wellness: A Sociological Approach*, 2nd edn, Mosby, Marrickville, NSW.

McNair, R., Anderson, S., and Mitchell, A. 2001, 'Addressing health inequalities in Victorian lesbian, gay, bisexual and transgender communities', *Health Promotion Journal of Australia*, vol. 11, no. 1, pp. 32–8.

Meyer, I. H. 2001, 'Why lesbian, gay, bisexual, and transgender public health?', *American Journal of Public Health*, vol. 91, no. 6, pp. 856–9.

Michie, S. 1992, 'Evaluation of a stress management service', *Health Manpower Management*, vol. 18, no. 1, pp. 15–17.

Miller, G. 1981, 'Putting Lady Mary in her place: a discussion of historical causation', *Bulletin of the History of Medicine*, vol. 55, no. 1, pp. 2–16.

Miller, G. E. and Cohen, S. 2001, 'Psychological interventions and the immune system: a meta-analytic review and critique', *Health Psychology*, vol. 20, no. 1, pp. 47–63.

Miller, G. T. 2000, *Living in the Environment: Principles, Connections, and Solutions*, Brooks/Cole Publishing Company, Pacific Grove, California.

Miller Jones, J. 1998, *Food Safety*, 2nd edn, American Association of Cereal Chemists Inc., St Paul, MN.

MindMatters 2001, *Community Matters: Working with Diversity for Wellbeing*, Department of Health and Aged Care, Canberra.

Mokdad, A. H., Bowman, B. A., Ford, E. S., Vinicor, F., Marks, J. S., and Koplan J. P. 2001, 'The continuing epidemics of obesity and diabetes in the United States', *Journal of American Medical Association*, vol. 286, no. 10, pp. 1195–2000.

Montgomery, H. E., Marshall, R., Hemingway, H., Myerson, S., Clarkson, P., Dollery, C., Hayward, M., Holliman, D. E., Jubb, M., World, M., Thomas, E. L., Brynes, A. E., Saeed, N., Barnard, M., Bell, J. D., Prasad, K., Rayson, M., Talmud, P. J., and Humphries, S. E. 1998, 'Human gene for physical performance', *Nature*, vol. 393, pp. 221–2.

Mooney, G. and Johnstone, K. 2002, 'Big problems versus best buys and does gender matter?', *Australian and New Zealand Journal of Public Health*.

Morbidity and Mortality Weekly Report 1997, 'Alcohol consumption among pregnant and childbearing-aged-women: United States, 1991 and 1995', *Morbidity and Mortality Weekly Report*, vol. 46, no. 16, pp. 346–50.

Mullins, R., Trotter, L., and Letcher, T. 2000, 'Environmental Tobacco Smoke: Public Opinions and Behaviour in 1998–99', in L. Trotter and T. Letcher (eds), *Quit Evaluation Studies No. 10*, Victorian Smoking and Health Program, Melbourne.

Murphy, B. 2003, *Women's Participation Program Evaluation Report*, Melbourne.

Murphy, B, and Keleher, H. 2003, *Framework for Health Promotion Action: A Discussion Paper for Course Development*, School of Health and Social Development, Deakin University, Melbourne.

Murphy, L. R. 1988, 'Workplace Interventions for Stress Reduction and Prevention', in C. L. Cooper and R. Payne (eds), *Causes, Coping and Consequences of Stress at Work*, John Wiley & Sons, Chichester.

Murray, C. J. M. and Lopez, A. 1996, 'Assessing the burden of disease that can be attributed to specific risk factors. Investing in health research and development', Ad Hoc Committee on Health Research Relating to Future Intervention Options, World Health Organization, Geneva.

Murray, C. J. M. and Lopez, A. D. 1996, *The Global Burden of Disease: A Comprehensive Assessment of Mortality and Disability from Diseases, Injuries and Risk Factors in 1990 and Projected to 2020*, Harvard University Press, Cambridge.

Murray, S. O. 1992, 'Components of the gay community in San Francisco', in G. Herdt (ed.), *Gay Culture in America*, Beacon Press, Boston.

Naidoo, J. and Wills, J. 1994, *Health Promotion: Foundations for Practice*, Bailliere Tindall, London.

National Centre in HIV Epidemiology and Clinical Research 2001, *HIV/AIDS, Viral Hepatitis and Sexually Transmissible Infections in Australia Annual Surveillance Report 2001*, vol. 12, no. 4, National Centre in HIV Epidemiology and Clinical Research, Sydney.

NHMRC 1986, *Effects of Passive Smoking on Health*, National Health and Medical Research Council, Australian Government Publishing Service, Canberra.

NHMRC 1997, *Effective School Health Promotion: Towards the Health Promoting School*, National Health and Medical Research Council, Australian Government Publishing Service, Canberra.

NHMRC 2000, *Current State of Research on Illicit Drugs in Australia*, National Health and Medical Research Council, Canberra.

NHMRC 2001, *Australian Alcohol Guidelines: Health Risks and Benefits*, National Health and Medical Research Council, Canberra.

NHMRC 2001a, *Dietary Guidelines for Australian Adults (draft)*, National Health and Medical Research Council, Canberra.

NHMRC 2001b, *Dietary Guidelines for Children and Adolescents in Australia, Incorporating Infant Feeding Guidelines for Health Workers, Infant Feeding Guidelines (draft)*, National Health and Medical Research Council, Canberra.

National Heart Foundation of Australia & Australian Institute of Health and Welfare 1990, *Risk Factor Prevalence Study: Survey no. 3*, Risk Factor Prevalence Study Management Committee, National Heart Foundation of Australia & Australian Institute of Health and Welfare, Canberra.

National Public Health Partnership, Preventing Chronic Disease: A Strategic Framework Background Paper 2001, <www.nphp.gov.au>, 30 November 2002.

Navarro, V. 1998, 'Comment: whose globalization?' *American Journal of Public Health*, vol. 88, no. 5, pp. 742–3.

Netherlands Institute of Mental Health and Addiction—the Trimbos Institute, National Drug Monitor 2001. Annual Report: CANNABIS, <www.trimbos.nl/ndm-uk/ndm_uk_cannabis_2001_4.html>, 29 January 2001.

New South Wales Health, 2003, <www.health.nsw.gov.au/public-health/ehb/aborig>, 15 February 2003.

New Zealand Network Against Food Poverty 2000, *Hidden Hunger—Food and Low income in New Zealand*, The Downtown Community Ministry, Wellington.

Nizette, D. and Creedy, D. 1998, 'Women and Mental Illness', in *Women's Health: A Primary Health Care Approach*, Maclennan & Petty, Sydney.

Noblet, A. J. and Murphy, C. P. 1995, 'Adapting the Ottawa Charter for Health Promotion to the workplace setting', *Health Promotion Journal of Australia*, vol. 5, no. 3, pp. 18–22.

NRC 1999, *Our Common Journey: a transition toward sustainability*, National Academy Press, Washington, D.C.

Nurses Board of Victoria 2000, 'Substance abuse and nursing', *Nexus*, vol. 6, no. 1, p. 7.

Nutbeam, D. 1998, 'Evaluating health promotion—progress, problems and solutions', *Health Promotion International*, vol. 13, no. 1, pp. 27–44.

O'Grady, H., Kelly, C., Bouchier-Hayes, D., and Leahy, A. 2002, 'Homocysteine and occlusive arterial disease', *British Journal of Surgery*, vol. 89, no. 7, pp. 838–44.

Pallotta-Chiarolli, M. 1991, *Someone You Know: A Friend's Farewell*, Wakefield Press, Adelaide.

Pallotta-Chiarolli, M. 1998a, *Girls Talk: Young Women Speak Their Hearts and Minds*, Finch Publishing, Lane Cove, Sydney.

Pallotta-Chiarolli, M. 1998b, 'Cultural diversity and men who have sex with men', National Centre in HIV Social Research, University of New South Wales and the Commonwealth Department of Health and Family Services, Sydney.

Pallotta-Chiarolli, M. 1999a, *Tapestry: Italian Lives Over Five Generations*, Milson's Point, Random House, Sydney.

Pallotta-Chiarolli, M. 1999b, 'Diary Entries from the "Teachers' Professional Development Playground" Multiculturalism Meets Multisexualities in Education', in G. Sullivan and P. Jackson (eds), *Multicultural Queer: Australian Narratives*, Haworth Press, New York.

Pallotta-Chiarolli, M. 2000, 'What do they think? Queerly raised and queer friendly students', *Youth Studies Australia*, vol. 19, no. 4, pp. 34–40.

Pallotta-Chiarolli, M., Van de Ven, P., Prestage, G., and Kippax, S. 1999, 'Too busy studying to have sex?: homosexually active Asian male international students and sexual health', National Centre in HIV Social Research, University of New South Wales and the Commonwealth Department of Health and Family Services, Sydney.

Palmer, G. and Short, S. 2000, *Health Care and Public Policy: An Australian Analysis*, 3rd edn, Allen & Unwin, Sydney.

Pantry, S. (ed.) 1995, *Occupational Health*, Chapman & Hall, London.

Parker, R. 1996, 'Empowerment, community mobilization and social change in the face of HIV/AIDS', *AIDS*, vol. 10 (supp. 3), pp. S27–S31.

Parker, R. 2002, 'The global HIV/AIDS pandemic, structural inequalities, and the politics of international health', *American Journal of Public Health*, vol. 92, no. 3, pp. 343–6.

Parker, R., Easton, D., and Klein, C. 2000, 'Structural barriers and facilitators in HIV prevention: a review of international research', *AIDS*, vol. 14 (supp. 1), pp. S22–S32.

Patterson, J. 2002, 'Integrating family resilience and family stress theory', *Journal of Marriage and Family*, vol. 64, no. 2, pp. 349–61.

Pearsall, J. (ed.) 1999, *The Concise Oxford Dictionary*, 10th edn, Oxford University Press, Oxford.

Pierce, J. P., Macaskill, P., and Hill, D. 1990, 'Long-term effectiveness of mass media led anti-smoking campaigns in Australia', *American Journal of Public Health*, vol. 80, pp. 565–9.

Pill, R. and Stott, N. 1990, *Making Changes: A Study of Working Class Mothers and the Changes Made in their Health Related Behaviour over 5 Years*, University of Wales College of Medicine, Cardiff.

Pimental, D., Tort, M., D'Anna, L., Krawic, A., Berger, J., Rossman, J., Mugo, F., Doon, N., Shriberg, M., Howard, E., Lee, S., and Talbot, J. 1998, 'Ecology of increasing disease: population growth and environmental degradation', *BioScience*, vol. 48, no. 10, pp. 817–26.

Plummer, K. 1989, 'Gay and lesbian youth in England', *Journal of Homosexuality*, vol. 17, pp. 195–223.

Plummer, D. 2001, 'Policing Manhood', in C. Wood (ed.), *Sexual Positions*, Hill of Content, Melbourne, pp. 60–75.

Plummer, D. C. In press, 'Parallel worlds: what the great sexual laboratory of Oceania reveals about homophobia'.

Plummer, D. C. 1999, *One of the Boys: Masculinity, HOMOPhobia and Modern Manhood*, Haworth Press, New York.

Plummer, D. C. 2001, 'The quest for modern manhood: masculine stereotypes, peer culture and the social significance of homophobia', *Journal of Adolescence*, vol. 24, no. 1, pp. 15–23.

Plummer, D. C. 2002, 'Parallel worlds: what the great sexual laboratory of Oceana reveals about homophobia', Monograph, School of Health, University of New England, Armidale, NSW.

Porter, D. and Porter, R. 1988, 'The politics of prevention: anti-vaccinationism and public health in nineteenth-century England', *Medical History*, vol. 32, no. 3, pp. 231–52.

Premier's Drug Advisory Committee 1996, *Drugs and our Community: Report of the Premier's Drug Advisory Council*, Victorian Government Printer, Melbourne.

Prestage, G., Kippax, S., Crawford, J., Noble, J., Campbell, D., Van de Ven, P., Baxter, D., and Cooper, D. 1995, *Sydney Men and Sexual Health (SMASH) Report B.2: A Demographic and Behavioural Profile of Young Men, 25 and Under, in a Sample of Homosexually-Active Men in Sydney*, HIV, AIDS & Society Publications, Sydney.

Prochaska, J., DiClimente, C., and Norcross, J. C. 1992, 'In search of how people change', *American Psychologist*, vol. 47, pp. 1102–14.

Public Health Association of Australia 2000a, 'Alcohol 2000', in *PHAA Policy Book*, Public Health Association of Australia, Canberra.

Public Health Association of Australia 2000b, 'Improving Aboriginal and Torres Strait Islander people's access to the food they need for health', in *2000 Policy Book*, Public Health Association of Australia, Canberra.

Public Health Association of Australia 2003, 'The regulation of abortion in Australia: public health perspectives', <www.phaa.net.au/abkit/abkit.htm>, 27 January 2003.

Public Health Association of Australia (Victorian Branch) 1997, *Images of Public Health in Victoria*, PHAA with the Public Health Division of the Department of Human Services, Victoria.

Quinlan, M. and Bohle, P. 1991, *Managing Occupational Health and Safety in Australia: A Multidisciplinary Approach*, The Macmillan Company of Australia, South Melbourne.

Reid, J. and Trompf, P. 1991, *The Health of Aboriginal Australia*, Harcourt Brace Jovanovich Group, Sydney.

Reidpath, D. D., Burns, C., Garrard, J., Mahoney, M., and Townsend, M. 2002, 'An ecological study of the relationship between social and environmental determinants of obesity', *Health and Place*, vol. 8, pp. 141–5.

Reiger, D. A., Farmer, M. E., Rae, D. S., Locke, B. Z., Keith, S. J., Judd, L. L., and Goodwin, F. K. 1990, 'Comorbidity of mental disorders with alcohol and other drug abuse: results from the epidemiologic catchment area (ECA) study', *Journal of the American Medical Association*, vol. 264, pp. 2511–18.

Reiger, K. 2000, 'Understanding the Welfare State', in P. Beilharz and T. Hogan (eds), *Social Self, Global Culture: An Introduction to Sociological Ideas*, 2nd edn, Oxford University Press, Melbourne.

Remafedi, G., Farrow, J. A., and Deisher, R. W. 1991, 'Risk factors for attempted suicide in gay and bisexual youth', *Pediatrics*, vol. 87, no. 6, pp. 869–75.

Reynolds, R. 'Is gay passé?', *The Age*, 20 September 2002, pp. 1, 3.

Richman, J. 1987, *Medicine and Health*, Longman, Harlow, UK.

Ridge, D. 1997, 'Why men still have unsafe sex: meanings, dynamics & contexts among younger gay men in Australia', PhD thesis, Latrobe University, Melbourne.

Ridge, D. and Murphy, B. 2002, *Consultancy On Youth for the United Nations Inter-Agency Working Group Final Report*, Melbourne.

Ridge, D., Hee, A., and Minichiello, V. 1999, 'Asian men on the scene: challenges to "gay communities"', *Journal of Homosexuality*, vol. 36, no. 3/4, pp. 43–68.

Ridge, D., Marshall, B., Northfield, J., Maher, S., St Leger, L., Sheehan, M., and Elisha, D. 2000, 'Health Promoting Schools Project: An evaluation', Deakin University, Melbourne.

Rifkin, J. and Perlas, N. 1984, *Algeny: A New Word—A New World*, Penguin Books, New York.

Rigby, K. 2002, *A Meta-Evaluation of Methods and Approaches to Reducing Bullying in Pre-Schools and Early Primary School in Australia*, Crime Prevention Branch, Commonwealth Attorney-General's Department, Canberra.

Robertson, A. E. 1998, 'The mental health experiences of gay men: a research study exploring gay men's health needs', *Journal of Psychiatric and Mental Health Nursing*, vol. 5, no. 3, pp. 33–40.

Roesler, T. and Deisher, R. W. 1972, 'Youthful male homosexuality: homosexual experience and the process of developing homosexual identity in males aged 16 to 22 years', *Journal of the American Medical Association*, vol. 219, no. 8, pp. 1018–23.

Rose, G. 1992, *The Strategy of Preventive Medicine*, Oxford University Press, Oxford.

Rosen, G. 1993, *A History of Public Health*, Johns Hopkins University Press, Baltimore.

Rothman, K. J., Hans-Olov A., and Trichopoulos, D. 1998, 'Should the mission of epidemiology include the eradication of poverty?', *The Lancet*, vol. 352, pp. 810–13.

Rowling, L. 1996, 'From health promotion in schools to health promoting schools', *The Journal of the Health Education Association*, Autumn HEAV Quarterly (Victoria), pp. 22–5.

Rowling, L. 1996, 'The adaptability of the health promoting schools concept: a case study from Australia', *Health Education Research*, vol. 1, no. 4, pp. 519–26.

Royal College of Physicians of London 1992, *Smoking and the Young— A Report of a Working Party*, Royal College of Physicians, London.

Royal College of Physicians of London 1995, *Alcohol and the Young— A Report of a Working Party*, Royal College of Physicians, London.

Royal New Zealand Plunket Society Inc. 2003, <www.plunket.org.nz>, 27 January 2003.

Ryan, S. and Travis, J. 1988 *The Wellness Workbook*, 2nd edn, Ten Speed Press, Berkeley, CA.

Rydell, C. P. and Everingham, S. S. 1994, 'Controlling cocaine: supply versus demand programs', <www.rand.org/publications/MR/MR331/mr331.html>, 25 January 2003.

Sallis, J. and Owen, N. 1997, 'Ecological Models', in K. Glanz, F. M. Lewis, and B. Rimer (eds), *Health Behaviour and Education*, Jossey-Bass Publishers, San Francisco.

Sallis, J. F., Hovell, M. F., Hofstetter, C. R, Elder, J. P., Hackley, M., Caspersen, C. J., and Powell, K. E. 1990, 'Distance between homes and exercise facilities related to frequency of exercise among San Diego residents', *Public Health Reports*, vol. 105, no. 2, pp. 179–85.

Sallis, J. F., Johnson, M. F., Calfas, K. J, Caparosa, S., and Nichols, J. F. 1997, 'Assessing perceived physical environmental variables that may influence physical activity', *Research Quarterly for Exercise and Sport*, vol. 68, no. 4, pp. 345–51.

Sallis, J. F. and Owen, N. 1999, *Physical Activity and Behavioural Medicine*, Sage Publications, Thousand Oakes, CA.

Salmon, J., Owen, N., Crawford, D., Bauman, A., and Sallis, J. F. 2003, 'Physical activity and sedentary behavior: a population-based study of barriers, enjoyment, and preference', *Health Psychology*, vol. 22, pp. 178–88.

Samorodov, A. 1996, 'Indicators of cost-effectiveness of policy options for workers with disabilities', International Labour Organization, Geneva.

Sandfort, T. G. M., de Graaf, R., Bijl, R. V., and Schnabel, P. 2001, 'Same-sex sexual behavior and psychiatric disorders—findings from the Netherlands Mental Health Survey and Incidence Study (NEMESIS)', *Archives of General Psychiatry*, vol. 58, no. 1, pp. 85–91.

Sarafino, E. P. 1998, *Health Psychology: Biopsychosocial Interactions*, 3rd edn, John Wiley & Sons, Brisbane.

Schrader, T. 2003, 'Australia, the Current Round of GATS Negotiations, and Health', submission to Department of Foreign Affairs and Trade on Australia's Offers and Requests for Opening Sectors in the Current Round of GATS Negotiations, <www.drs.org.au/new_doctor/79/Schrader.htm>.

Scollo, M. and Borland, R. 2002, 'Taxation reform as a component of tobacco control policy in Australia', WHO, December.

Scull, J. 2001, 'Reconnecting with nature', *Encompass*, vol. 5, pp. 1–5.

Seal, I. 1999, 'Fix the school–not the student', *Journal of the Health Education Association of Victoria*, Summer edition, February, pp. 17–18.

Seligman, M. E. P. 1975, *Helplessness: On Depression, Development, and Death*, Freeman, San Francisco.

Seligman, M. E. P. 1993, *Learned Optimism*, Random House, Sydney.

Sen, A. 2000, 'Social exclusion: concept, application and scrutiny, social development papers No. 1', Office of Environment and Social Development, Asian Development Bank, <www.adb.org/Documents/Books/Social_Exclusion/default.asp>, 6 January 2003.

Sheehan, M., Marshall, B., and Sunderland, K. 2000, *School Matters: Mapping and Managing Mental Health in Schools*, Mental Health Branch, Department of Health and Aged Care, Canberra.

Sindall, C. 1997, 'Resource review of C. Barker, R. Hogg and C. McGuire (eds) "Health Promotion and the Family"', *Health Promotion International*, vol. 12, no. 3, pp. 259–60.

Skiold, L. (ed.) 2000, *A Look into Modern Working Life*, National Institute for Working Life, Stockholm.

Smith, F. B. 1979, *The People's Health: 1830–1910*, Croom Helm, London, p. 233.

Smith, K. R. and Desai, M. A. 2002, 'The Contribution of Global Environmental Factors to Ill-health', in P. Martens and A. J. McMichael (eds), *Environmental Change, Climate and Health. Issues and Research Methods*, Cambridge University Press, Cambridge.

Snow, J. (ed.) 1936, *Snow on Cholera*, The Commonwealth Fund, New York, p. xxxvi.

Soskolne, C. L. and Bertollini, R. 1998, *Global Ecological Integrity and 'Sustainable Development': Cornerstones of Public Health*, International workshop, European Centre for Environment and Health, World Health Organization, Rome, Italy.

Spector, P., Dwyer, D., and Jex, S. 1988, 'Relation of job stressors to affective health and performance outcomes: a comparison of multiple data sources', *Journal of Applied Psychology*, vol. 73, pp. 11–19.

Spielberger, C. D. 2002, 'Stress, Anger-Hostility, Hypertension and Heart Disease', paper presented at Stress and Anxiety Research Society Conference, Melbourne, Australia.

St Leger, L. 1998, 'Australian teachers' understandings of the health promoting school concept and the implications for the development of school health', *Health Promotion International*, vol. 13, no. 3, p. 223.

Stahl, T., Rutten, A., Nutbeam, D., Bauman, A., Kannas, L., Abel, T., Luschen, G., Rodriquez, D. J., Vinck, J., and ven der Zee, J. 2001, 'The importance of the social environment for physically active lifestyle—results from an international study', *Social Science Medicine*, vol. 52, no. 1, pp. 1–10.

Stephen Jay Gould, Quotation Page, <www.quotationspage.com/quotes/Stephen_Jay_Gould>, 29 January 2003.

Stephens, C. 2000, 'La globalisacion nos matan', Globalisation is killing us, <www.health-matters.org.uk>, 23 January 2003.

Stephenson, J., Bauman, A., Armstrong, T., Smith, B., and Bellew, B. 2000, 'The costs of illness attributable to physical inactivity', Commonwealth Department of Health, Canberra.

Stephenson, P. 2001, 'Environmental health action in Indigenous communities', *Environmental Health*, vol. 1, no. 1, pp. 72–81.

Stephenson, P. 2002, 'Mainstreaming the agenda: Indigenous environmental health at a crossroads', *Environmental Health*, vol. 2, no. 3. pp 53–65.

Stewart, J. 2002, 'A small world: environmental health', *Journal of the UK Chartered Institute of Environmental Health*, vol. 110, no. 3, pp. 68–70.

Stewart, J. A. 2000, 'Women's psychosocial well-being following a major life transition', unpublished manuscript, Deakin University, Geelong.

Stilgoe, J. R. 2001, 'Gone barefoot lately?', *American Journal of Preventative Medicine*, vol. 20, pp. 243–4.

Stone, E. J., McKenzie, T. L., Welk, G. J., and Booth, M. L. 1998, 'Effects of physical activity interventions in youth: review and synthesis', *American Journal of Preventative Medicine*, vol. 15, no. 4, pp. 298–315.

Stuart, R. B. 1974, 'Teaching facts about drugs: pushing or preventing?', *Journal of Educational Psychology*, vol. 66, pp. 189–201.

Svensson, P. G. 1988, 'The 2nd International Conference on Health Promotion: Healthy Public Policy, 5–9 April 1988, Adelaide, Australia', *Health Promotion: An International Journal*, vol. 3, no. 3, pp. 237–9.

Swerissen, H. and Duckett, S. 2002, 'Health Policy and Financing', in H. Gardner and S. Barraclough (eds), *Health Policy in Australia*, Oxford University Press, Melbourne.

Swinburn, B. A. 1995, 'The thrifty genotype hypothesis: concepts and evidence after 30 years', *Asia Pacific Journal of Clinical Nutrition*, vol. 4, pp. 337–8.

Tai, Y., Saunders, J., and Celermajer, D. 1998, 'Collateral damage from alcohol abuse: the enormous costs to Australia', *Medical Journal of Australia*, vol. 168, pp. 6–7.

Takacs, D. 1996, *The Idea of Biodiversity: Philosophies of Paradise*, Johns Hopkins University Press, Baltimore.

Takala, J. 1995, 'Worldwide View of Occupational Health', in S. Pantry (ed.), *Occupational Health*, Chapman & Hall, London.

Taylor, R. and Guest, C. 2001, 'Protecting health, sustaining the environment', in D. Pencheon, C. Guest, D. Melzer, and J. A. Muir Gray (eds), *Oxford Handbook of Public Health Practice*, Oxford University Press, Oxford, UK, pp. 206–17.

Thomas, C., Parsons, C., and Stears, D. 1998, 'Implementing the European Network of Health Promoting Schools in Bulgaria, the Czech Republic, Lithuania and Poland: vision and reality', *Health Promotion International*, vol. 13, no. 4, pp. 329–38.

Troiden, R. 1989, 'The formation of homosexual identities', *Journal of Homosexuality*, vol. 17, no. 1–2, pp. 43–73.

Trotter, L. and Mullins, R. 2003, 'Environmental Tobacco Smoke: Public Opinions and Behaviour in 2000–01', in T. Letcher and L. Trotter (eds), *Victorian Tobacco Control Studies: Quit Evaluation Studies Volume No. 11*, Victorian Smoking and Health Program, Melbourne.

Turrell, G., Oldenburg, B., McGuffog, I., and Dent, R. 1999, *Socioeconomic Determinants of Health: Towards a National Research Program and a Policy and Intervention Agenda*, School of Public Health, Queensland University of Technology Ausinfo, Canberra.

UNDP 2002, *Human Development Report 2002: Deepening democracy in a fragmented world*, United Nations Development Program, Oxford University Press, New York.

UNEP, UNICEF & WHO 2002, *Children in the New Millennium*, United Nations, Geneva.

UNICEF, UNAIDS & WHO 2002, *Young people and HIV/AIDS: Opportunity in Crisis*, United Nations, Geneva.

United Nations (combined agencies) 1996, *Time to Act: The Pacific Response to HIV and AIDS*, United Nations, Suva.

United Nations 2002, *Global Challenge Global Opportunity, Trends in Sustainable Development*, UN Department of Economic and Social Affairs, New York.

US Department of Health and Human Services (USDHHS) 1996, 'Physical activity and health: a report of the Surgeon General', USDHHS, Centres for Disease Control and Prevention, Atlanta, Georgia.

VicHealth 1996, 'Older people celebrating health ageing', *VicHealth Letter Issue 5*, Victorian Health Promotion Foundation, Melbourne.

Victorian Gay and Lesbian Rights Lobby 2000, 'Enough is enough: a report on discrimination and abuse experienced by lesbians, gay men, bisexuals and transgender people in Victoria, <http://home.vicnet.net.au/~vglrl>, 15 September 2002.

Victorian Health Promotion Foundation, 1999 'Rural partnerships in the promotion of mental health and wellbeing: Mental Health Promotion Plan 1999–2002', VicHealth, Carlton South, Victoria.

Vocational Rehabilitation Branch—International Labour Organization (ILO) 1999, 'ILO policies and activities concerning vocational rehabilitation', ILO policy paper, International Labour Office, Geneva.

Voisey, H. and O'Riordan, T. 2001, 'Globalization and Localization', in *Globalism, Localism and Identity*, Earthscan Publications Ltd, London.

Vos, T. and Begg, S. 1999, *Victorian Burden of Disease Study: Mortality*, Health Intelligence Series, Melbourne: Public Health Division, Department of Human Services, Victoria.

Wadsworth. M. 1999, 'Early Life', in M. Marmot and R. Wilkinson (eds), *Social Determinants of Health*, Oxford University Press, Oxford.

Wagner, G. 2002, 'Health Promoting Schools Evidence for Effectiveness Workshops Report', *Promotion and Education: International Journal of Health Promotion and Education*, vol. 9, no. 2.

Walpole, R. 1987, *Community Health in Australia*, Penguin, Ringwood, Victoria.

Wass, A. 2000, *Promoting health: the primary health care approach*, Harcourt Brace, Sydney.

Weatherburn, D. and Lind, B. 1999, 'Heroin harm minimisation: do we really have to choose between law enforcement and treatment?' *Crime and Justice Bulletin, no. 46*, Bureau of Crime Statistics and Research, NSW.

Werner, D. 1997, 'Questioning the solution: the politics of primary health care and child survival with an in-depth critique of oral rehydration therapy', *HealthWrights*, Palo Alto, CA.

Western Australia Health Department 1995, *The Western Australian Aboriginal Environmental Health Survey, Survey Report*, Aboriginal Health Policy and Programs Branch, Health Department of Western Australia, Perth.

Whatmore, L., Cartwright, S., and Cooper, C. 1999, 'United Kingdom: evaluation of a Stress Management Programme in the Public Sector', in M. Kompier and C. Cooper (eds), *Preventing Stress, Improving Productivity: European Case Studies in the Workplace*, Routledge, London.

White, V.M., Hill, D.J., and Effendi, Y. 2003, 'Patterns of alcohol use among Australian secondary students: results of a 1999 prevalence study and comparisons with earlier years', *Journal of Studies on Alcohol*, January, pp. 15–22.

WHO 1946, 'Constitution of the World Health Organization', reprinted in *Basic Documents*, 37th edn, World Health Organization, Geneva.

WHO 1978, Declaration of Alma Ata. International conference on primary health care, Alma Ata, USSR, 6–12 September 1978', <www.who.int/hpr/archive/docs/almaata.html>, 4 February 2003.

WHO 1981, Global strategy for health for all by the year 2000, Geneva, <www.who.int/archives/hfa>, 4 February 2003.

WHO 1984, Concepts and principles of health promotion: report of a working group, <http://whqlibdoc.who.int/euro/-1993/ICP_HSR_602__m01.pdf >, 4 February 2003.

WHO 1986a, 'The Ottawa Charter for Health Promotion', World Health Organization, Geneva, <www.who.int/hpr/archive/docs/ottawa.html>, 5 March 2003.

WHO 1986b, Ottawa Charter for Health Promotion, International Conference on Health Promotion, World Health Organization, Geneva.

WHO 1986c, 'Ottawa 1986: Report of an International Conference on Health Promotion, November 17–21 1986, Ottawa, Ontario, Canada', *Health Promotion: An International Journal*, vol. 1, no. 4, pp. i–v, 405–60.

WHO 1986c, Logo of the Ottawa Charter for Health Promotion, <www.who.int/hpr/archive/pconference/first/logo.html>, 2 February 2003.

WHO 1988, Second International Conference on Health Promotion: Recommendations on Healthy Public Policy <www.who.int/hpr/archive/docs/adelaide.html>, 2 February 2003.

WHO 1991, Third International Conference on Health Promotion, Sundsvall Statement on Supportive Environments for Health, <www.who.int/hpr/archive/docs/sundsvaal.html>, 4 February 2003.

WHO 1992, 'Our Planet, Our Health', *WHO Commission on Health and Environment*, World Health Organization, Geneva.

WHO 1993a, 'The urban health crisis. Strategies for health for all in the face of rapid urbanization', Report of the Technical Discussions at the 44th World Health Assembly, World Health Organization, Geneva.

WHO 1993b, *WHO Global Strategy for Health and Environment*, World Health Organization, Geneva.

WHO 1993c, *Health, Environment and Development: Approaches to Drafting Country-Level Strategies for Human Well-Being Under Agenda 21*, World Health Organization, Geneva.

WHO 1996, 'Health Promoting Schools—Regional Guidelines: A Framework for Action', World Health Organization, Western Pacific Regional Office, Manila.

WHO 1997a, Fourth International Conference on Health Promotion. Jakarta Declaration on Health Promotion into the 21st century, <www.who.int/hpr/archive/docs/jakarta/english.html>, 5 March, 2003.

WHO 1997b, *Health and Environment in Sustainable Development, Five Years after the Earth Summit*, World Health Organization, Geneva.

WHO 1998a, Health Promotion Glossary, <www.who.int/hpr/backgroundhp/glossary/glossary.pdf>, 12 February 2003.

WHO 1998b, World Health Assembly Resolution on Health Promotion. 51st World Health Assembly, WHA 51.12, World Health Organization, Geneva.

WHO 2000, Fifth International Conference for Health Promotion. Ministerial statement on Health Promotion, <www.who.int/hpr/conference/products/products.html>, 6 January 2003.

WHO 2002, *World Health Report 2002: Reducing Risks, Promoting Healthy Life*, World Health Organization, Geneva.

WHO 2003a, 'Measle vaccines', <www.who.int/vaccine_research/diseases/measles/en>, 1 November 2003.

WHO 2003b, 'Polio eradication', <www.polioeradication.org>, 27 January 2003.

WHO 2003c, Health promotion developments within the Western Pacific region of WHO, <www.wpro.who.int/hpr/default.htm>, 6 January 2003.

Wilkinson, R. and Marmot, M. (eds) 1998, *Social Determinants of Health: The Solid Facts*, World Health Organization, Europe.

Wilkinson, R. G. 1996, *Unhealthy Societies: The Affliction of Inequality*, Routledge, London.

Williams, G. 2001, 'Theorizing Disability', in G. Albrecht, K. Seelman, and M. Bury (eds), *Handbook of Disability Studies*, Sage, Thousand Oakes.

Williams, L. 2002, 'Beating bullies at their own game', *Melbourne Star*, 31 October, p. 6.

Wilson, E. O. 1984, *Biophilia*, Harvard University Press, Cambridge, Massachusetts.

Wilson, E. O. 1993, 'Biophilia and the Conservation Ethic', in S. R. Kellert and E. O. Wilson (eds), *The Biophilia Hypothesis*, Shearwater Books/Island Press, Washington, D. C., pp. 31–41.

Wilson, E. O. 2001, 'The ecological footprint', *Vital Speeches*, vol. 67, pp. 274–81.

Winstanley, M., Woodward, S., and Walker, N. 1995, *Tobacco In Australia: Facts and Issues*, 2nd edn, Victorian Smoking and Health Program, Australia.

Woodward, A., Hales, S., Litidamu, N., Phillips, D., and Martin, J. 2000, 'Protecting human health in a changing world: the role of social and economic development', *Bulletin of the World Health Organization*, vol. 78, no. 9, pp. 1148–55.

World Information Transfer 2002, *Towards Earth Summit 2002: Health and Environment: Supporting sustainable livelihoods*, World Health Organization.

Wright, R. 2002, 'The Dissolution of "Significant" Relationships Among Gay Men: Implications for Mental Health Promotion', unpublished Honours thesis, Deakin University, Melbourne.

Yagil, D. 1998, 'If anything can go wrong it will: occupational stress among inexperienced teachers', *International Journal of Stress Management*, vol. 5, no. 3, pp. 179–88.

INDEX

Page references in *italics* refer to illustrations and to Figures and Tables outside of text discussions